HOME REMEDIES
FROM A
COUNTRY DOCTOR

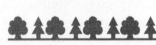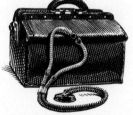

BY JAY HEINRICHS, DOROTHY BEHLEN HEINRICHS, AND THE EDITORS OF *YANKEE* MAGAZINE

Skyhorse Publishing

Copyright © 2011 by Yankee Publishing, Inc.
Illustrations © 2011 by Yankee Publishing, Inc.
Published by arrangement with Rodale, Inc.

All Rights Reserved. No part of this book may be reproduced in any manner without the express written consent of the publisher, except in the case of brief excerpts in critical reviews or articles. All inquiries should be addressed to Skyhorse Publishing, 307 West 36th Street, 11th Floor, New York, NY 10018.

Skyhorse Publishing books may be purchased in bulk at special discounts for sales promotion, corporate gifts, fund-raising, or educational purposes. Special editions can also be created to specifications. For details, contact the Special Sales Department, Skyhorse Publishing, 307 West 36th Street, 11th Floor, New York, NY 10018 or info@skyhorsepublishing.com.

Skyhorse® and Skyhorse Publishing® are registered trademarks of Skyhorse Publishing, Inc.®, a Delaware corporation.

Visit our website at www.skyhorsepublishing.com

12 11

Library of Congress Cataloging-in-Publication Data is available on file.
ISBN: 978-1-60239-973-0

Printed in the United States of America

HOME REMEDIES *from a* COUNTRY DOCTOR

YANKEE PUBLISHING STAFF

Publishing Director: Jamie Trowbridge

Book Editor: Sharon Smith

Writers: Jay Heinrichs, Dorothy Behlen Heinrichs, the editors of *Yankee* magazine

Editorial Consultants: Gregory Baker, D.D.S.; Lawrence Bernstein, M.D.; Laurence Bouchard, D.O.; Gerard Bozuwa, M.D.; Linda B. Dacey, M.D.; Mary-Catherine Gennaro, D.O.; Dale Gephart, M.D.; Brewster Martin, M.D.

Book Designer: Jill Shaffer

Illustrators: Susan Carlson, Michael Gellatly

Fact-Checkers: Robina Gangemi, Paris Mihely-Muchanic

Copy Editor and Proofreader: Barbara Jatkola

Indexer: Nanette Bendyna

Computer Keyboarder: Sheryl Fletcher

Editorial Assistants: Sue MacEwan, Nancy Trafford

To Greg Baker, Larry Bernstein, Larry Bouchard,
Gerard Bozuwa, Linda Dacey, Mandy Gennaro,
Dale Gephart, and Brewster Martin:
healers, storytellers, friends.

Contents

Contents

Introduction

O ver the past couple of centuries, country doctors have earned themselves a pretty enviable reputation. Think of country doctors, and words such as *trustworthiness, determination, selflessness,* and *no-nonsense wisdom* come to mind.

And for good reason: Having just spent two years interviewing hundreds of doctors in rural New England, we at *Yankee* magazine can confirm that the caring country doctor tradition is hale and hearty. This is a region where you can still find family physicians making house calls, and where doctors often know the folks they're treating not just as patients but also as friends and neighbors.

This thriving Yankee doctor tradition was born out of the character of the land and its people. New England's rocky fields and craggy hills shelter a rugged and independent population who can't skip over to the doctor's office for every little nick or scratch. (And they wouldn't be caught dead complaining about their minor ills, either. That just wouldn't do for a true Yankee.) And so rural doctors teach their patients how to minister to hundreds of common ailments themselves. Whether you live in a farmhouse or a high-rise, we suspect you'd like that empowering information, too.

Some of the techniques that doctors teach their country patients are secrets known to physicians of an earlier era—secrets that we can still use today. Well, you may not want to use *all* of them. You'll want to avoid dosing yourself with ashes of snails to treat diabetes, or stuffing your nostrils with wool to cure a headache, as New England doctors used to recommend in colonial days.

But country doctors also used to tell their patients some pretty useful stuff: to sprinkle red pepper in your socks for cold feet, for instance—a cure that modern doctors say actually works. And did you know that spiderwebs really can help stop a cut from bleeding (page 137)? Or that willow bark tea can relieve arthritis pain (page 19)?

It's not easy to separate the medical wheat from the chaff, the still-effective cures from nostrums that can be useless or even harmful. But you don't have to. *Home Remedies from a Country Doctor* does it for you. Based on interviews with more than 250 doctors, dentists, nurses, midwives, and other medical professionals, this book offers the old-time ways as well as the best of more contemporary at-home remedies. And every single tip has been carefully reviewed by qualified Yankee doctors.

The physicians in *Home Remedies from a Country Doctor* tell you what to do if your tongue gets frozen on a pump handle or sled runner (yeth, it really happens!), how to heal a foot that's been stepped on by a cow or horse, and the best technique for getting over a barbed wire fence. And even if you haven't met up with a pump handle, a farm animal, or a vicious strand of barbed wire lately, you'll find plenty of information you can use when your back is aching or an accidentally hammered thumb is throbbing. Our Yankee doctors offer thousands of up-to-date, down-home cures that don't cost a lot of money—everything from superglue for a cut (page 386) to the "paper clip trick" for a smashed thumb (page 231).

You'll also find the latest in medical advice for the most modern of ailments, from stress to repetitive motion injury. Whereas many of the first Yankee doctors were also ministers who were just as likely to give you remedies for your soul as for your body, these days country doctors are as rigorously trained and up-to-date on modern ailments as the ones in the big city. But they're closer to the old-time country ways. They're closer to the old-time country stories, too, and we couldn't resist including some of the best.

Introducing a Few of Our Country Doctors

Speaking of the best, we picked up many cures—and a bookful of those great stories—from four of our favorite

New England doctors. You'll get to know them much better throughout the book, but we'll introduce you to them now.

LAWRENCE H. BERNSTEIN, M.D., used to make house calls by bicycle during his 22 years as a family doctor in the town of Storrs, Connecticut. "My father, Joseph Bernstein, was a family doctor in Springfield, Massachusetts, and I started going on house calls with him when I was five or six," Dr. Bernstein says. "I just never stopped." House calls are easier for him these days, though: He now practices at a total-care facility in Longmeadow, Massachusetts. You'll see him throughout the book as "Dr. Larry."

GERARD BOZUWA, M.D., spent 36 years as the sole town doctor for Wakefield, New Hampshire, before he retired in 1994. There's a plaque honoring him outside the house he worked in—a house that doctors began occupying in 1849. Dr. Bozuwa has a plaque of his own inside his home office: a collection of fishing lures he pulled out of hapless fishermen over the years. "Dr. B.," as we call him, came to America from Holland, where he completed his medical studies after being freed from a World War II Japanese prison camp in Indonesia. Now he's a dyed-in-the-scratchy-wool, self-reliant New Englander: He read this book's manuscript by candlelight when an ice storm knocked out his electricity for four days.

MARY-CATHERINE GENNARO, D.O. ("Dr. Mandy"), is a family osteopath in private practice in Warren, New Hampshire. (An osteopath has graduated from an osteopathic medical school—learning a medical philosophy that's slightly different from that of common modern medicine—and must go through the same rigorous training as an M.D.) The busy mother of two and the wife of a fellow osteopath, Dr. Gennaro supplements her private practice by serving as a staff physician at Cottage Hospital in Woodsville, New Hampshire, and as an adjunct professor of community medicine at Dartmouth Medical School in Hanover, New Hampshire. Oh, and she makes house calls, too.

BREWSTER MARTIN, M.D., was born in Pittsfield, Vermont. The governor of the state recruited him to start a practice right out of medical school. Dr. Martin stayed in the little town of Chelsea (population 1,166) as the town doctor for 40 years before retiring in 1993. You can still find him, telling stories about country doctoring, three houses down and across the first branch of the White River from the health center he founded. No wonder Dr. Brewster was named Vermont Doctor of the Year in 1991.

Besides providing their best stories and their own preferred remedies, these four—and a host of other country doctors—helped ensure this book's factual accuracy. Drs. Martin, Bozuwa, and Bernstein read the entire manuscript before it went to press. So did osteopathic family physician Laurence Bouchard, D.O., of Narragansett, Rhode Island, along with Dale Gephart, M.D., a doctor in Hanover, New Hampshire, who's an expert on herbal remedies. Gregory L. Baker, D.D.S., an orthodontist in Woodstock, Vermont, and West Lebanon and New London, New Hampshire, reviewed all of the dental remedies. And every medical person quoted in this book reviewed the copy in which his or her comments were included. All of them gave generously of their time as if they were advising an extended family of patients—which, come to think of it, they are.

How to Use This Book

You will undoubtedly find this accumulated wisdom invaluable, but this book is not meant to replace your own family physician. If you're unsure about how to handle your symptoms, see your doctor before your problems worsen. If, however, you wish to find the perfect home remedy to treat a minor ailment—or to understand better what your doctor has diagnosed—this is the book for you, with more than 200 symptoms organized in alphabetical order. Folks often use different names for the same diseases, so if you can't find what you're looking for in the chapter headings, check the index. Look in the index, too, even if you've found the alphabetical entry for the subject you want. You'll find additional information there. For example, you'll find great remedies under "Cold Hands and Feet," but you'll also want to look for even more descriptions and cures in the section "Poor Circulation."

Keep this book by your bed or in your bathroom, and peruse it even when you're feeling fine. It'll seem as though you're receiving a house call from an old-time country doctor—and that can be good for both body *and* soul.

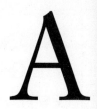

AFTERNOON SLUMP
Nip the need to nap

Do you find yourself nodding off around midafternoon? Join one big sleepy club: The afternoon is a normal low point in humans' daily sleep/wake cycle. Although the research is inconclusive, some scientists think that a big lunch high in carbohydrates can make you drowsy by increasing the amount of sleep-causing serotonin in the brain. Therefore, a light lunch might be a good idea before a job interview or a final exam.

Still, most of our heavy-lidded afternoons are the result of wide-eyed evenings the night before, according to Michael Sateia, M.D., director of the Sleep Disorders Clinic at the Dartmouth-Hitchcock Medical Center in Lebanon, New Hampshire. "As a society we are sleep-deprived," Dr. Sateia says. "Most people receive less than the optimal amount of sleep, and many are grossly sleep-deprived. Any sleep deficit will exaggerate afternoon slump."

What *is* an optimal amount of sleep? "Enough to wake feeling fully rested and to stay alert through the entire day," Dr. Sateia says. "If you've had enough sleep, you should be able to wake up in the morning without an alarm. For most adults, that is 7½ to 8 hours every night." Some people can get by on 6 hours or less, while others need at least 10 hours of shut-eye.

If you're getting plenty of sleep at night and still find yourself nodding off the next afternoon, you might have sleep

The Governor's Health Care Plan

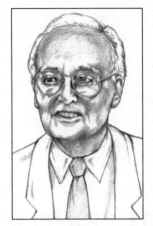

WHEN I was in my last year of medical school at the University of Vermont, the dean called a classmate of mine, Luke Howe, and me into his office. We thought we were in serious trouble. Deans don't call you into their offices for nothing.

Turns out the governor of Vermont planned to talk his little town of Chelsea into buying the building next to the governor's house. He wanted to equip it as a community health center. The governor had asked the dean to come up with a couple of doctors to staff it. "Are you interested?" the dean asked us. We said yes. Dr. Howe stayed 10 years. I stayed 40. I still live just three houses down and across the first branch of the White River from that health center.

That's the best kind of health care improvement: just as local as you can get it.

BREWSTER MARTIN, M.D., *a retired family doctor in Chelsea, Vermont (population 1,166), and cofounder of the Chelsea Family Health Center. He was named Vermont Doctor of the Year in 1991.*

apnea, in which interrupted breathing disrupts sleep. See a doctor if your slumps become habitual or if they're hurting your performance on the job.

Otherwise, here's what you can do to slay the occasional afternoon draggin'.

Get the Blood Up

"Five minutes of exercise can help to wake you up," says Lawrence H. Bernstein, M.D., a former family doctor who is the medical director at Jewish Geriatric Services in Longmeadow, Massachusetts. If you're feeling draggy, get up and walk around briskly, go up and down a flight of stairs a couple of times, or nip outside for a breath of air. "Get the blood stirring," Dr. Bernstein says.

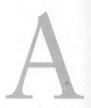

Steal a Few Winks

On the theory that if you can't fight sleep, join it, Dr. Bernstein recommends an afternoon catnap. "The medical literature shows that people benefit from a 5- to 10-minute nap," he says. "I often sit in my desk chair after lunch and just shut down for a few minutes before I see my afternoon patients. It works like a charm."

Or Sip Some Joe

"People have used caffeine to wake up for a long time now," Dr. Sateia says. "It may be helpful for the occasional afternoon slump to drink a little coffee or cola judiciously."

ALTITUDE SICKNESS
A risk of getting high

It's the ski vacation you've been dreaming about. You fly to the resort town and hit the ski lifts, soaring up to dizzying heights—literally. All of a sudden, your balance is off, you have a terrific headache, and you're at risk of losing your airline lunch.

You probably have a case of altitude sickness, also known as mountain sickness. The bad news is, you can get it anytime you go higher than a mile above sea level—5,280 feet. The good news is, there's an almost instant cure for mild cases: Just go down.

Nearly anyone can suffer from altitude sickness, from highly conditioned athletes to vacationing couch potatoes. The faster and higher you ascend, the worse you are likely to suffer. Researchers are not entirely sure what causes the misery high up, but they theorize something like this: The air is thinner at high altitudes because of the reduced atmospheric pressure. Because oxygen molecules are spread out more than they are at more moderate heights, you take in less oxygen with every breath.

Without sufficient oxygen, your body's cells burn fuel—food—less efficiently. Your brain tries to compensate by ordering faster breathing, which in turn washes carbon dioxide out of blood. Above 8,000 feet, fluid starts to leak from your blood vessels and capillaries into the surrounding tissues.

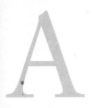Your face, hands, and feet may look puffy. In extreme cases, fluid can get into the lungs, hampering breathing. Sometimes the brain swells—an extremely dangerous condition called cerebral edema.

Perk Up by Getting Down

For such a mysterious disease, the main cure is remarkably simple. "All forms of altitude sickness are improved simply by going down a few thousand feet," says Charles Houston, M.D., professor emeritus of medicine and environmental health at the University of Vermont College of Medicine and author of *High Altitude Illness and Wellness.*

Down Water When You're Up

When mountain guide Nick Yardley led climbs of 20,320-foot Mount McKinley in Alaska, he gave each of his clients two liter-size bottles of water when they went to bed. "They had to drink it all before morning," says Yardley, who directed the International Mountain Climbing School in North Conway, New Hampshire, before becoming national sales manager of the Climb High catalog in Shelburne, Vermont. "The best way to prevent altitude sickness is to drink water. Avoid alcohol or caffeine, which are diuretics that will dry you out. Water, juice, a little hot chocolate, and some hot Jell-O are best. I love hot Jell-O—it's one of the best drinks ever invented for the outdoors. It warms you right up, and the sugar gives you instant energy."

Dr. Houston confirms that water is extremely important.

Climb Socially

"Different people under similar conditions sometimes respond quite differently to altitude," Dr. Houston says. "We know little about why." He notes,

A Deadly Risk on High

MOST people who go up to a mile or more above sea level leak some fluid from the blood vessels into the tissues surrounding the veins and capillaries in the lungs. You might develop an annoying cough, but there's usually no cause for alarm. The body readily reabsorbs the fluid, especially once you get back down to more moderate elevations.

Sometimes, however, enough fluid gathers that it begins to leak into the lung's air sacs. Breathing becomes difficult, and the victim is in danger of drowning in his own fluid. If you or a companion shows any signs of this ailment, called high-altitude pulmonary edema, or HAPE, descend immediately. Here are six danger signals to watch out for, according to Charles Houston, M.D., professor emeritus of medicine and environmental health at the University of Vermont and author of *High Altitude Illness and Wellness*.

- Shortness of breath and increasingly labored breathing
- Coughing up blood
- Confusion and anxiety
- Rapid pulse
- Extreme fatigue
- An inability to walk in a straight line

Sometimes altitude can affect the brain, too, resulting in a condition called high-altitude cerebral edema, or HACE. As with HAPE, a person with HACE staggers around as if drunk.

"Either condition can come up very fast," notes longtime mountain guide Nick Yardley of Shelburne, Vermont. "You can go from looking okay to being unconscious in two hours. If you have swelling in your hands, face, or feet, these could be early warning signs of pulmonary or cerebral edema. The only real cure is descent." Dr. Houston concurs with this.

however, that one important factor is how fast a person ascends.

Doctors recommend that you try to get two days' worth of rest to "acclimatize," or get accustomed to high altitudes, before doing any strenuous exercise. "Take it a little at a time" if you want to ascend still farther, advises Murray Hamlet, D.V.M. Hamlet is chief of the Research Support Division at the U.S. Army Research Institute of Environmental Medicine in Natick, Massachusetts. He advises the army on cold-weather and high-altitude conditions. "Go up a little, then rest. Go up more, then rest some more. In the meantime, drink plenty of water."

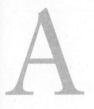

ANEMIA
Help while your problem is being ironed out

If your body is getting rid of iron faster than it's taking it in—a problem that affects about 3 percent of all adult women—you may have iron-deficiency anemia. You need iron to carry oxygen in the blood and to dispose of waste carbon dioxide. Too little iron can result in a variety of ailments, from headache to loss of appetite to ringing in the ears. Some iron-poor people feel constant fatigue; others get a strange craving for ice or even clay.

Most people who have anemia feel worn-out and draggy. "The hallmarks of anemia are fatigue, a pale complexion, and an intolerance of exercise," says Mark Greenberg, M.D., a cardiologist at the Dartmouth-Hitchcock Medical Center in Lebanon, New Hampshire. "Anemia is especially common in menstruating women. They lose iron along with the menstrual blood." Women also need more iron when they're pregnant or breastfeeding.

How do you get that iron? Your doctor can prescribe supplements if necessary, but the best treatments you can give yourself—under a doctor's supervision—are a proper diet and a daily multivitamin.

Once your doctor has diagnosed your iron deficiency, here's how you can get back to being a red-blooded American.

Eat Like Popeye

"If a woman comes in with anemia and she is still menstruating, I usually recommend that she take a multivitamin that has extra iron," says F. Daniel Golyan, M.D., a former New Englander who is now an electrophysiologist on Long Island. "She should also include plenty of iron-rich vegetables and grains in her diet, such as spinach and beans, in addition to meats."

Be a Carnivore

"Good sources of iron to combat anemia are raisins and red meat," says Brewster Martin, M.D., a retired family doctor in Chelsea, Vermont. Other iron-rich foods include fish, liver, and cereals and breads that have been fortified with iron.

Eat Slow Food

An old-time remedy for iron-poor blood is blackstrap molasses. "It's not often sold anymore in regular grocery stores," says herbalist Jane Smolnik, owner of Crystal Garden Herbs in Springfield, Vermont. "You might have to look for this kind of molasses in a health food store." A teaspoon a day of blackstrap molasses, gulped down straight, gives you a powerful dose of iron, Smolnik adds.

ANIMAL SCRATCHES
Cures for when Puss gives you the business end of her boots

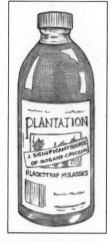

Iron-packed blackstrap molasses is an old cure that still works to treat anemia.

The cutest little kitten can pack some powerful weaponry in the form of sharp claws. Sure they're tiny, but that only makes them that much sharper.

You should be concerned about more than a surprise booboo when a kitten rakes you. Besides breaking the skin, the creature brings unwanted gifts in the form of viruses and bacteria. If a wild animal scratched you or your child, you probably wouldn't hesitate to head for a doctor. That's a good idea, says Robert F. Wilson, M.D., a pediatrician who is retired from his practice in Dover, New Hampshire. "You'll want to make sure you're up on your tetanus booster shots," he explains. But what harm is there in a little kitty's scratch?

Lots, potentially, says Dr. Wilson. "Cats—especially young ones—can carry cat scratch disease, a bacterial infection. What originally looks like a minimal scratch can develop as a big lump near where you were scratched." The first thing you get is a blister where the cat got you. Often you'll find a swollen gland around the same area—in your armpit if you were scratched on the arm, in your groin if you were scratched on your leg, on your head or neck if the scratch was higher up. Cat scratch disease also can bring a fever (in fact, the illness is commonly known as cat scratch fever), and you might feel draggy and headachy as well. In rare cases, cat scratch disease can cause sores and other problems on the eyes. In extremely rare cases, people develop convulsions.

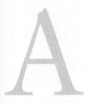

Cats aren't the only carriers of cat scratch disease. Doctors think you also might be able to get it from dogs and monkeys.

"If you get an animal scratch that starts to swell, you should see a doctor," Dr. Wilson says. But don't get *too* nervous. Cat scratch disease is rarely dangerous except in people with immune system illnesses, such as AIDS. People can't spread the disease to each other. Once you've had the illness, you're usually entirely recovered within a month, and your body develops an immunity. And even your cat will end up with a clean bill of health. Cats only *carry* the disease; they don't suffer from it. A carrying cat is contagious for only a short time, and the disease is rare in adult cats. So you don't need to be overly leery of your kitty.

A WORD FROM DR. B.

The Girl Who Loaned an Ear

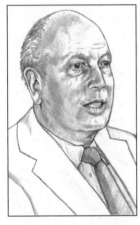

ONE time a girl called me saying a horse had just bitten off a piece of her ear. "Yeah, sure," I said, thinking she was exaggerating. She came over to show me, and, sure enough, a piece was missing.

There was little I could do but clean the wound, put on a bandage, and give her a tetanus shot. The girl didn't seem to be overly traumatized by the experience. She returned to her horse and eventually became my office nurse. Years later, I attended her wedding.

But there's a lesson here. You should never get too snuggly with an animal that can scratch or bite you. Doctors see lots of chomped pet owners. For years we kept horses, and we used to invite the local Pony Club over to our place. I'd get nervous when the girls would snuggle up to their horses. I'd tell them to be careful. After all, animals aren't humans; they can scratch or bite. But then again, so can humans. I'd be careful about snuggling up to them, too.

GERARD BOZUWA, M.D., *retired after 36 years as the sole family doctor for the town of Wakefield, New Hampshire.*

The scratch itself, though, is cause for caution. Here's what you should do.

Wash, Wash, Wash

"The single best thing you can do for an animal scratch is to wash it with soap and water," says Peter Mason, M.D., a family doctor in Lebanon, New Hampshire. "Flush the wound with plenty of water. Then soak the scratch in hot, soapy water for 10 to 15 minutes, swishing the water on the scratch to improve the blood flow to the wound. If you flush all the bacteria out of the wound, you're less likely to need antibiotics."

Add a Cleanser

"If your scratch is bleeding, rinse it in equal parts hydrogen peroxide and water," says Everett Orbeton, M.D., a retired pediatrician in South Portland, Maine.

Find the Scratcher

"Cat owners say that one kitten out of every litter is the one that does all the scratching," Dr. Wilson says. "If you're planning not to keep them all, the scratcher is the first one you should give away."

ANKLE SPRAIN
New twists on an old injury

The most common problem that throws a wrench into an exercise program is a sprained ankle. A sprain is most likely to occur when you're walking or running over an uneven surface, such as an old sidewalk. That's when you unintentionally put too much weight on the rubber-band-like ligaments, causing them to stretch to the tearing point. "A sprain is a tear in your ligaments," says Hugh P. Hermann, M.D., a family physician in Woodstock, Vermont. That's different from a strain, which is an overstretched muscle.

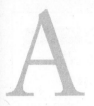

It's sometimes hard to tell whether you have a strain, a sprain, or even a broken bone. If you suspect anything but a minor twist or the pain persists for more than two or three days, have your doctor take a look at that aching ankle. In most cases, you'll be back to your old jog within a few weeks. Here's how to speed things up with a minimum of pain.

Get Some RICE

RICE is a four-pronged remedy whose initials stand for rest, ice, compression, and elevation. The "rest" part? "You should stay off your injury for a day or two," says John Dunn, M.D., an emergency room physician at the Northwestern Medical Center in St. Albans, Vermont. Then there's the ice: "Put a plastic bag with crushed ice against the injury and hold it there for 15 minutes at a time." Compression: "Wrap the ankle with an elastic bandage, which you can get at any drugstore and most sporting goods stores." And elevation: "Put your leg up above the level of your heart for the first 24 to 48 hours, applying ice during this period. Use a walking stick or crutches if you need to walk to the bathroom."

Boot Up

A good way to provide the "compression" part of your RICE treatment is to wear lace-up boots, Dr. Hermann advises.

Swallow a Pill

"Take an anti-inflammatory drug such as ibuprofen to reduce the pain and swelling for the first day or two after a sprain," Dr. Dunn says.

But Don't Keep Swallowing

After the swelling goes down, stick to mild painkillers, advises Dr. Dunn. "Pain is your body's way of making you treat

---

Take an Ankle in Stride

A SPRAINED ankle usually heals itself within a few weeks, says Daniel Wing, M.D., who practices rehabilitation medicine throughout Vermont. But if you keep injuring the same spot, the problem may not be faulty healing. A study of college athletes at the University of Vermont showed that most ankle injuries are not caused by "weak ankles," as is commonly thought, but by an unbalanced gait. "The feet of some people flop one way or another," Dr. Wing explains. "The important thing is to keep the foot and ankle stable while you walk or run." If you suspect a problem with your gait, he adds, see a podiatrist or physical therapist, who can examine your walk and prescribe orthotic devices for your shoes or ankles.

your sprained ankle gently," he says. "A mild painkiller is okay, and so is a moderate amount of walking—a mile or two a day. But prescription drugs and narcotics are not such a bright idea." The strong stuff makes you more likely to put too much stress on your injured ligaments.

Heat Up

After the first 48 hours, Dr. Dunn says, the bulk of your internal bleeding should have stopped, making ice no longer necessary. "After that, apply heat to the injury," he advises. "Heat reduces the pain and speeds healing."

Then Get Up

Once the swelling has gone down, your best bet is to move around. "Doctors used to tell you to baby your ankle for a couple of weeks," Dr. Dunn notes. "We used to be horrified watching football trainers just tape up their players' ankles and send them back out onto the field after a day or two. Now there is evidence that the trainers were right: Sprained ankles get better faster if you use them."

ARTHRITIS
What are joints like that doing in a person like you?

The pain and stiffness you feel around your joints may just be a sign that you're getting on in years. Then again, your arthritis may mean something else altogether. Doctors use *arthritis* as a catchall term for inflammation of the joints. "The word has come to mean that something is wrong with the materials that hold us together," says John Bland, M.D., a rheumatologist in Cambridge, Vermont. The most common kind, osteoarthritis, is the result of wear and tear on bone and cartilage over time. More than 15 million people over the age of 45 complain of osteoarthritis. It causes a deep,

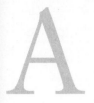achy pain in the joints, and you may sometimes feel stiff and sore when you lie in bed at night—especially after a game of touch football or a wrestling match with your granddaughter.

Then there's rheumatoid arthritis, the other major form of joint inflammation. "The rheumatiz" tends to strike earlier in life—the peak time is in your forties. Doctors think that this poorly understood disease stems from the body's own immune system acting against itself to break down bone and cartilage. Rheumatoid arthritis generally tends to make your joints feel warm and sore, and they can be swollen and tender as well.

There are numerous other forms of arthritis as well—more than 100 varieties, including gout, intestinal problems, infections, and even skin disorders. Once your doctor has pinpointed the root of your joint problems, you can ease the aches and pains at home with these remedies.

Take Good Ol' Aspirin

"As long as you are not allergic to it and it doesn't bother your stomach, aspirin is a great, great drug," says Laurence Bouchard, D.O., an osteopathic family physician in private practice in Narragansett, Rhode Island. "It will help alleviate joint pain and decrease the inflammation of arthritis." Dr. Bouchard notes that if aspirin upsets your stomach, you can buy over-the-counter buffered varieties, such as Bufferin.

Do a Preemptive Strike

"A lot of people wake up in the morning stiff with arthritis," Dr. Bouchard says. "The inactivity of sleep allows the joints to stiffen up at night. To prevent that nighttime stiffening, take an anti-inflammatory drug such as aspirin or ibuprofen before going to bed. Eat a little something with your pills, or take them with a glass of milk, so the medicine won't irritate your stomach."

Put Up a Cold Front

"If you have arthritis and still enjoy activities like gardening, ice your affected joints right after coming inside. Don't allow them to become inflamed," says Sarah Johansen, M.D., an internist and medical director of emergency services at New London Hospital in New London, New Hampshire.

Heat with Chili Peppers

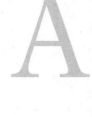

Scientific studies show that capsaicin—the "hot" chemical in chili peppers—can relieve the pain of arthritis. When you smear it onto your skin, the theory goes, you short-circuit the pain signals and keep them from traveling to your brain. You can find capsaicin over the counter at drugstores, contained in such popular remedies as Capzasin-HP and Zostrix. "Use just a little at first," says Daniel Caloras, M.D., a family doctor in private practice in Charlestown, New Hampshire. "Some people find these remedies irritating."

Dr. Caloras says that many of his patients use a lotion that has capsaicin in a lower potency. Look for brands that have 0.025 percent capsaicin. And don't get carried away with this idea and try smearing yourself directly with chili peppers, Dr. Caloras says. That's a higher potency than most skin will tolerate.

Catch This

For years, arthritis sufferers have sworn that eating lots of fish helped ease their aches and pains. In fact, researchers at

---

A WORD FROM DR. MARTIN

My Favorite Painting

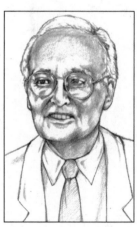

ON THE bedroom wall in my home, there's a beautiful painting of a winter scene. The snow-covered trees are just beginning to show the blush of swelling buds—a sign of the coming spring.

One of my patients did the work. Crippled by rheumatoid arthritis, she painted the scene holding a brush between her teeth.

I think of that painting whenever I feel a little ache in my joints. Life begins with hope and courage; it doesn't end with a body's limitations.

BREWSTER MARTIN, M.D., *a retired family doctor in Chelsea, Vermont (population 1,166), and cofounder of the Chelsea Family Health Center. He was named Vermont Doctor of the Year in 1991.*

Brigham and Women's Hospital in Boston have confirmed that fish oil does appear to relieve the morning stiffness of rheumatoid arthritis. Other studies have shown similar results. You can take advantage of this by increasing the amount of fish in your diet or by taking fish oil pills. You will find the pills at most health food stores. Follow the dosage directions on the label.

Power Up

"People with either rheumatoid arthritis or osteoarthritis profit enormously from regular exercise programs," Dr. Bland says. "Walking is far and away the best exercise for these people. Joint stiffness and pain decline and power increases after you get in the habit of walking at least two miles a day."

Travel Light

Overweight people are more likely to develop osteoarthritis as they get older. To reduce the strain on your joints, lose weight, doctors say.

Get Longer

"A major part of the management of arthritis is stretching," Dr. Bland says. "Stretch for 18 to 20 minutes each day." Focus your stretching where it hurts the most, though it's a good idea to increase flexibility all over, he says. To increase the range of motion in your shoulder, for example, Dr. Bland recommends this stretch: Keeping your right arm straight, slowly rotate it to make as large and complete a circle as possible. Think in terms of spinning a giant hula hoop. It should take about 5 seconds to complete the circle. Make another circle with the same arm, then do two 5-second circles with the other arm. Dr. Bland describes this and other stretches in his book *Live Long, Die Fast: Playing the Aging Game to Win.*

Raise a Cane

"One of the problems with arthritis is that it can make you unsteady on your feet," Dr. Johansen

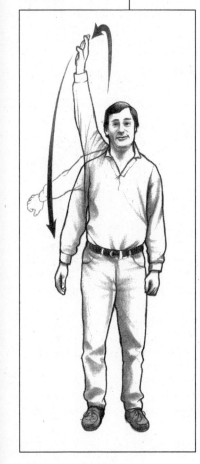

To stretch an aching shoulder, keep your arm straight while slowly rotating it in a circle.

says. "Use a cane or a walker to relieve the weight borne by the affected joints. If you have arthritis in one knee, hold the cane in your opposite hand. That relieves the stress."

Drown Some Raisins

"Here's a remedy I have used for my own arthritis," says Harry Bird, M.D., a retired anesthesiologist in Hanover, New Hampshire, and the former commissioner of health and human services for the State of New Hampshire. "Pack a small jar with golden raisins and cover them with gin. Eat nine raisins every morning, squeezing the extra gin back into the jar." Dr. Bird uses this cure even when he's not feeling arthritis discomfort. "I think it works for both prevention and treatment," he says. He's not sure why it works; "it just does."

To Bee or Not to Bee?

If you suffer from arthritis, you've probably heard of the old bee sting remedy. Does it work? Ask Charles Mraz, a nonagenarian beekeeper who has been stinging himself for most of his life. "I was hit by rheumatic fever in 1934," he says. "My knees were so painful I could barely walk. I had been keeping bees since I was 14, and for years old-timers had told me that bee venom was good for arthritis. So I held a couple of bees to the insides of my knees, they stung me, and I went to bed. The next morning I got up, and it was a miracle: My knees didn't hurt a bit!"

Since then, says Mraz, "I've treated thousands of people. Folks just come over to the hives I keep behind my house. They put a few bees in a mayonnaise jar with holes punched in the lid and a little honey for food. They keep my bees up to a week, then use them when they need them." Mraz recommends using forceps or large tweezers to remove bees from the jar. "Pick them up by the head or thorax. They don't

---

ANNALS OF MEDICINE
How Bark Eased the Bite of Arthritis

OLD-TIME New Englanders still swear by "rheumatiz" remedies that most doctors won't get near: carrying buckshot or a potato in your pocket, drinking turtle shell ashes mixed with water, rubbing your joints with snake oil. From ancient times until World War II, some doctors thought arthritis was the result of bad teeth; their treatment was to extract the offenders.

One old-time remedy—tea made from willow bark—actually works. The bark contains salicin—chemically similar to the great painkiller salicylic acid, which was discovered by scientists in 1899 and quickly became known as aspirin.

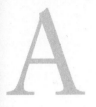

like that, so you don't have to convince them to sting you." Hold the bee right where it hurts, he says.

"Bee venom is great stuff," confirms Bradford Weeks, M.D., a family doctor who moved from New Hampshire to Clinton, Washington. "It contains anti-inflammatory peptides that act against the pain and inflammation of arthritis." If you are allergic to bees, Dr. Weeks cautions you not to use this remedy without the supervision of a doctor. "And even if you aren't highly allergic, buy a bee sting kit from your pharmacy and keep it handy."

ASTHMA
Methods for easing the wheezing

If you occasionally find it hard to breathe—getting wheezy or gaspy or having sudden fits of coughing—you may be among the 1 in 10 Americans who suffer from asthma. People under the age of 18 are just as likely as adults to have the wheezes; about 4 million children are asthmatic, a figure that makes asthma the most common chronic childhood illness in this country.

Why some people develop asthma and others don't is something of a medical mystery. Oh, doctors know what the illness *is:* "It's an obstructed and irritable airway," says Edward Kent, M.D., a pediatric allergist with Timberlane Allergy and Asthma Associates in South Burlington, Vermont. "People with asthma have periods of difficult breathing, and the chest feels irritable. The symptoms include coughing that fails to produce any phlegm, a feeling of tightness in the chest, shortness of breath, and wheezing."

Some people have cough-variant asthma; their breathing appears normal, but they have periods of hacking that can last for weeks. "Cough-variant asthma is pretty common in children," Dr. Kent says. "An asthmatic child will often get a cold and then cough for another two or three weeks after the initial infection goes away. Then he'll get another cold, and the cough will start all over again." A cough that lingers for more than a week should trigger a trip to the doctor, he says.

There are even more triggers for an asthma attack than there are varieties of asthma. "Allergies are a major cause,"

Dr. Kent says. "Inhaled irritants such as dust, dust mites, pet dander, plant pollen, and molds can cause breathing troubles in asthmatics." Stepping outside on a cold day also can start an asthmatic wheezing, he says. So can a glass of wine, aspirin, an emotional upset, even a whiff of a date's cologne. Food allergies have been suspected in asthma attacks. The latex gloves used in hospitals and doctors' offices can cause breathing problems in some wearers. And some people find their asthma getting worse when there's a change in the weather, such as a decrease in barometric pressure before a thunderstorm.

Why some people get the wheezes on these occasions while others breathe just fine—and why allergies cause asthma in some people while causing entirely different symptoms in

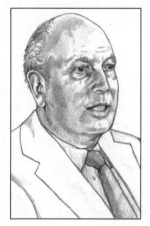

Sedate Isn't Always Good

WHEN I was starting out as a full-time doctor in Wakefield, I had a patient who came in with a bad attack of asthma. He was a very nervous, excitable man. The trouble he had breathing only made him more nervous, and his panic took his breath away even more. It was a vicious cycle.

I admitted him to our local hospital, but nothing I did could get him out of his attack. Finally, I gave him a sedative and got an ambulance to take him to the big medical center two hours away. I went with him, of course. Well, at the big hospital, the doctors laid me out in lavender—they chewed me out because sedatives suppress the breathing center in the brain. I had my tail between my legs for weeks, but the patient didn't bear a grudge. He and I became good friends.

There are two lessons in that story. First, doctors are fallible, especially when they're rookies. (I'm living proof.) Second, if you're having trouble staying calm during an asthma attack, don't take a tranquilizer.

GERARD BOZUWA, M.D., *retired after 36 years as the sole family doctor for the town of Wakefield, New Hampshire.*

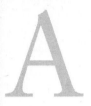others—is still beyond the ken of medical science. But doctors have a pretty good bag of tricks for making you breathe easier. Here are some of the best.

Sit Easy

"If you're beginning to have an asthma attack, sit down," says David Goodman, M.D., a pediatric allergist at the Dartmouth-Hitchcock Medical Center in Lebanon, New Hampshire. Breathe slowly and try to stay calm, he says. "When the wheezing starts, some people become anxious and hyperventilate, which further restricts the airways."

Floor It

"If you have an asthmatic in the family, get rid of your rugs," says Lawrence H. Bernstein, M.D., a former family doctor who is the medical director at Jewish Geriatric Services in Longmeadow, Massachusetts. "Your carpeting is a great habitat for dust mites, which are among the worst asthma triggers. Keep your bedroom free of things that accumulate dust—skip the dust ruffles and minimize the stuffed animals. And encase your bed's pillow and mattress in plastic." Put the pillowcase and bedclothes over the plastic, which helps keep dander and dust mites out of contact with your lungs, he says.

Don't Bed with Kitty

"Pets are a tough issue for families with asthma," Dr. Bernstein says. "Keep pets out of the bedroom and close the door at night. If asthma becomes a serious health issue, you might have to give your pets up to relatives and friends."

Dry Up

If in summertime you're living with wheezing, consider getting central air-conditioning. "Keep the humidity down," Dr. Bernstein says. "That's a trigger. And air-conditioning helps filter pollen and dust from the air, making breathing easier."

ANNALS OF MEDICINE

But the Taste Took Your Breath Away

BACK in colonial times, doctors called asthma "the phthisic." A common cure: the urine of a red cow, downed with a generous amount of beer. Although the current term for the ailment isn't much easier to spell, modern remedies are easier to wrap your tongue around.

Put Out Fires

"If you heat your house with wood and your child starts wheezing when the cold weather begins, he could be sensitive to soot," Dr. Bernstein notes. "For a couple of weeks, try using an alternative source of heat and see what happens. If the child gets better, you might want to keep the woodstove cold."

Guard Your Air

"Smoking doesn't cause asthma, but it certainly exacerbates the problem," says Stephen Blair, M.D, a pediatrician in private practice in Claremont, New Hampshire. "If your airway is mildly sensitive, smoke can turn that sensitivity into asthma." This applies to secondhand smoke as well. "Stay away from smokers in general," he advises.

Learn to Inhale (the Right Way)

Many asthmatics find instant relief in inhalers—small tubes with aerosols attached that deliver medicine right to the airway and are available by prescription. But as many as half the people who turn to inhalers use them improperly, getting smaller doses than they need. A common mistake is to inhale before squeezing the aerosol. Doctors say the correct approach is to hold the inhaler to your mouth, squeeze it, and then breathe in, holding your breath for 10 seconds.

It takes practice to use an inhaler correctly. Sometimes an adapter can help to get the medicine where it will do the most good.

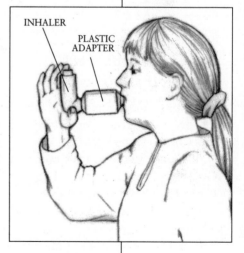

INHALER

PLASTIC ADAPTER

"It's not easy to get the technique right," Dr. Goodman says. "The medicine comes out of the inhaler at 60 miles an hour. Even with good coordination, a lot of the medicine winds up on the tongue or the back of the throat, where it doesn't do you any good. To keep that from happening, you can buy a plastic adapter from your drugstore. Put your mouth over one end of the tube. Puff the inhaler into the other end, then take a long, slow, deep breath. The tube will slow down the medicine, allowing you to breathe it into your airway."

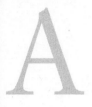

Bean Your Breath

A cup of coffee or two 12-ounce bottles of cola can cause the bronchial passages to dilate, offering more room for breathing. If you're having an asthma attack, consider giving yourself a jolt or two.

Go Fish

Doctors have long suspected that a diet rich in fish oil might reduce the number and severity of asthma attacks. Some studies suggest that a fish dinner at least once a week might be good for asthmatics.

ATHLETE'S FOOT
Bringing your itchy dogs to heel

If your feet feel as if they're taking on a life of their own—getting itchy between the toes, with peeling skin that might blister occasionally—chances are your hooves are infected with the fungus *Tinea pedis,* which is a kind of ringworm.

The common name is athlete's foot, but you don't have to be a jock to get the itch. "Just about everyone gets athlete's foot at one time or another," says Charles Hammer, M.D., a dermatologist with the North Country Outreach Program of the Lahey Hitchcock Clinic in St. Johnsbury, Vermont. "The fungal spores are everywhere in the environment. Some people are more susceptible than others. People whose feet tend to sweat a lot are at the highest risk." That's because the fungus loves warm, moist places, such as sweaty socks.

Not only does athlete's foot affect more than athletes—it's not always limited to the feet. "You can get athlete's foot on your hands," says Owen Reynolds, M.D., a dermatologist in private practice in North Andover, Massachusetts. "You can also get the fungus in your groin."

AN OUNCE OF PREVENTION

Give Your Feet Their Just Deserts

To help keep from getting athlete's foot, keep your feet dry," says Charles Hammer, M.D., a dermatologist with the North Country Outreach Program of the Lahey Hitchcock Clinic in St. Johnsbury, Vermont. "Change your socks whenever they get wet or sweaty—you might carry extra socks in your pocketbook or briefcase. And wear sandals, or shoes that breathe easily, whenever possible."

Wherever your fungus is afoot, here are some ways to stamp it out.

Spare a Change

"If you have athlete's foot, avoid wearing the same shoes every day," says Brewster Martin, M.D., a retired family doctor in Chelsea, Vermont. "Kids and their beloved sneakers are hard to treat for athlete's foot. Their sneakers never dry out completely, which makes them an ideal habitat for the fungus."

Wear White

"White cotton socks are a must if you have athlete's foot," Dr. Reynolds says. "White cotton absorbs moisture best."

Go Informal

"Sandals are the ideal footwear for athlete's foot sufferers," Dr. Reynolds says. "They keep your feet off the ground, preventing the fungus from spreading, while allowing your skin to breathe."

Kill the "Worm"

"Most over-the-counter foot powders contain miconazole nitrate as the active ingredient, and that usually works well," Dr. Hammer notes. "An even better treatment—one that used to be available only by prescription but now comes over the counter—is Clotrimazole cream. Apply it twice a day for 7 to 10 days, and that should clear up the problem."

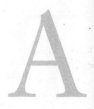

B

BACKACHE

Fighting pain that attacks from behind

It just doesn't seem fair: You were only lifting a bag of groceries from the car or helping your child tape her favorite artwork to the fridge. Or maybe you were just putting in some overtime at the office. So why are you being punished with an aching back?

That depends on which part of your back hurts, says Daniel Wing, M.D., a doctor who practices physical rehabilitation medicine throughout Vermont. "Most backaches are caused by strains in the joints and ligaments, or less often, the muscles," he says. You usually know when it happens—the pain comes on suddenly right after you move your back in a direction it isn't used to going. When you bend, twist, or lift something heavy, you sometimes tear muscles or ligaments or jam a joint, causing a bit of bleeding and swelling. "It feels like something has collapsed in your lower back," Dr. Wing says.

Movement isn't the only cause of a backache, though. A slipped disk—one of the flexible spacers that cushion the vertebrae—can be extremely painful. And so can problems in the joints of the lower back. "A common source of back pain is an injury to the sacroiliac joint, which is just below the bump above your buttocks," Dr. Wing says. One sign that it's your sacroiliac: You feel pain in that area when you sit down, walk down stairs, or twist getting out of a car, he says.

A joint or muscle problem often responds well to home remedies, Dr. Wing notes, but "an injured disk needs medical attention if the pain lasts longer than two weeks or causes muscle weakness in your legs." How can you tell the difference? Lie on your back and pull your knees toward your chest. If your back feels better, you probably have a joint or muscle problem, he explains. If the pain gets worse, suspect a disk injury and make a doctor's appointment.

In most cases, though, it's better to leave a backache alone. "If this is your first episode of back pain and you don't have a great deal of leg pain with it, go on with your life," Dr. Wing says. "Ninety percent of people with backaches will return to normal activity in two to three weeks without doing anything special. Just step down your activity to a comfortable level."

And in the future, Dr. Wing says, follow these back-saving steps.

- Take frequent breaks during car trips.
- "Avoid prolonged standing. If you do have to stand in one place for more than 10 minutes, put one foot up on an object five or six inches high, such as the brass rail at a bar or a small block."
- Don't lift an object right after rising from a chair. "Stand up straight before scooching down to lift anything."
- When you lift, keep your back straight and your knees bent to transfer the weight to your legs, not your spine. If you're lifting something light, such as a piece of litter from the ground, keep your back straight and stand on one leg, letting the other leg come up behind you.

(continued on page 30)

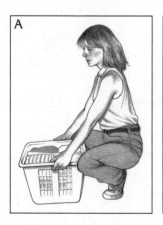
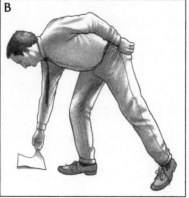

When lifting, keep your back straight (A). Stand on one leg to pick up something light (B).

Go for the Home Stretch

You can relieve muscular back pain, or prevent it from appearing in the first place, with these simple stretching exercises, says Sarah Johansen, M.D., an internist at New London Hospital in New London, New Hampshire.

Be sure to perform these exercises slowly, as gentle stretches. "You're not doing them to get stronger but to get more flexible," notes Linda B. Dacey, M.D., an internist at the Dartmouth-Hitchcock Medical Center in Lebanon, New Hampshire. "By doing them slowly and gently, you can get a good stretch without injury."

1. Lie flat on your back on the floor, using a firm pad or a rug as a cushion. Draw both knees up to your chest and hold them there for two minutes, breathing deeply.

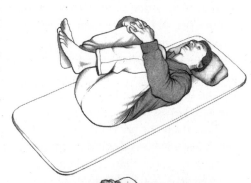

2. Then pull up your right leg alone, holding it for two minutes. Now switch to your left leg, holding it for two minutes.

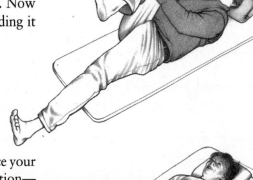

3. Still lying on your back, place your feet in the "butterfly" position—your knees out and feet together, touching at the soles. Tilt your pelvis up so that your lower back is against the floor. Hold for two minutes.

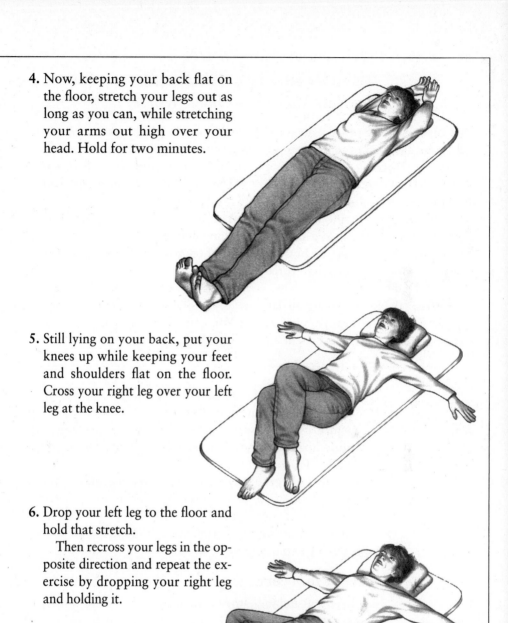

4. Now, keeping your back flat on the floor, stretch your legs out as long as you can, while stretching your arms out high over your head. Hold for two minutes.

5. Still lying on your back, put your knees up while keeping your feet and shoulders flat on the floor. Cross your right leg over your left leg at the knee.

6. Drop your left leg to the floor and hold that stretch.

Then recross your legs in the opposite direction and repeat the exercise by dropping your right leg and holding it.

Does Rest Make Your Back Worse?

Y ou don't have to see a doctor if your back aches when you get up in the morning," says Daniel Wing, M.D., a doctor who practices physical rehabilitation medicine in towns throughout Vermont. A little morning stiffness now and then is normal. But if you wake up hurting every morning for more than three weeks, get a checkup.

Also see a doctor if you hurt all day long, he adds. "And if the pain wakes you up at night, get medical attention fairly soon." Other reasons to take your back to a physician, according to Dr. Wing, include the following:

• The pain increases the longer you rest your back.
• You're experiencing weight loss along with back pain.
• Your backache is accompanied by a fever.
• The pain radiates from your back down to your leg.
• You can't control your bowel or bladder.

• Before you get out of bed in the morning, "roll onto your belly and get up on your elbows for a minute or two. That squeezes excess water out of your disks, preventing injuries that can arise from standing up with an unprepared back."
• "When you get out of a car, swivel your legs and body out before you stand. Do the reverse getting into a car: Sit first, then swivel your legs in."

If it's too late for prevention this time, here are some ways to get more comfortable.

Douse the Flame

"Take anti-inflammatories, such as aspirin or ibuprofen," says Sarah Johansen, M.D., an internist at New London Hospital in New London, New Hampshire. "You need relatively high doses over a few days to two weeks to do any good. For example, take 800 milligrams of ibuprofen every eight hours for one week." Then go cold turkey from the pills for a few days to avoid side effects such as stomach or kidney problems, Dr. Johansen says. But as long as you're on the pills, "it is very important to maintain the medication level by taking it regularly, in order to gain the anti-inflammatory benefit."

Experiment with Temps

"Try both ice and heat on your back pain," Dr. Johansen says. "Make an ice pack by filling a small plastic bag with ice and wrapping a towel around it. You can make a warm compress by soaking a face towel under the hot-water tap and then wringing out the water. Be sure you don't get the water so hot that you burn yourself. Apply the cold and then the heat to your sore back and see which feels better. Then use the winner of the experiment for 20 minutes at a time, four times a day."

Get in Touch

"Gentle massage is good for the kind of backache that arises from muscle strain," Dr. Johansen says. "You don't need any fancy techniques—just have a partner gently rub or press where it hurts."

This Cure Has a Familiar Ring

"A tubful of warm water feels great on the back," says Daniel Caloras, M.D., a family doctor in private practice in Charlestown, New Hampshire. "A whirlpool is even better."

Take Laps of Luxury

"Swimming is excellent for a backache," says Laurence Bouchard, D.O., an osteopathic family physician in private practice in Narragansett, Rhode Island. "Immersion in water takes the weight off your back and gives it a nice break."

BAD BREATH
Is your mouth rude?
Here's how to get fresh with it

If you notice that friends are waiting anxiously for you to inhale, chances are the problem is in a specific part of your mouth: your tongue if you're younger than middle-aged, your gums if you're middle-aged or older. Bacteria form chemical reactions with food particles and other wastes on the surface of your tongue, giving off gaseous sulfur compounds much like an unregulated factory smokestack. The result: Your breath smells like a blighted industrial area.

The Five-Minute Floss

Five minutes of flossing every day will help to reduce bad breath, according to Gregory Colpitts, D.M.D., a dentist who practices in Franklin, New Hampshire. But flossing helps only if you do it right. Here's how, according to Dr. Colpitts.

- Wrap the floss around the last three fingers of each hand, keeping your index finger and thumb free. That will help you handle the floss more easily.
- Insert the floss between the teeth, then make sure to go down both sides of the inverted V between the teeth. Don't just pull it straight in and out.

"It is the edge of the floss that does the work," Dr. Colpitts says.

- Floss each tooth, using floss or tape (either waxed or unwaxed). Keep the up-and-down motion going until you hear the tooth squeak. "That lets you know you've removed all the plaque."

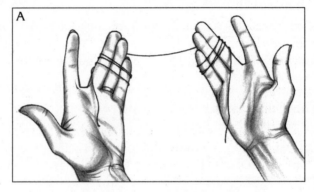
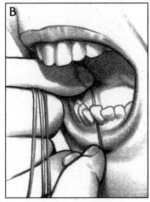
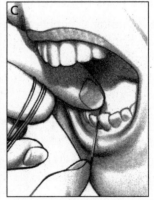

Wrap the floss around the last three fingers of each hand (A). Then use your forefingers to press the floss between the teeth (B) and work it up and down (C) until the teeth are squeaky clean.

But your gums can be your mouth's biggest air polluters. If you haven't followed your dentist's advice about brushing and flossing regularly, bacteria can build up on your gums and go to work on old food particles. The chemical reactions can actually cause gum tissue to deteriorate. This odor of decay is what causes bad breath in most people, according to Gregory L. Baker, D.D.S., an orthodontist in private practice in Woodstock, Vermont, and West Lebanon and New London, New Hampshire. "Simple brushing and flossing habits can cure a lot of breath problems," Dr. Baker says.

Your dragon breath may not be your fault, however. Just sleeping at night can raise a stink, as every newlywed has discovered to his horror. That's because you salivate less at night, giving mouth bacteria a chance to do their scavenging work on the wastes in your mouth—not just leftover food but also dead skin cells and the previous day's saliva. A good morning brushing usually clears up the problem, though some people suffer from a kind of permanent morning breath in which the salivary glands don't produce as much as they should.

Other causes of bad breath can include tonsillitis, tooth problems, acid reflux (in which acid backs up from your esophagus into your mouth, especially while you sleep at night), drugs such as some antidepressants that suppress saliva production, and stress. "People who have sinus problems and breathe through their mouths are also more likely to have bad breath," Dr. Baker says. And he notes that the mouths of diabetics often have a faintly sweet odor that could be offensive to some people.

Bad breath can be the sign of a serious disease such as liver or kidney failure. "Any bad breath that you can't explain and that won't go away in response to basic oral hygiene techniques should be examined by a doctor," Dr. Baker notes.

But first make sure that your breath really is bad. Lab research shows that people aren't very good at judging their own mouth smells. Ask a very, very close friend to take a whiff (a stranger in the street or, say, your boss might object to the experiment). If the diagnosis is grim or your friend faints dead away, try these home remedies.

Give Breath the Brush-Off

"To prevent bad breath, brush your teeth," says Gregory Colpitts, D.M.D., a dentist in private practice in Franklin, New Hampshire. "If you don't brush your teeth, plaque forms. The bacteria on the plaque form gases that can stink." Technique is important in effective brushing. "Brush from side to side at the gum line, where bacteria tend to live the most. Brush the upper and lower jaws separately," Dr. Colpitts

Tired of Breathing Smoke? The Answer Looms Ahead

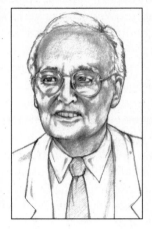

I SMOKED for about eight years—long enough to know that I was probably addicted. When I decided to stop, my wife went to a needlework store and bought me a little four-inch laptop loom to occupy my hands and mind. I made four afghans that winter and didn't smoke a single butt. You can see the afghans in my living room instead of ashtrays.

Since then I've convinced a lot of men to give up smoking, and some of them have made beautiful afghans. A neighbor of mine had smoked for 40 years until I got him to quit the smoking habit and take up knitting. He knitted like mad until the day he died.

If you're thinking of quitting, buy a loom or take knitting lessons at the same time you stop smoking. You'll be proud of the double accomplishment of not smoking and learning a craft.

BREWSTER MARTIN, M.D., *a retired family doctor in Chelsea, Vermont (population 1,166), and cofounder of the Chelsea Family Health Center. He was named Vermont Doctor of the Year in 1991.*

says. He notes that a good sign of proper brushing is teeth that feel like glass. "Teeth are meant to be smooth. That mossy feeling isn't supposed to be there."

String It Along, Too

A good toothbrushing isn't complete without a diligent round of flossing, says Dr. Colpitts, who notes that 80 percent of people fail to floss. "Good flossing requires five minutes of focused time, which sounds like a lot but can save you a lot of hassles later, including bad breath."

Lash Your Tongue

"Brush your tongue as well as your teeth," Dr. Baker says. "The tongue is a source of a lot of evil smells. Also brush the roof of your mouth."

Give Your Mouth No Butts

"Smoke coats your breathing passages with a film that smells," Dr. Colpitts notes. "Bad breath is one of many reasons to stop smoking."

Segregate Your Food

"If you still have chronic bad breath even if you exercise good oral hygiene, examine your diet," says Rosemary Gladstar, an herbalist in East Barre, Vermont, and author of *Herbal Healing for Women*. "Try not to eat carbohydrates and proteins in the same meal. That doesn't bother most people, but carbohydrates tend to get digested quickly, and proteins digest slowly, which makes a rotten smell in some people's mouths."

Go to Seed

"Chewing the seeds of fennel, dill, or anise will help freshen the breath, and, of course, peppermint leaves will always sweeten the breath," Gladstar says. All are available at grocery stores.

BAGS UNDER THE EYES
Stop being dogged by the bloodhound look

Do you see a stranger—a baggy-eyed, not-altogether-attractive stranger—when you look in the mirror in the morning? You're not having an out-of-body experience, just an under-the-skin cosmetic crisis. "Bags are caused when fluid collects in the skin under the eyes," says Charles Hammer, M.D., a dermatologist with the North Country Outreach Program of the Lahey Hitchcock Clinic in St. Johnsbury, Vermont. "This happens primarily when you lie flat for long periods, such as when you sleep at night. The prone position redistributes the fluids in your body. During the day, gravity pulls fluids toward your legs. At night, fluids are spread equally throughout the body, including the skin under your eyes." Bags also can result from allergies and from irritating chemicals, Dr. Hammer says. Here's what you can do to bag them.

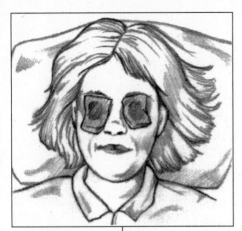

Wet tea bags can tighten baggy skin.

Suit Yourself to a Tea

"If you have bags under your eyes, try putting a cool, wet tea bag on each eye for 15 minutes," says Valerie Major, a licensed cosmetologist and manager of Beth's Salon in Woodstock, Vermont. The tannin in tea is an astringent, causing skin to tighten.

Scope Out Your Salad

"Take thinly sliced cucumbers and place one over each eye," Major advises. "Let them sit for 15 minutes." The cool moisture of cucumbers helps relieve the swelling. "It feels great," she adds.

Read Your Bags Away

"Start reading labels on your cosmetics, sunscreens—anything you put on your face—if bags under the eyes are your problem," Dr. Hammer says. "Avoid products containing propylene glycol and the fragrances cinnamyl alcohol and cinnamaldehyde. These ingredients don't bother everyone, but if you have a problem, eliminate them all. If the bags go away, you'll know that one of the products you were using was causing an allergic reaction. Add back one product each week until you find the culprit."

Scrub Some Soaps

"Certain soaps—particularly antibacterial soaps—may cause irritation in some people," Dr. Hammer notes. "Try switching brands to see if the bags under your eyes disappear."

Make a Splash

"Leave off all of your regular moisturizers and soaps for a few days," Dr. Hammer says. "Wash your face with plain water and use plain petroleum jelly to moisturize your face. If your bags clear up, soap or a moisturizer is your problem."

Shake the Salt

"If you wake up one morning with bags under your eyes, ask yourself, 'Did I eat pizza within the past 24 hours?'" Dr.

Hammer says. "If you eat a very salty meal such as pizza, it makes your body retain more water. This can cause fluid to collect under the skin beneath your eyes."

Cover the Bags

"If you want to disguise the bags under your eyes, use a concealer under your makeup," advises Cara Calomb-Down, co-owner of the Keene Beauty Academy in Keene, New Hampshire. "If the circles are purple, use yellow concealer. If the circles are reddish, use green."

BARBED WIRE CUTS
Let sharp fences point you to these remedies

You're out for a pleasant walk through the woods when sharp teeth suddenly seize you and won't let go. Chances are, it's not some wild animal that got you but old barbed wire, left from the time when these woods were fenced-in pastures. "Much of the barbed wire around here was put in in the early to mid-1900s to keep cattle in," says Roger Thrall, a

Take the Sting out of the Barbs

I GREW up on a farm in California," says Rosemary Gladstar, a nationally known herbalist who lives in East Barre, Vermont. "My Armenian grandmother would make many herbal remedies from plants growing around the yard. I learned from her and became an herbalist myself. I make a wonderful salve that is my disinfectant of choice around our house. In fact, I took it with me when my two-year-old son and I spent four and a half months riding horses up the Pacific Crest Trail on the West Coast. I still take it with me whenever I go mountain climbing in the Andes."

To make Gladstar's favorite liniment, mix together 1 teaspoon goldenseal (available at health food stores), 1 teaspoon myrrh (also available at health food stores), ½ teaspoon cayenne pepper, and 1 cup rubbing alcohol. "Let the mixture sit for two to four weeks. Then strain it into a bottle marked 'External Use Only,'" Gladstar says. "It will sting a little bit, because of the alcohol in it. But we use it on every cut, insect bite, and pitchfork injury we have."

surveyor in East Thetford, Vermont. "The old fencing will rust away entirely in a generation or two, but in the meantime, it's nasty to be around."

As a country surveyor who must tramp a lot of woods and old fields, Thrall has tangled with barbed wire more times than he can count. He doesn't bear a grudge against the sharp fencing, though; he even collects it. "More than 1,000 varieties of barbed wire have been patented since it was invented in the mid-1800s," he says. "I find it fascinating."

Thrall notes that manufacturers rate barbed wire by degrees of "viciousness," according to the fence's ability to inflict harm on trespassers. "The most vicious fences are made to keep other people either in or out," he says with a touch of irony.

Even relatively mild-mannered cattle fencing can act pretty ornery around the unwary hiker. "Barbed wire always seems to get you when you're wearing new clothes," Thrall says. To unsnag yourself from a clinging fence, "use patience. Look closely to see how you're caught up, then pick your way out barb by barb. Sudden movements will only make things worse."

Here's how to make things better.

Use Elbow Grease

"Scrub the heck out of a barbed wire cut with soap and water," says Brewster Martin, M.D., a retired family doctor in Chelsea, Vermont. "I mean really scrub it; don't just pat it. A washcloth is good for the extra abrasion."

Get Shot

"If you haven't had a tetanus booster within five years, it's time for another one," Dr. Martin says. "Get one within 24 hours of getting cut." Contrary to popular belief, tetanus doesn't come from the rust on barbed wire; the tetanus bacteria live mostly in the ground. Still, says Dr. Martin, play it safe by checking the date of your last booster whenever

You'd Think It Would Have Bombed

In 1811, the French emperor, Napoleon Bonaparte, hired the chemist Bernard Courtois to make nitrate for gunpowder. While working on the project, Courtois discovered the element iodine. Alcohol had already become popular in Europe as an antiseptic as doctors began to understand the importance of fighting germs, and iodine's germ-killing properties soon become apparent. To this day, iodine is a common treatment for scratches.

you've been cut outdoors. Any open wound can expose you to the harmful stuff on the ground.

Watch the Crotch

The unkindest cut of all, fence-wise, is the kind that gets you when you're trying to step through barbed wire. It has happened more than once to Timothy Bent, a farmer and emergency medical technician for the town of Hanover, New Hampshire. "Most of the time, it's your shirt that gets caught first," he says. "When you pay it too much attention, that's when you tend to duck, and the bottom strand gets you in the pants." If your shirt gets stuck between strands of barbed wire, Bent says to use one hand to push down the bottom strand—the one that threatens your crotch. "With the other hand, reach behind you and try to untangle yourself. If that doesn't work, go ahead and rip your shirt. Anything to keep from getting caught in the crotch."

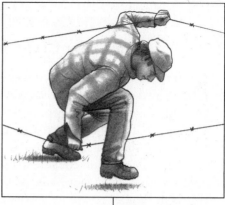

If your shirt gets stuck on a barb, use one hand to fend off the lower wire and the other to disentangle the shirt.

BED-WETTING
Steps to a well-disciplined bladder

It is a true test of a parent's understanding and patience. You've just settled into a sound sleep when your soggy child comes into your bedroom saying, "I've wet the bed."

If your kid is younger than 5 years old, the best response is to replace the sheets and PJs and go back to bed. No other special treatment is usually needed before age 5, says Stephen Rous, M.D., chief of urology at the Veterans Administration Medical Center in White River Junction, Vermont. "Infants urinate automatically when the bladder feels full. There is no voluntary control," Dr. Rous says. "Fifteen percent of all children still wet the bed beyond the age when other children are dry at night—age 2 or 3 for girls, 3 or 4 for boys. The problem tends to go away by itself. At age 18, only 1 percent of boys are still wetting the bed."

What makes bed wetters let fly? "Usually these kids have a normal bladder capacity, and their sphincter tone—the

Does Your Child Snore as Well as Wet?

SOME bed wetters have two ways to deny themselves (and their parents) of a good night's sleep: nighttime urination and breathing disorders—such as snoring and its close and dangerous cousin, sleep apnea. If your child snores *and* wets the bed, home remedies haven't worked, and your doctor has ruled out urinary or hormonal problems, consult an ear-nose-throat doctor, says Dudley Weider, M.D., an otolaryngologist at the Dartmouth-Hitchcock Medical Center in Lebanon, New Hampshire. Your child's bed-wetting may be related to a fixable breathing problem. "We've done more than 200 adenoids operations and tonsillectomies since 1978 for bed-wetting," Dr. Weider says.

"Typically, one month after the operation, 75 percent of those kids have significantly decreased their bedwetting. Twenty-five percent have stopped entirely."

This does not mean that if your child wets the bed, she's automatically a candidate for surgery. "A wet bed can be the signal that there are other physical problems, such as breathing disorders, that can affect the child later in life," Dr. Weider explains. "Many kids who are severe snorers are irritable during the day. A few will be excessively sleepy during the day, while some will develop orthodontic problems because of constant mouth breathing." Any of these problems *may* be a reason for surgery.

strength of the muscle that controls urination—is normal," says Dudley Weider, M.D., an otolaryngologist at the Dartmouth-Hitchcock Medical Center in Lebanon, New Hampshire. "What is different about bed wetters is that they make more urine at night than is normal. They don't secrete enough antidiuretic hormone to slow urine production at night."

Respiratory problems such as sleep apnea also can cause bed-wetting in children. "These kids are snorers," Dr. Weider says. "Those with sleep apnea tend to hold their breath during sleep, taking 4- to 5-second pauses between breaths and sometimes holding their breath for up to 10 seconds." This disrupted breathing prevents deep sleep, which is when the body secretes the antidiuretic hormone, according to Dr. Weider.

Genetics seem to play a role as well. "Seventy percent of the time, a child who is a bed wetter has a parent who was a bed wetter," says Peter Brassard, M.D., a family doctor in private practice on Block Island, Rhode Island.

A urinary tract infection may be another cause. An infection may be especially likely if a child with a history of dry sheets suddenly begins wetting them, Dr. Rous says. "If you suspect a urinary tract infection, take your child to the doctor to culture the urine and take a bathroom history," he advises. Also seek medical attention if your child tends to wet her pants during the day, he adds.

Although doctors say that psychological problems are usually not at the root of bed-wetting, punishment *can* lead to troubles. "In the old days, it was thought you had to teach a kid not to wet the bed," says Everett Orbeton, M.D., a pediatrician who is retired after 44 years of private practice in Portland, Maine. "In those days, if they wet the bed, you made them get up, strip off the sheets, and wash them in the middle of the night." Doctors no longer recommend blaming bed wetters. "There shouldn't be any punishment," Dr. Orbeton says. "These children are probably anxious enough about their habit already."

So what *do* you do besides constantly changing the sheets? Here are some answers.

Set the PJs on Automatic

Many doctors recommend bed-wetting alarms, which use a sensor on the crotch of the pajamas to alert the wearer to a nighttime accident. "I believe in alarms," says Patricia Edwards, M.D., a pediatrician in private practice in Concord, New Hampshire. "They are effective 95 percent of the time if the parents are willing to do the work." Dr. Edwards says that the child must be at least seven years old before his brain is sufficiently developed for the alarm to work. "Even then," she says, "the alarm often wakes up everyone but the bed wetter. The parents have to get the child up and to the bathroom."

After about six months, the child should be able to stay dry without the alarm. "It is like getting into the habit of waking up with an alarm clock," Dr. Edwards says. "After a while, even if the

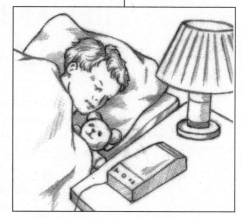

Consider a bed-wetting alarm for a child age seven or older.

power goes out, you still wake up at the right time. A bed-wetting alarm works on the same principle."

Medical studies have shown that the alarms really work and may be superior to other methods, such as drug therapy. You can buy a bed-wetting alarm at a medical supply store.

Don't Top Off the Tank

Let the child have her milk with supper but nothing else to drink after supper, Dr. Orbeton recommends.

Steer the Kid to a Pit Stop

"Taking the child to the bathroom late at night is a common home remedy, and it can help keep the bed dry," Dr. Weider says. "But the kid won't wake up, and he won't remember you took him either. So while it works as a short-term solution, you can't count it as effective long-term training."

Or You Can Fill 'Er Up

Sometimes a urologist will diagnose a too-small bladder in a bed wetter. The child can't get through the night without feeling the pressure of the evening's accumulation of liquid. "In that case," Dr. Weider says, "the doctor might recommend giving the child a lot to drink to stretch the bladder." Just don't provide the extra liquid right before bedtime.

Go with the Flow

"Most kids get over bed-wetting on their own," Dr. Orbeton says. "Let the child sleep."

BEE AND OTHER INSECT STINGS
The latest buzz on sweet relief

One of the downsides to summer, bee stings can be pretty painful annoyances. And there are plenty of other flying attackers ready to zap you when you step outdoors in the summer, too. "The stinging insects that can cause reactions are the honeybee, the bumblebee, the yellow jacket, the yellow hornet, the white-faced hornet, and any of several varieties of wasp," says Wilfred Beaucher, M.D., an internist,

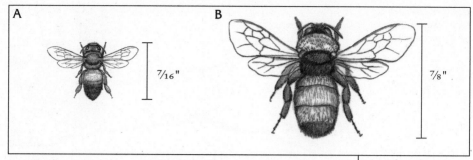

A | B

7/16"

7/8"

allergist, and immunologist in Chelmsford, Massachusetts, and Nashua, New Hampshire. The honeybee—a brownish, hairy creature—usually loses its stinger when it gets you. The other stinging insects, which have stingers that they can withdraw from your flesh, can attack repeatedly.

We failed to mention the killer bee, didn't we? Actually, killer bees are a breed of African honeybees that have interbred with American varieties to form an unusually aggressive insect. Africanized bees defend their nests zealously, and people who come too close occasionally get multiple stings. The bees are widespread in Arizona and Texas and have entered California. The best protection from their sting is to stay away from bees' nests in general, doctors say.

If you have been stung and the reaction hasn't spread to the rest of your body, here's what you can do to relieve the pain and itching.

A honeybee (A) usually loses its stinger when it gets you. A bumblebee (B) can sting again.

How Bad Is the Reaction?

IF YOU get a bit of redness and swelling where a bee has stung you, you're probably safe in taking care of it yourself, according to Wilfred Beaucher, M.D., an internist, allergist, and immunologist in Chelmsford, Massachusetts, and Nashua, New Hampshire. But if the reaction affects the rest of your body, it could be life threatening.

Here are signs that you need medical attention as soon as possible, according to Dr. Beaucher.

- A large part of your body itches, or you get hives all over your skin.
- You have trouble breathing or have a tight feeling in the throat or chest.
- You feel dizzy or sick to your stomach.
- The reaction continues for more than 72 hours after you were stung.

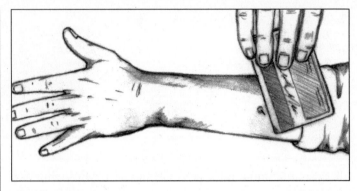
Use a credit card to flick away a stinger and venom sac.

Get the Stinger

The first thing you should do after you've been stung by a bee is try to extract the stinger and venom sac, says Edward Kent, M.D., a pediatric allergist with Timberlane Allergy and Asthma Associates in South Burlington, Vermont. "The venom sac looks like a tiny bag," Dr. Kent says. "If the bag is in place, you probably have a honeybee sting. Don't squeeze or smash it—you could end up injecting more poison into yourself. Instead, take a credit card and flick the sac away with a light scraping motion."

Try the Little Chill

"Once you've made sure the stinger is out and the area is clean, put an ice cube directly on the sting for a few minutes," says Ronald Lentz, M.D., medical director of the Block Island Medical Center in Rhode Island.

Soothe the Allergy

"Take an antihistamine such as diphenhydramine—the active ingredient in Benadryl—to reduce the itching and swelling of a bee sting," Dr. Kent says. Diphenhydramine is available over the counter at drugstores.

Rub on Ammonia

Here's an old-time bee sting remedy: ammonia. Ammonia is alkaline, making

---

AN OUNCE OF PREVENTION

Avoid Turf Battles

You should be especially careful when you paint the windows and shutters of your house. "Bees, hornets, and wasps seek out these places," says Wilfred Beaucher, M.D., an internist, allergist, and immunologist in Chelmsford, Massachusetts, and Nashua, New Hampshire. "They're good homes, protected from the wind and rain." Also watch out when you're working around the mulch in your yard. Stinging insects such as hornets and yellow jackets often make nests in compost piles or in mulch that's piled up around bushes.

BEE AND OTHER INSECT STINGS

it counteract the acidic toxins in insect venom. "It works," Dr. Beaucher says.

Don't Be Attractive

How do you avoid a repeat performance? "If you are going to be outside where bees are, wear non-floral-print clothing," Dr. Beaucher says. "Bees are attracted to flowers. They're also attracted to pictures of flowers." Avoid wearing such flowerlike colors as yellow, red, orange, and green. "Pink, blue, and white are good to wear," he says. "Bees don't like those colors."

Be careful not to smell too nice, either. "Don't wear perfume or scented products like hair spray," Dr. Beaucher says.

BELCHING
Defending against aerial attacks

There may have been a time in your life when belching was considered an asset, even a skill. To this day, you can command the respect of second-graders by reciting a major part of the alphabet in a single eructation, as doctors call a burp.

In the grown-up world, however, you probably won't win the respect of your peers by letting fly with a good one. And yet even when we're healthy, our bodies continue to issue forth air—an average of 11 times in 20 hours—whether we want them to or not. The reason is that our ordinary habits tend to trap air in the upper gastrointestinal tract, according to Linda B. Dacey, M.D., an internist at the Dartmouth-Hitchcock Medical Center in Lebanon, New Hampshire. "Often your belching is due to eating or drinking too fast," she says. "In gulping your food, you also gulp air, which eventually has to come back up." Carbonated beverages can give you burpable gas, and anxiety can cause you to swallow air unconsciously, she says.

So how do you quiet the 'urp? Here are some remedies.

Take a Fizz

Good old bicarbonate of soda—known to every cook as baking soda—can help reduce a belching episode, according to Dr. Dacey. Just mix a teaspoon of baking soda with water. "If you're on a salt-restricted diet, though, avoid bicarbonate of soda," Dr. Dacey advises. "This remedy contains a lot of sodium."

Use the Simethicone of Silence

Over-the-counter remedies containing simethicone, such as Mylanta, can help reduce an uncomfortable bout of belching, Dr. Dacey says.

Proceed Gingerly

"If belching is a problem, try ginger to relieve your stomach and stop the burping," says Corinne Martin, a certified clinical herbalist in Bridgton, Maine. Martin says you can take powdered ginger in a capsule, brew ginger tea, or eat fresh ginger. All of these forms are available at health food stores. "Ginger is great for stomach problems, including belching," confirms Sarah Johansen, M.D., medical director of emergency services at New London Hospital in New London, New Hampshire.

Eat Like a Bird

Chewing on anise, fennel, and celery seeds—all available in grocery stores—can relieve belching, Martin says. You can chew just one variety at a time or mix them up.

Don't Be Greedy

"Chew your food carefully," says Laurie Duncan, M.D., an internist who moved from Cooperstown, New York, to Washington, D.C. "Don't gulp your food. It's like eating air."

Can Pop

"If belching is a problem for you, avoid carbonated drinks," Dr. Duncan advises.

TIME TO SEE THE DOCTOR

Not All Burping Is Benign

BELCHING may be indicative of underlying medical problems," says Laurie Duncan, M.D., an internist who moved from Cooperstown, New York, to Washington, D.C. Here are some signs that you need medical help, according to Dr. Duncan.

- Your belching is getting worse.
- You vomit a bit of your stomach contents when you belch.
- You also feel bloated or sick to your stomach.
- You feel a burning sensation in your chest.
- The belching continues for more than three days.
- Your belches have a foul smell.
- You find yourself losing weight and belching a lot.
- Your bowel habits change.

Be Blander

"Some hot or spicy foods, green peppers, or onions can cause you to belch," Dr. Duncan says. "See if abstaining from them helps your belching problem."

BIRTHING PAINS
Ensuring a special delivery

It wasn't so long ago—just a few generations—when birthing was mostly a home event, without benefit of painkilling drugs and fancy equipment. Only a third of the babies born in this country in 1935 came into the world in a hospital. But then medical care and attitudes changed dramatically, and two decades later only 1 baby out of 20 was born at home. Anesthesia for deliveries was around long before that, of course. Queen Victoria made it fashionable to be knocked out with chloroform when she used it to deliver her own babies in the 1850s.

Now the pendulum has swung the other way, and health care practitioners are increasingly recommending natural childbirth—labor with a minimum of drugs. "I don't routinely give drugs to patients in labor unless absolutely necessary," says Eric A. Sailer, M.D., an obstetrician-gynecologist at the Dartmouth-Hitchcock Medical Center in Lebanon, New Hampshire. "Drugs can slow delivery and increase the risk of complications. And the drugs can affect the baby."

"Easy for him to say," a mother-to-be might think. But experienced mothers, doctors, and midwives alike say that there are ways to deal with the pain that avoid the use of drugs. "Women often figure out how to deal with their own pain in childbirth," says Deborah Drew, C.N.M., a certified nurse-midwife in Westerly, Rhode Island. "Mothers will get agitated when the worst contractions hit, and the first response is to medicate them. But if you leave them alone for 20 minutes, they'll figure out how to handle the pain and may decide against medication."

Just what is that pain? During childbirth itself, what you're feeling is the powerful contraction of your uterus, a muscular

B womb that holds the fetus. The contractions gradually expel the baby through the birth canal. Early contractions may be uncomfortable but not extraordinarily painful. It's when the contractions begin in earnest, feeling strong and frequent, that labor has really started.

Not all birthing pain comes from contractions. At the end of a mother's term, the baby's head moves down toward the birth canal and presses against the cervix at the top of the canal. "It's like taking a loaf of bread and holding the bag it's in by the back end," says Thomas J. O'Connor III, M.D., an obstetrician-gynecologist in private practice in Rockport, Maine. "Hold the bag, and the loaf pushes down against the twist tie. That's what the baby's head is doing against the cervix, causing what we call engagement pain." In addition, about a tenth of all labors involve "back labor," when the back of the baby's head pushes against the mother's spine, Dr. O'Connor says.

No matter which kind of birthing pain you're feeling, over the centuries people have come up with tactics to make the childbearing process, well, bearable. They include ways to deal with the sources of the pain, techniques to distract yourself from the contractions, and tactics for confronting the pain itself. We give some of the best methods below.

Improve Your Morale Fiber

"Treat labor like a marathon," suggests Hope Ricciotti, M.D., an obstetrician-gynecologist in Boston and coauthor of *The Pregnancy Cookbook*. "You want to carbo-load like an athlete when you think you're about to go into labor." Dr. Ricciotti explains that carbo-loading means eating lots of food high in carbohydrates, such as potatoes, bread, pasta, and cereal. "Begin bulking up on carbs the week before your due date," she suggests. "This will give you the energy you are going to need for labor."

And Keep Eating

"The first thing I tell my patients is to eat what they feel like eating," Drew says. "Eat whatever sounds good. You might want to avoid eating anything too heavy, since you're likely to throw up during labor. But definitely eat, and drink fluids, too. Herbal tea, water, and juice are good."

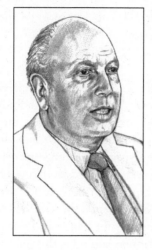

Human Stirrups Work Just Fine

SOME years ago, the phone rang just as my wife, Titia, and I were finishing supper. It was a midwife. "Please come. I'm having trouble," she said.

Like most country doctors, I had my own delivery kit with syringes, gloves, basin, a clamp, that sort of thing. I brought it and Titia with me. The midwife met us at a modest house where music was booming out of the stereo. The living room was filled with men drinking beer. The mother was in the bedroom, having a difficult labor. Her cervix was fully dilated, but there was no sign of the baby.

Fortunately, I'd been trained in Holland, which has a long tradition of home deliveries. I put the mother on her back across the width of the bed and told the midwife and Titia each to hold one leg. They acted as stirrups, you see. They gave the mother something to push against while holding the legs out of the way. The mother pushed, Titia and the midwife held on, and I caught a tiny three-pound baby that immediately did what it was supposed to do: cry. The mother went to the bathroom, and that's when we discovered it was twins. She had the second baby on the bathroom floor.

All the while the music blared. "What kind of situation is this?" I asked myself. But when the midwife showed the men the babies, they all broke out in applause. They were there to support the mother.

We took her and the babies to the hospital, where we were met with hostility by the medical staff, who couldn't believe the woman would risk a home delivery. That was before home deliveries had become fashionable again.

I learned something that day. Mothers need emotional support during childbirth, not just medical support. I recommend having a loved one (you might skip the beer and the music) along during your delivery.

GERARD BOZUWA, M.D., *retired after 36 years as the sole family doctor for the town of Wakefield, New Hampshire.*

Go Tubbing

"A warm bath may be helpful in relaxing the mother and helping her deal with the contractions," Drew notes.

Assume Your Position

American women traditionally lie on their backs to deliver babies, but "a woman can use whatever position she finds comfortable," Drew says. "This is extremely variable, and you just have to see what works for you. Some women do best in a sitting position, some on their backs, some on their hands and knees."

To ease the pain of back labor, Dr. O'Connor recommends the knee-chest position. Get on your hands and knees and stick your rear end up in the air. For engagement pain, when the baby's head presses against the birth canal, lie down and put your legs up on pillows. "Try a heating pad for your lower back as well," Dr. O'Connor says.

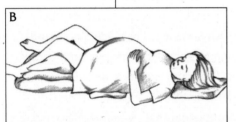

To ease back labor, try the knee-chest position (A). For engagement pain, boost your legs with pillows (B).

Try Different Strokes

"Ask your partner or caregiver to massage whatever hurts," Drew says. "For some women, this is very soothing." This won't work in all cases, however. Some women hate to be touched during labor. But others like to have their backs or stomachs rubbed.

Whistle While You Labor

"Some women find it helpful to sing in labor, and some mothers whistle," Drew says. "This can help take your mind off the pain." Drew recalls one woman who had recently taken a class in German. "She counted to 20 in German over and over with every contraction, all through her labor. It seemed to help."

Learn the Keys to Ease

"It is great if mothers can take relaxation classes to prepare for the birth of the baby," Drew notes. Your doctor or midwife can recommend classes that are right for you.

BLACK EYE

Cures for a minor shiner

Impressive as a black eye may look, it's usually nothing more than a bruise, says Eugene J. Bernal, O.D., an optometrist in White River Junction, Vermont. "The eye is pretty well cushioned to protect it from injury," Dr. Bernal says. "The orbital bones—the ones that surround your eyes—are set up as protection, and there is a lot of fat around the eye as well." A hard knock can damage the small blood vessels in the tissue around the eye, causing blood to leak out and create the characteristic discoloration of a shiner. "A black eye means the protection worked. You've bruised the surrounding tissue, which absorbs much of the blow; the globe of the eye is less affected."

But Dr. Bernal says it's a good idea to have your eye checked out at any rate. "An eye doctor will want to examine you for three possible forms of injury. First, you might have small tears in the retina, the membrane in the back of the eye. Second, your doctor will check for bleeding in the anterior, or front portion, of the eye. And third, you might have a fracture in one of the tiny bones surrounding the eye that could trap a muscle and alter your ability to see."

If you have a run-of-the-mill black eye, the ultimate cure is time. "It can take a black eye weeks to go away," says Lawrence H. Bernstein, M.D., a former family doctor who is the medical director at Jewish Geriatric Services in Longmeadow, Massachusetts. "As with any bruise, the blood under the skin has to be reabsorbed by the tissue, and that's a long process."

Although it's impossible to speed up the healing, here's what you can do to reduce the pain and discoloration.

TIME TO SEE THE DOCTOR

Are You Seeing Stars?

THE first thing to check for with any injury to the eye is any indication of damage to the globe," says Stephen Blair, M.D., a pediatrician in Claremont, New Hampshire. Here are some signs Dr. Blair says you should watch for.

- Blood or redness in the eyeball
- Seeing stars, spots, or other specks
- A sudden narrowing in your field of vision
- Blurry or double vision
- Sensitivity to light
- Pain in the eye itself

"If any of these symptoms is present, see a doctor," Dr. Blair says. "But it's always a good idea to have a hurt eye examined, even if you don't see any obvious damage."

B

Pack on the Ice

"To help reduce any swelling, apply a bag of ice to your black eye for 10 minutes every hour for the first day after the injury," says Henry Kriegstein, M.D., an ophthalmologist in private practice in Hingham, Plymouth, and Sandwich, Massachusetts. "Ice won't affect how black the eye becomes, and it won't make the blackness go away any faster, but it can reduce the swelling and make you feel better."

Put on Shades

"Sunglasses are very good at covering up black eyes," Dr. Kriegstein says. "Foundation makeup will help, too."

Save Steak for Eating

What about the time-honored remedy of putting a nice juicy steak on your eye? Save the steak for the dinner table, our sources say. "You do not put steak on a black eye, because the steak isn't clean," explains Stephen Moore, M.D., an ophthalmologist in Great Barrington, Massachusetts. "It could introduce bacteria to the eye. The key thing is to put something cold (such as an ice pack) on the eye."

BLEMISHES

Clearing skin that grows bumps in the night

It's your own personal horror movie. You look in the mirror in the morning and discover that your face has received visitors overnight: a pimple, or two or three, or a whole rash of the little monsters, each one a tiny pore that has managed to get infected.

Join the crowd: Of all the skin diseases, acne—the outbreak of blackheads, whiteheads, and pimples—is the most common. More than half the teenagers in the United States find acne when they look in the mirror.

That Old Black(head) Magic

IN 1752, the duchess of Chartres, cousin of the French king Louis XV, was so embarrassed by her acne that she paid legendary lover and part-time magician Giovanni Giacomo Casanova a fortune to cure her. Casanova consulted a secret oracle, which spelled out a magical cure: Eat less, get lots of rest, exercise, and wash the skin regularly. The duchess obeyed Casanova and his oracle, and her complexion soon improved. Casanova's "occult" healing powers became famous throughout Europe.

Doctors say that Casanova's inspired sense of hygiene was ahead of its time. "Keeping clean is an important part of preventing acne," says Jorge Crespo, M.D., a dermatologist who left New England to work with the Clark & Daughtrey Medical Group in Lakeland, Florida.

Acne occurs in specialized hair follicles called sebaceous follicles—tiny, oily depressions in the skin. You have some 5,000 of them, mostly on your back, your chest, and (of all the dumb luck) your face. Acne comes from the sebaceous glands under the skin, which pump the oil that keeps your skin from drying out. When everything is working right, the oil flows through pores and out over your skin, along with dead cells. Sometimes, though, the oil and dead cells back up in a pore and solidify, forming a whitehead. The tip on the surface of the skin can blacken, becoming a blackhead. If the plug bursts the walls of the pore, bacteria can get in and cause an infection; in other words, the dreaded pimple.

You don't have to let acne get under your skin. Despite the old folktales, you can't get acne from constipation or from having sex. Doctors now say that even chocolate—a longtime suspect in acne—does not seem to cause pimples.

In normal skin (A), the sebaceous glands pump the body's natural oils out to the surface of the skin through hair follicles. A blocked follicle can lead to a whitehead or blackhead (B). It's when bacteria get in that a pimple forms (C).

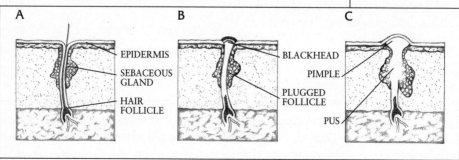

A
EPIDERMIS
SEBACEOUS GLAND
HAIR FOLLICLE

B
BLACKHEAD
PLUGGED FOLLICLE

C
PIMPLE
PUS

B

"We used to tell teenagers that chocolate and fried foods were causing their problems, while all along it was really bacteria," says Gerard Bozuwa, M.D., a retired family practitioner in Wakefield, New Hampshire.

The real trick to zapping zits, say our country sources, is to control the bacteria.

Get Acquainted with Uncle Benz

"Treat pimples on your face with an over-the-counter wash, cream, or gel containing benzoyl peroxide," says Charles Hammer, M.D., a dermatologist with the North Country Outreach Program of the Lahey Hitchcock Clinic in St. Johnsbury, Vermont. Benzoyl peroxide is an antiseptic that kills bacteria and opens the pores of the skin to control whiteheads and blackheads. The gel form of benzoyl peroxide pimple remedies helps cure blemishes without drying out your skin.

"Many products contain benzoyl peroxide," Dr. Hammer notes. "Oxy and Oxy 10 cream have benzoyl peroxide as an active ingredient. Apply the product to your face two times a day after washing. And be very careful not to get it on dyed clothing. It can take the color out."

This Remedy Will Wash

"Wash your face with plain soap that has no fragrance in it," Dr. Hammer recommends. "Dove and Dial are as good as the more expensive brands."

Watch for "Pimples" That Aren't

Some blemishes aren't pimples but small, pus-free welts on the skin. In that case, says Dr. Bozuwa, you could be having an allergic reaction. "See your doctor or an allergist to find out what might be causing the allergy." Your blemishes might also be a mild skin infection. "You often see a skin infection in young men who are just starting to shave," Dr. Bozuwa says. To clear up an infection, he recommends an over-the-counter topical antibiotic such as Bacitracin or Polysporin.

Try an Herb for a Spell

A classic cure for pimples is witch hazel, a liquid herbal extract that you can buy over the counter at most drugstores. "Witch hazel is a good drying agent," says Mark Quitadamo, M.D., a staff dermatologist at the Lahey Hitchcock Clinic in Bedford, New Hampshire. "It is sometimes used as an astringent on the face following other forms of acne treatment, such as benzoyl peroxide."

Did witches clear up their complexions with witch hazel in the old days? Possibly—people have been using the stuff for centuries. Early New England colonists learned many uses for witch hazel from Native Americans. But the name has nothing to do with necromancy, say etymologists. The "witch" in witch hazel comes from the Middle English *wych* or *wyche*, which means "pliable." According to Michael Castleman, author of *The Healing Herbs,* the branches of the witch hazel bush bend easily, making them good material for Indian bows.

BLISTERS
Skin-saving facts
to counter pain from friction

Did you get a bit too ambitious with the garden rake or hike too far in too-new boots? If so, your skin might show some interesting friction blisters, caused by the heat of tool or boot rubbing against you. "Blisters are fluid-filled cavities lined with skin," says Kathryn A. Zug, M.D., a dermatologist at the Dartmouth-Hitchcock Medical Center in Lebanon, New Hampshire. Dr. Zug notes that friction isn't the only cause of blisters, by a long shot. "A sunburn or kitchen burn can raise blisters. So can poison ivy or other allergy-causing substances. Some rare skin diseases produce blisters, as can drug reactions or diseases caused by viruses such as herpes or shingles."

If your blisters are especially large—more than two inches in diameter—it's best to get medical attention, Dr. Zug says. Otherwise, what's a tenderfoot (or hand) to do? "In most cases, nothing," Dr. Zug advises. "Leave a blister alone. Don't pop it unless it's extremely tender."

Ah, there's the rub. For the bothersome blister, here are some simple treatments.

Spread Some Jelly

"The best thing for a blister is to wash it with soap and water, keep it clean, and apply plain old petroleum jelly to lubricate the site and prevent further rubbing," Dr. Zug says. "Petroleum jelly is a dermatologist's wonder remedy. It is inexpensive. It has no additives, so it won't sting or burn. You are very unlikely to be allergic to it. And it is excellent for keeping the skin moist, which helps in healing."

Give It an "H"

Preparation H, an over-the-counter hemorrhoid remedy, is a common soother for blisters from allergic reactions to things such as poison ivy. "It has hydrocortisone in it, which helps reduce any inflammation," Dr. Zug says.

Get Silky

Dr. Zug recommends wearing silk against roughed-up areas. "It slides easily against the skin and decreases friction," she says. If you can't afford silk, nylon will do in a pinch, she adds.

Zap the Germs

If your blister becomes oozy, pussy, or painful, try applying an over-the-counter antibiotic ointment such as Bacitracin. Dr. Zug warns, however, that some people become allergic to topical antibiotics. "If the blister gets redder or itchier after you use the ointment, stop using it."

Pop the Balloon

"If your blister is building up and getting rubbed a lot," Dr. Zug notes, "ster-

---

AN OUNCE OF PREVENTION

What to Do if Trouble's Afoot

Do you get blisters on your heels? Your shoes might be too loose, says Ralph McCoy, a certified orthotic shoe technician and owner of the Shoetorium shoe store in Lebanon, New Hampshire. "You can buy liners, called heel grips, in your shoe store," McCoy says. "Or you can make your own liners. Stick a piece of cardboard under the shoe's insole."

To prevent blisters when you hike or play sports, McCoy recommends wearing two pairs of socks—good, absorbent athletic socks over a thin pair made of polypropylene, available at sporting goods stores.

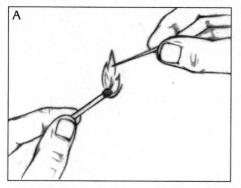

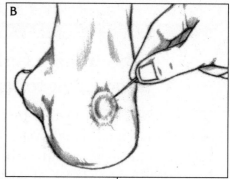

ilize a sewing needle with rubbing alcohol or a burning match. Sterilize the blister itself with alcohol, too. If you use a sterilized needle, be sure it's cool. Then poke a small hole in the blister and let it drain. That'll relieve the pressure. Leave the loose skin intact. The skin is nature's covering, and it is the best there is."

You can sterilize a needle with a burning match (A), then use the needle to poke a small hole in the blister and relieve the pressure (B).

BLOODSHOT EYES
Whitening those crimson orbs

Have you looked in the mirror and seen the makings of a horror movie—crimson eyes that need only a fur-covered face and fangs to complete the effect? The full moon probably isn't the cause of bloodshot eyes, but there are plenty of other possibilities. "The flu or a high fever can redden eyes," says Eugene J. Bernal, O.D., an optometrist in White River Junction, Vermont. "When your temperature is up, your blood vessels dilate, and you can see that in the eyes."

A swim in a chlorinated pool, an all-night study session, allergies, or dry air also can put the red in your eyes, according to Dr. Bernal, who adds that an alcoholic's eyes often are chronically bloodshot. Alcohol dilates the blood vessels, he explains, leading to the bloodshot eyes that often accompany an alcoholic's characteristic flushed cheeks and red nose. Even a teetotaler can get a harmless red spot in an eye from a burst blood vessel—caused by a sneeze or the strain of lifting something heavy. Nothing to worry about—the spot should go away after a week. But "if bloodshot eyes keep coming back, see your doctor," Dr. Bernal says.

The Teenage Girl Who Came to See

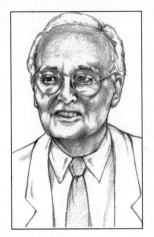

IN THE weeks before I retired from running my town's community health center, I told my patients one by one that this would be the last time they'd see me as their doctor. Albert was one of my patients. I'd treated him for 40 years. He was 56 and born without eyes. Albert still lived at home with his parents, spending his days in the living room rocking chair while his parents took turns reading to him. I had been seeing him monthly, because he had had heart surgery and I was monitoring his medication. When I told Albert I was retiring, he said, "I have no idea what you look like, but I'm going to miss seeing you." Then he reached up and touched my face and felt the tears there.

I took Albert to the waiting room to wait for his brother, who had arranged to pick him up. Then I went back to my examining room to see my next patient: a girl from a nearby private high school who had a bit of the head of a nail in her cornea. I numbed the eye, took out the sliver of metal, applied some ointment, and told her she'd have to wear a patch for 48 hours. She burst into tears. The school Christmas party was the next night, she said, and she couldn't possibly go wearing a patch.

I took her by the hand and led her into the waiting room, where I introduced her to Albert and told her his story. Back in the examining room, she said to me, "Dr. Martin, you don't have to say anything more."

Two days later, she came back so I could check her eye. A friend of hers had painted an eye on the patch, and she had gone to the dance. I got a beautiful note from her later, thanking me for taking the time to teach her one of life's most important lessons.

BREWSTER MARTIN, M.D., *a retired family doctor in Chelsea, Vermont (population 1,166), and cofounder of the Chelsea Family Health Center. He was named Vermont Doctor of the Year in 1991.*

The most common cause of bloodshot eyes is conjunctivitis, or pinkeye. If you have this condition, your eyes will not only turn pinkish or red but often will discharge a yellowish or greenish guck and feel crusty and itchy when you get up in the morning. Pinkeye can be caused by irritation from allergies such as hay fever. Or you might get the kind caused by bacteria or a virus. The viral kind can be very contagious. Your tears can give other people pinkeye for up to two weeks after you get it.

Although you might not appreciate the monster look, bloodshot eyes usually are not serious. One problem, however, can cause permanent damage: keratitis, an inflammation or infection of the cornea. Improperly washed contact lenses can cause the disease, which requires a doctor's care.

Whatever the cause, try to avoid rubbing your red eyes if they also feel itchy and sore. That just fans the fire. What should you do instead? Thomas Palmer, a seventeenth-century Massachusetts doctor, recommended smearing the blood of pigeons and swallows onto your eyes. Modern country doctors tell us you shouldn't try this remedy. But they have given us a few alternatives.

Lend Them a Tear

"Over-the-counter eyedrops, such as Tears Naturale II and Hypotears, can be used to keep the eyes lubricated and make them less irritated," says Stephen Moore, M.D., an ophthalmologist in Great Barrington, Massachusetts. "Dry eyes often become bloodshot." Read the product label before you buy. "I don't recommend drops that contain vasoconstrictors," Dr. Moore says. "These drops constrict the blood vessels in your eyes, making them look less red. But they can have a rebound effect, causing your blood vessels to dilate permanently." Some eyedrops contain preservatives that can irritate sensitive eyes. "If you need to

Seeing More Than Red?

RED eyes accompanied by pain or blurred vision should be seen by a doctor," says Henry Kriegstein, M.D., an ophthalmologist in Hingham, Plymouth, and Sandwich, Massachusetts. "The pain could signal a number of serious conditions that need early treatment." Dr. Kriegstein also recommends seeing a doctor if you feel as if you have something in your eye, "even if you can't see it."

Also see a doctor if your eyes are red for more than two days at a time, are sensitive to light, stay red for more than two hours after you remove your contact lenses, or discharge a yellow or greenish goo.

use drops chronically, look for preservative-free brands, such as Bion Tears and Refresh Plus."

Sink the Pink

"The itchiness that often accompanies red eyes can be relieved by a cool cloth," says Henry Kriegstein, M.D., an ophthalmologist in Hingham, Plymouth, and Sandwich, Massachusetts. "A cool compress, such as a washcloth soaked in cold water, also can help constrict the blood vessels, making your eyes look less red."

React to the Reaction

"Over-the-counter antihistamines can be used for an entire season if your bloodshot eyes are the result of an allergy," Dr. Kriegstein says. "To get rid of the allergic reaction, including bloodshot eyes, you can use Vasocon-A, Naphcon-A, or Opcon-A four times a day throughout the allergy season."

Shut Them Up

"The best cure for the bloodshot eyes that come from fatigue is sleep," Dr. Bernal says. "Nothing works better."

BODY ODOR
Putting a runaway smell in neutral

It may be hard to believe when you're standing in a locker room, but sweat—the pure sweat that runs off you in the gym—does not smell. Sweat can spread odors around, such as aromas caused by meals you've eaten, but the moisture itself is inoffensive. So what is that odor coming from under your arms in the middle of a job interview?

Chances are, your embarrassing smell is caused not by the wetness seeping through your shirt but by an odoriferous cocktail with two ingredients: bacteria and tiny secretions from a kind of sweat glands called apocrine glands. These glands are concentrated under your arms, in your groin, and on your perineum—the skin between the anus and the genitals. Bacteria that thrive in the tropiclike environments of underarms and skin folds act on the milky droplets secreted by the apocrine glands to produce body odor. Stress makes the apocrine glands rev up into high gear.

Heat and physical activity, on the other hand, stimulate a different kind of sweat—the clear, odorless liquid that comes from the eccrine glands. A well-bathed farmer getting the hay in on a hot day may smell as sweet as the hay itself, while a tax evader sitting before a lie detector might make his interrogator dizzy with the odor. "Your genetic inheritance can help determine whether or not you have a strong body odor," says Jorge Crespo, M.D., a dermatologist who left New England to work with the Clark & Daughtrey Medical Group in Lakeland, Florida. "Some people's native bacterial flora cause more odor than others'."

Why are we burdened with glands that make us stink? The secretions from the apocrine glands have been shown in the laboratory to be chemically similar to odors that other species

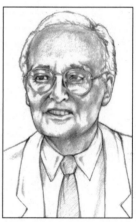

of mammals use to communicate. Some scientists speculate that BO was once a kind of aphrodisiac, a musky perfume that attracted the opposite sex.

Assuming that your nose does not have quite those romantic inclinations, here are some specific remedies from our rural doctors.

Declare War on Germs

Without bacteria, your sweat won't smell as much, doctors say. "Antibacterial soaps like Dial and Lever 2000 are effective against body odor," says Mark Quitadamo, M.D., a dermatologist at the Lahey Hitchcock Clinic in Bedford, New Hampshire. "Wash daily with one of these soaps, as long as you don't have sensitive skin."

Stalk Your Pits with Corn

"Try to avoid antiperspirants," says Gerard Bozuwa, M.D., who is retired after 36 years as a family doctor in Wakefield, New Hampshire. "Antiperspirants close off the sweat glands, and that stops up a natural process. Instead, soak up the sweat before you go out by sprinkling your underarms with cornstarch, which you can buy at any drugstore or grocery store. Baby powder works as well."

Go Sour to Smell Sweet

Dr. Quitadamo recommends Domeboro, an old-time, over-the-counter powder that forms the basis for an astringent. "It works quite well," he says. Mix Domeboro with cool or lukewarm water and apply it by soaking a washcloth with the mixture and applying the washcloth as a compress to problem areas. Domeboro is available at drugstores and grocery stores.

Spice May Not Smell Nice

"Spicy foods definitely can cause body odor," Dr. Crespo warns. "Garlic is the most notorious. It is excreted through the skin almost entirely unchanged. People who are sensitive to the smell can detect it on someone else's body two, even three days after the garlic was eaten. Curries and other foods in Indian cuisine also cause body odor. It isn't because the person is unclean. The odor simply comes from what he or she has eaten." Dr. Crespo says that if you're feeling self-conscious about your smell, it's best to avoid spicy foods that trigger odors.

BOILS

What to do when your skin is having a swell time but you're not

A boil—an infected, pus-filled hair follicle—is more annoying than dangerous. Staphylococcus bacteria invade your skin, and your body's defenses fend off the attacking germs. Pus and painful swelling result. Boils often appear on the back of the neck and on moist parts of the body that are frequently chafed by clothing or other parts of your anatomy.

	EPIDERMIS
	BOIL
	SEBACEOUS GLAND
	HAIR FOLLICLE

When bacteria invade a hair follicle, you end up with pus and a painful red bump in the skin. Above: A simple boil with a single center.

"There are two kinds of boils," says Gerard Bozuwa, M.D., who is retired after 36 years as a family doctor in Wakefield, New Hampshire. "A simple boil is a painful red bump that eventually gets a yellow center. The second kind, also called a carbuncle, is a boil with numerous centers. Both kinds are very common on the back of the neck if it's

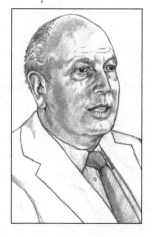

A WORD FROM DR. B.

The Problem Could Be Blood Sugar

BOILS are not a natural thing in healthy people. If you get boils frequently, ask your doctor to look at the underlying cause.

Your doctor might test you for diabetes. Diabetics are much more likely than other people to get boils. If someone comes in with boils, diabetes is the first thing we doctors check for.

GERARD BOZUWA, M.D., *retired after 36 years as the sole family doctor for the town of Wakefield, New Hampshire.*

frequently shaved. Clothing can rub against the area and irritate it, inviting infection."

Avoid the temptation to squeeze a boil. Without proper medical treatment, a burst boil could spread the staph infection to other parts of your body. "The danger in a boil is if, through squeezing, the boil bursts the wrong way, forcing the infection in where it can't drain," Dr. Bozuwa says. "That can cause a first-stage infection of the lymph system, which you can see as red streaks radiating from the boil on your skin. The lymph system drains into your bloodstream, which can then lead to a second-stage infection—that is, true blood poisoning, and it is life threatening."

So we're not squeezing, are we? Here's what you can do instead.

Heat until the Boil's Over

"You can usually bring a small boil to the surface and make it drain on its own if you use warm compresses, such as warm washcloths," says Charles Hammer, M.D., a dermatologist with the North Country Outreach Program of the Lahey Hitchcock Clinic in St. Johnsbury, Vermont. "Apply the warm compresses to the boil twice a day for 15 minutes at a time. If the boil fails to drain in a week, you should see a doctor."

Bring Your Boil to a Tea

A warm, moist tea bag can help as a compress, says Mark Quitadamo, M.D., a dermatologist at the Lahey Hitchcock Clinic in Bedford, New Hampshire. "The tannic acid in a tea bag is antibacterial, which can be useful for relieving the infection."

Hit the Hurt

Besides applying compresses, "the other thing you should do for a boil is take a painkiller, such as aspirin or ibuprofen," Dr. Quitadamo says. "Pain is the worst

TIME TO SEE THE DOCTOR

When It's a Big Bubble, Your Boil Could Be Trouble

IF A boil is larger than half an inch in size, or deep and pus-filled, have a doctor look at it. Red lines emanating from a boil are a sign that the infection could be spreading—another good reason to get medical attention. Also see your doctor when a fever accompanies a boil. In addition, "if a boil is red, angry, and painful, you should go right to the doctor to have it lanced and drained," says Charles Hammer, M.D., a dermatologist with the North Country Outreach Program of the Lahey Hitchcock Clinic in St. Johnsbury, Vermont.

part of a boil." If compresses and painkillers fail, "see a doctor. You may need to have it lanced, and you may need antibiotics to deal with the infection." Don't give aspirin to children because of the risk of Reye's syndrome.

BREAST ACHES
Saying no thanks to painful mammaries

During the week or so before your period, your breasts may want to tell you about the monthly hormonal changes you're going through. They may become lumpy, sore, and tender, giving you a twinge every time they bounce. The problem usually goes away soon after your period starts.

What's going on? As your body prepares every month to become pregnant, releasing an egg to be fertilized, your breasts do their own form of preparation, readying the milk glands and growing extra fibrous tissue to support the extra weight of an eventually milk-filled breast. Sometimes the process gets carried away with itself. Fluids collect in the milk ducts and glands, and fiber growth causes the breast tissue to thicken. The result: those monthly lumps and aches in one or both breasts.

Take heart in the knowledge that your breasts won't always suffer. "One of the few advantages to getting older is that women with breast aches usually find the problem easing with age," says Hope Ricciotti, M.D., an obstetrician-gynecologist at the Beth Israel Deaconess Medical Center in Boston. "As women age, the fibrous tissue converts to fat, and the lumps and aches disappear."

Here's what you can do while you're still in the achy period.

> ### TIME TO SEE THE DOCTOR
> ## *Check for Lumps*
>
> IF YOUR breast aches are associated with a lump, redness, tightened skin, or a bloody or pink discharge from a nipple, see a doctor right away," says Thomas J. O'Connor III, M.D., an obstetrician-gynecologist in private practice in Rockport, Maine. "Your symptoms could be a sign of fibrocystic disease or more serious problems."

Keep Midol in Mind

"Women were taking Midol for breast aches before all these other painkillers, such as acetaminophen and ibuprofen,

B

came on the market," says Mardrey Swenson, a certified lactation consultant and La Leche League leader for the Upper Connecticut Valley in West Lebanon, New Hampshire. "Midol is a nonaspirin analgesic and a diuretic, and it still works fine. It helps reduce breast aches."

Take Arctic Refuge

"Ice helps with breast aches," says Brewster Martin, M.D., a retired family doctor in Chelsea, Vermont. Dr. Martin says to fill an ice pack or a washcloth with ice cubes and apply the cold compress to your achy parts for 10 to 20 minutes several times a day. "Ice decreases the rapidity with which the pain message is sent to the brain," he explains.

Add Dandelion to Your Diet

Rosemary Gladstar, an herbalist in East Barre, Vermont, and author of *Herbal Healing for Women*, recommends taking dandelion greens to regulate the amount of fluid in your breasts. "The dandelion leaf is a mild, natural diuretic. Taking it will help with breast tenderness caused by water retention in your body." She suggests buying it in capsule or tea form at a health food store. "You could make a tea of the leaves, but the taste is bitter," she says.

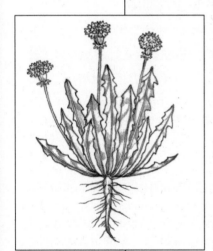

Tea or a capsule made from the green leaves of the dandelion plant can help regulate the amount of fluid in your breasts.

Skip the Valentine's Day Chocolates

"If you suffer from breast aches, avoid caffeine and chocolate altogether," Dr. Ricciotti says. Caffeine and some other ingredients in chocolate, tea, and coffee are members of a family of compounds known as methylxanthines. Eliminate their use entirely, and you could find your breast problems going away, says Dr. Ricciotti.

Refresh Your Bras

"Large breasts can weigh as much as four pounds each, putting a real strain on your ligaments and causing pain," says Lawrence H. Bernstein, M.D., a former family doctor who is the medical director at Jewish Geriatric Services in Longmeadow, Massachusetts. "Buy a new bra if the elastic in your old one seems stretched. I know some women who have been wearing the same bra for ten years. They're not doing themselves a favor."

Get a New Lift

"Underwire bras, especially the 'wonder' bras that push your breasts up, aren't great for women with breast problems," Dr. Ricciotti says. "Supportive exercise bras are best."

Let Nature Call

"Lactating mothers suffering from breast aches will find relief if they nurse their babies on demand," Dr. Ricciotti advises.

BREASTFEEDING PROBLEMS
Ways to get you and your baby back in sync

"A pair of substantial mammary glands has the advantage over the two hemispheres of the most learned professor's brain, in the art of compounding a nutritious fluid for infants." This bit of poetic wisdom has been attributed to Oliver Wendell Holmes, the great nineteenth-century physician and writer.

Research is increasingly proving Holmes right: We now know that breastfed babies suck in their mothers' immunities as well as milk. "Breastfed babies get sick, but their illnesses are milder than those of formula-fed babies," says Mardrey Swenson, a certified lactation consultant and La Leche League leader in the Upper Connecticut Valley of New Hampshire.

When they grow up, breastfed babies may even qualify as learned professors; some studies seem to show that they score higher on IQ tests than their counterparts.

Mothers benefit, too. "Letting babies suckle immediately after delivery makes the uterus contract, helps the placenta pass, and can help stop the bleeding," Swenson says.

Then there is the downside: Your breasts may feel heavy, lumpy, and swollen, and your nipples may feel as though they've been attacked by an animal—which, in a way, they have. Here's how to go with the flow in comfort.

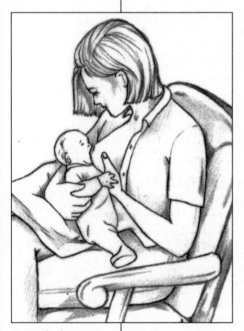

Breastfeed tummy to tummy, chest to chest.

Belly Up to the Bar

"The vast majority of breastfeeding problems have to do with proper positioning and getting the baby to latch on," Swenson says. "The baby should be held tummy to tummy, chest to chest with the mother. Only a few mothers are built so the crook of the arm lines the baby up properly with the nipple. Try holding the baby's head more toward your forearm and tucked against you with your arm supporting the baby's back and neck."

Try It Down Under

Swenson also recommends the Australian nursing position if you tend to let out milk forcefully. Lie on your back with your baby on top. "The milk goes to the front of the baby's mouth, making choking less likely."

Avoid a Chomp

"Babies can bite before they have teeth," Swenson warns. "Look for a pattern. It could be that the baby is getting impatient waiting for your milk to eject and may bite down. When the milk slows, other babies may get distracted and turn to look at something interesting without letting go."

How you react can determine whether the biting becomes a problem. "When a baby bites, it hurts," Swenson says in what nursing mothers know is an understatement. "A mother's reaction of shock or anger may make some babies upset, and they may go on a nursing strike. Other babies like the reaction and try biting again." The solution: Learn when the baby is most likely to bite and have your finger ready to keep the mouth from closing. "If the biting tends to come near the end of feeding on one side, switch to the other breast before the baby bites," Swenson advises.

Rest the Pesto

Rosemary Gladstar, an herbalist in East Barre, Vermont, and author of *Herbal Healing for Women,* says to avoid eating too much parsley while breastfeeding. "A little garnish won't hurt. But a lot of it, such as what you get in parsley-based pesto, will interfere with milk production."

Take Your Nipple to Tea

"Tea bags make a good treatment for nipple infections when nursing," says Mark Quitadamo, M.D., a dermatologist at the Lahey Hitchcock Clinic in Bedford, New Hampshire. "Apply a cool, wet tea bag to your sore nipple. It'll have a soothing effect, and the tannic acid in tea may be antibacterial, preventing infection."

Empty Out

If your breasts ache from being engorged with milk, nurse your baby every time he asks, says Hope Ricciotti, M.D., an obstetrician-gynecologist in Boston and coauthor of *The Pregnancy Cookbook.* "Switch the breast you offer first so that each breast is thoroughly emptied of milk."

Ice Up

If your engorged breasts still ache, Dr. Ricciotti recommends putting a bag of ice against the swollen-feeling parts. "Don't

Yet Another Breastfeeding Problem: The Law

IN 1992, Deborah "Arnie" Arnesen became the first woman to be nominated by a major political party for governor of New Hampshire. She won the honor in spite of having publicly broken the law seven years before—right on the floor of the state legislature. "In 1985, when I was a state representative, I started taking my five-week-old daughter, Kirsten, with me to work," Arnesen says. "My seat was in the very last row, and I kept a portable crib behind me. I nursed Kirsten on the floor of the legislature and in committee meetings."

The Associated Press ran a nationwide story, and a local newspaper listed Arnesen as one of the "sights to see" when visiting the state capitol. "They listed the dome of the capitol building, the pictures of former governors, the wonderful collection of military flags—and me, breastfeeding," Arnesen says. She notes that the sight is much more common now. "Other women legislators have nursed their babies publicly since then."

Nonetheless, public breastfeeding can be viewed as illegal in New Hampshire, which is one of many states where the practice is considered a form of indecent exposure.

take a hot shower," she says. "That could make you feel worse."

Stay Dressed

"A nursing mother may find she is more comfortable if she sleeps with her nursing bra on," Dr. Ricciotti notes. The bra holds things in place, preventing uncomfortable jostling of the breasts.

Call for Milk

"A mother needs some help getting started," Swenson says. "Without training, she may be floundering at home, and it is easy to get discouraged. New mothers are very vulnerable." Swenson suggests contacting La Leche League, a group that provides support to breastfeeding mothers. To find a local branch of La Leche, look under Midwives in the Yellow Pages of your phone book, call one of the names listed there, and ask that person for the number of the group in your area. (The organization itself is not always listed in the phone book.) The group, by the way, gets its name from the Spanish for "the milk." When La Leche League was formed in the

1950s, newspapers would not print the word *breast*. One of the founding mothers took the group's name from a statue of the Madonna and baby Jesus at a shrine in Florida.

BRITTLE NAILS
How to cope with the tough breaks

Shock troops for your fingers, your nails take a lot of abuse. But the most damaging assault, surprisingly, comes from dry air, especially during the winter months. "Water normally makes up around 23 percent of your nails," says Charles Hammer, M.D., a dermatologist with the North Country Outreach Program of the Lahey Hitchcock Clinic in St. Johnsbury, Vermont. "Once the water content falls below 17 or 18 percent, your nails become dried out and cracked. Dry air in the winter is a big cause."

Frequent washing can dry out nails, Dr. Hammer says. So can irritating cleansers and solvents. "And, as we get older, our nails dry out along with our skin."

Here are some remedies to help keep the moisture in.

Block Those Suds

"Don't wash the dishes with your bare hands," Dr. Hammer says. "Don't just wear plain rubber gloves either. If you keep the gloves on for any length of time, your hands will sweat and water will drip into the gloves, causing the same effect as if you'd immersed them in water in the first place. To keep them dry, wear cotton-lined rubber gloves, available at most drugstores."

Split with the Polish

"Some fingernail polishes and nail hardeners contain formaldehyde, a widely used preservative, which can irritate skin and nails," Dr. Hammer says. "If you think your polish is causing problems, switch to a polish that doesn't contain formaldehyde, or avoid polish altogether."

Cream Up

"You can increase the moisture in your nails by using moisturizing creams," says Robert Averill, M.D., a dermatologist in private practice in western Massachusetts and northern New Hampshire. "It really doesn't matter which brand; ask your druggist for an over-the-counter emollient cream."

Rub It In

"To treat your brittle nails, rub some cuticle oil onto the nail itself," says Silvia Demedeiros, a manicurist and owner of Nails by Silvia in Pittsfield, Massachusetts.

Make Room for Jell-O

"Drink gelatin," advises Gerard Bozuwa, M.D., who is retired after 36 years as a family doctor in Wakefield, New Hampshire. "Just mix your favorite flavor of Jell-O and drink it while it's still warm. I've been telling patients that for years, and it must work, because they've always thanked me." Dr. Bozuwa adds that eating Jell-O has the same effect, if you feel like going to the extra trouble of refrigerating it.

Stay Watery

"Drink plenty of water to maintain the body's natural moisture levels," says Cara Calomb-Down, co-owner of the Keene Beauty Academy in Keene, New Hampshire. "If you're dry, your nails will be, too."

Get Slick in Bed

"Apply petroleum jelly to your nails at bedtime," Dr. Hammer advises. "Cover them with cotton gloves, and your nails will retain much more of their moisture."

BROKEN BONES
*Home treatments
for a cracked skeleton*

How do you know if you've broken one of the 206 bones in your body? Much of the time you don't. It's not always easy to tell if you have a fracture. But, doctors say, when in doubt, get immediate medical help. "You risk damaging the broken bone even more if you don't take it to a doctor," says John Dunn, M.D., an emergency room physician at the Northwestern Medical Center in St. Albans, Vermont, and author of the book *Winterwise: A Backpacker's Guide.* "Let pain and function be your guide. If it hurts a lot or it won't work right, take it in." What if you break a bone far from medical help—during a wilderness camping trip, say? If you can walk comfortably and don't have too far to go, Dr. Dunn recommends a "self-rescue," hiking your way out. But don't try a long trek on a broken leg, he warns. Your best bet in that case is to wait for help.

What can happen if you try to tough it out? Daniel Nelson is a self-rescuer who, having broken his leg, skied his way out of the wilderness. A former guide on Washington State's Mount Rainier, Nelson managed to break his leg while skiing down New Hampshire's wild Mount Moosilauke with his son's Scout troop. "I turned to avoid a stream and hit a tree with my leg," he says. "I couldn't put any weight on it. But I was three miles from the nearest road, and skiing seemed the fastest way out." Nelson skied on one foot, using his poles for balance, until he got back to his car. One of the other Scout leaders drove. "I was on crutches for the rest of the winter," he says. "The doctors said I was lucky the break wasn't made worse from skiing. So the lesson here is to immobilize a broken bone. If I'd been sure my leg was broken, I would have asked the Scouts to carry me out."

Although a break in a large leg bone can be dramatic, the most common breaks among children are in the arm, wrist, and collarbone, according to Stephen Blair, M.D., a pediatrician in private practice in Claremont, New Hampshire. "These breaks occur when the child falls off playground equipment or a bike, or falls out of a tree house, and puts an arm stretched out in front to stop the fall."

Afterward, They Could Repair Your House

UP UNTIL the late nineteenth century, if you broke a bone, you would go to a specialist called a bonesetter. This was no medical doctor with extra anatomical training. Most bonesetters were carpenters and blacksmiths picking up some extra money on the side. They could promise great skill with their tools; their knowledge of their patients' inner works was a chancier proposition.

These days, general practitioners are trained to fix broken bones. They'll send you to a specialist if your break is unusual, particularly difficult to fix, or accompanied by another medical problem. That specialist will be trained in medicine—not carpentry—so it's a much better idea than it was a century ago to seek immediate medical attention when you think you've broken a bone.

The Woman Who Refused a Pin

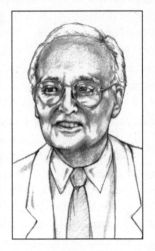

During the 40 years I worked at the Chelsea Family Health Center in Vermont, one of my favorite patients was an elderly woman named Elsie. One day, at the age of 96, Elsie had a fall. Her hip still hurt five days later, so her daughter called and had me come see her. I examined her and then called an ambulance to take her for an x-ray. It took some persuading to get Elsie to agree to the x-ray. She wasn't one for fancy medical procedures.

Sure enough, the test showed that her hip was broken. I told her that the usual procedure at that time was a simple operation to put a pin in the hip. "What did you do before those smart fellas came up with those pins?" she asked me. Twelve weeks of bed rest, I told her, followed by some weeks on crutches.

"Then I'm going home right now," Elsie said. "What's 12 weeks when you've lived 96 years?" Having skipped the operation, she was walking around again after a few months. She lived to be 103.

Sometimes a good attitude and inner strength are better than the best of modern medicine.

Brewster Martin, M.D., *a retired family doctor in Chelsea, Vermont (population 1,166), and cofounder of the Chelsea Family Health Center. He was named Vermont Doctor of the Year in 1991.*

Here's what you can do to minimize the pain and help with the healing.

Heal with RICE

"Before you can get to the doctor, you can help things along with RICE," says Lawrence H. Bernstein, M.D., a former family doctor who is the medical director at Jewish Geriatric Services in Longmeadow, Massachusetts. RICE stands for rest, ice, compression, and elevation. "Stay off the injury, put bags of ice on it for 10-minute periods, and keep it raised," Dr. Bernstein says. "Gently put a compress—a clean cloth will do—on the broken part. Skip the compression if it hurts."

Watch for a False "Break"

"I often see an injury in children ages one to four that we call nursemaid's elbow," Dr. Blair says. "It seems a lot like a broken arm, but it's actually a dislocated joint." Here's how it happens: Parent and toddler are walking along hand in hand, and suddenly the child decides to switch directions. "The radial head at the elbow pops out. The kid acts as if his arm is broken, complaining of the pain and refusing to use the arm." Your doctor can easily diagnose nursemaid's elbow by asking what happened just before the arm started hurting. If the answer is a sudden jerk on the arm, "then it's almost certainly nursemaid's," Dr. Blair says. Your doctor can pop the elbow back into place. "Some children have elbows that go out easily. I can teach the parents how to put the elbow back where it belongs." Ask your doctor if you can learn to do the "popping" move as well.

BRONCHITIS
Calming cures for angry lungs

If your cough just won't quit, you have an achy feeling in your chest, you're wheezing, and your coughing is bringing up some interesting-looking substances, you may have bronchitis.

"Bronchitis is an inflammation of the bronchi, the smallest branches in the lungs," explains Dudley Weider, M.D., an otolaryngologist at the Dartmouth-Hitchcock Medical Center in Lebanon, New Hampshire. Your air passages fight the inflammation by creating mucus, which makes you cough, which brings up all that colorful phlegm.

"Bronchitis can have any one of four causes," Dr. Weider says. "You can get it from an allergy; from environmental pollutants, especially glues and formaldehyde; from bacteria; or from viruses." If you're coughing up a lot of phlegm, Dr. Weider says, a virus or bacterial infection is the most likely cause.

Although bronchitis can make you feel pretty awful—fever and an all-over achy feeling are part and parcel of this

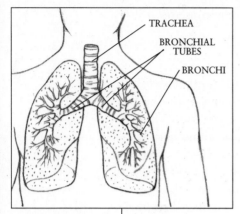

Bronchitis affects the bronchi, the smallest branches in your lungs.

illness—you can take comfort in the fact that the disease is common and not that serious. Get yourself to a doctor if your breathing has a rattle; you might have pneumonia. For run-of-the-mill bronchitis, your doctor can determine the best way to deal with the underlying cause. A bacterial infection, for example, can be treated with an antibiotic. In addition, our country physicians recommend some at-home remedies to make you rest easy and less wheezy.

Stay Juicy

"You want to keep the secretions from your lungs nice and liquefied," says Robert Fagelson, M.D., an otolaryngologist in Brattleboro, Vermont. "Drink a lot of fluids."

Slow the Cough . . .

A dry, unproductive cough can cause microscopic damage to the vocal cords, making you hoarse, Dr. Weider says. "You can reduce the amount of coughing by sucking on cough drops or drinking tea with honey." The action of swallowing helps to control the coughing reflex, he explains.

. . . And Make It Count

"Try over-the-counter medications that contain guaifenesin," Dr. Fagelson suggests. Guaifenesin is an expectorant found in many cough medications, including Robitussin and Triaminic Expectorant. It will help you expel the mucus.

Boost Your Bark

"If your bronchitis is accompanied by a dry, unproductive cough, try taking a teaspoon of slippery elm or marshmallow root mixed with lemon, honey, and hot water," says Rosemary Gladstar, an herbalist in East Barre, Vermont, who formulates teas for herbal companies. These herbs are available as powders at health food stores. "Slippery elm and marshmallow root don't dissolve easily in water," she notes. "Mix in a blender or stir vigorously before drinking."

Go for the Candy Plant

"Licorice, taken as a tea or tincture, helps reduce the inflammation that accompanies bronchitis," Gladstar says. One of the oldest cures for coughs and bronchitis, licorice is generally available at herbal stores and is considered safe by the U.S. Food and Drug Administration. But authorities warn against taking the herb in high doses. A pinch of powder in tea three times a day is enough. And make sure you're getting the real thing. Most "licorice" candies contain anise, not licorice.

But Skip This Weed

"Avoid cigarette smoke when you have bronchitis," Dr. Weider says. "Smoke makes bronchitis worse, whether you yourself are smoking or you're breathing in secondhand smoke." Dr. Weider explains that smoking destroys the tiny hairs, or cilia, on the lining of the lungs, which help remove mucus and other waste products. At the same time, the smoke irritates the lungs, stimulating production of mucus. "As a result, you have more mucus and fewer cilia to deal with it. That's why smokers cough a lot in the morning."

Be a Humid Being

"A problem here in New England—one that makes people with bronchitis suffer even more—is that the insides of our homes are too dry in the winter," Dr. Weider says. "We have the heat on and the windows closed, which drives the humidity way below what it should be." Dr. Weider recommends getting the humidity up to at least 33 percent by using a cold-water vaporizer from a drugstore.

Get Steamed

"If you have bronchitis, step into a hot, steamy shower and breathe the steam. It really helps." That's the advice of Julia

---

TIME TO SEE THE DOCTOR
Watch the Calendar When You're Coughing

IF YOUR bronchitis makes you cough for a month, see your doctor about getting a prescription for an antibiotic," says Dudley Weider, M.D., an otolaryngologist at the Dartmouth-Hitchcock Medical Center in Lebanon, New Hampshire. "Even if a virus was the original cause, chances are good that you have a secondary bacterial invasion that needs an antibiotic for a cure."

The Lord Giveth . . .

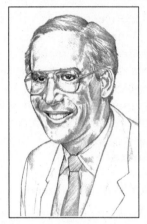

NOT long ago I became the proud owner of several photographs of waterwheels. The collection is one I've always admired, but these particular pictures have a greater meaning for me. They remind me of a family that's been a special part of my practice for more than 20 years.

Many years ago, a young woman who was a patient of mine gave birth to a baby she had to raise alone. Soon after, she developed multiple sclerosis. Within six months, she was completely bedridden and couldn't talk. Her elderly grandparents took her in and raised her little boy.

She developed pneumonia when her son was eight years old. When the little boy learned his mother was going to die, he came up to me and asked, "May I say goodbye to Mommy?" He did, and his mother died soon after.

The boy, named Jay, grew up and married. His great-grandfather, who had raised Jay, died a few years ago—the day after Jay's first son was born. I especially miss the older man. He was an outstanding photographer, and it's his pictures of waterwheels that I now cherish. Jay sent me those photos a month after his great-grandfather's death.

Call it a case of long-term care—only the care was on both sides.

LAWRENCE H. BERNSTEIN, M.D., *a family doctor who made house calls in Storrs, Connecticut, for 22 years. He now works at Jewish Geriatric Services in Longmeadow, Massachusetts.*

Foote, R.N., a retired nurse currently living in Norwell, Massachusetts.

"Abolutely, that works," Dr. Fagelson concurs.

Go Deep with Purple

Gladstar notes that "one of the best ways to fight bronchitis is to drink echinacea tea." Echinacea, or purple coneflower, is a perennial whose dried leaves and roots are available in tea form at most herbal stores. Skip this cure if you're allergic to ragweed, a close relative of the echinacea plant. But for other folks, the plant has been shown to be an immune system stimulant as well as a natural antibiotic.

BUNIONS
Saying so long to toes that get ahead of themselves

You may have been confronted lately by a staggering reality: Those fancy high heels that seemed perfect for a night on the town have become instruments of torture, forcing your weight against your big toe and turning your fancy dancing into gimpy limping.

You can blame both the toe and the shoe for your problem. Oh, and you can throw in a little genetic bad luck as well. The bone in some big toes has a tendency to slip toward the other toes, creating a toe that presses against the front of the shoe. Swelling starts at the base of the big toe where it rubs against the shoe and expands as it encounters obstacles—such as those elegant high heels you wear on Saturday nights. The swelling forces your toes to press on one another even more, increasing the pain.

Bunions are primarily a women's problem; men rarely get them. Some doctors think that unsensible shoes are a big reason. "We don't see many bunions in northern New England, because women wear comfortable shoes—flats, sandals, Birkenstocks, and the like," says Mary-Catherine Gennaro, D.O., a family osteopath in Warren, New Hampshire.

If you have a history of uncomfortable fashion and unbearable bunions, the only real solution is surgery. But if you're not at that painful point yet, here's how to get your feet to toe the line.

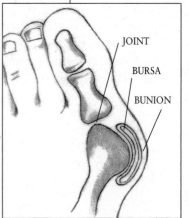

Bunions are often caused when the bone in a big toe slips out of position.

Sneak Up on Bunions

"A bunion in the early stages shouldn't bother you if you adapt the shoe to the foot instead of the foot to the shoe," says Gerard Bozuwa, M.D., a retired family doctor in Wakefield, New Hampshire. The most adaptable shoe is a sneaker made for walking, Dr. Bozuwa says. Get one with a wide "toe box," the part that nestles your buniony toes. "Why do you see old ladies in tennis shoes?" Dr. Bozuwa asks. "Bunions, that's why. They're sacrificing fashion to beat the surgeon."

Flatten Out

"Avoid wearing any shoes that lift your heels," Dr. Gennaro suggests. "That forces pressure against your toes, causing your bunions to get worse and increasing the pain. Your entire shoe wardrobe should be flat."

Hold the Toe

Dr. Mary-Catherine Gennaro's husband, Victor Gennaro, D.O., an orthopedic osteopath in Woodsville, New Hampshire, recommends over-the-counter orthotic devices made especially for people with bunions. "Dr. Scholl's makes an especially good device called a bunion cushion," Dr. Victor Gennaro says. "It holds your toes in the proper position to keep them from rubbing against each other."

Be a Softie

"Soak the bunion in warm water to soften the outer surface of the toe," says Rosemary Gladstar, an herbalist in East Barre, Vermont. "Then rub off the coarse skin with a pumice stone, available at most beauty supply stores and drugstores. By getting rid of excess skin, you reduce the amount of pressure and rubbing between your toe and your shoe."

TIME TO SEE THE DOCTOR

A Young Toe Needs a Good Look

IF YOU'RE already having bunion problems while you're still in your twenties, get your foot examined by your doctor, recommends Michael Ackland, M.D., an orthopedic surgeon in private practice in Hyannis, Massachusetts. "Bunions keep growing over the decades," Dr. Ackland says. "So if you're in your sixties, you can probably stay comfortable with proper shoes. But if you're still young, you'll eventually need surgery, and you might as well not wait too long." Surgery can correct the bone structure in your foot, preventing your bunion from getting any bigger, he explains.

BURNS

Turning down the skin's temperature

The sun is not the only cooker that fries the skin of the millions of Americans each year who get burned. Other forms of ultraviolet radiation, boiling liquids, steam, and hot objects are also common skin sizzlers. Most burns are of the relatively benign first-degree variety, in which the outermost cells of the skin get damaged. While the burn can be painful and red, the wound usually clears up within a week without any scarring.

The hotter your skin gets, and the longer it stays hot, the worse the burn. So the secret to fast burn healing is to cool down your outer layer as quickly as possible. After your skin's Fahrenheit falls, you can apply some soothing remedies recommended by our country contacts.

Chill, Man

As a glassblowing supervisor at the Simon Pearce Glass factory in Windsor, Vermont, Jerry McComas has seen his share of burns—on himself as well as his co-workers. McComas and his fellow master craftsmen hand-blow fine glassware by manipulating liquefied glass in furnaces heated to 2,000°F. One wrong move and molten glass can get on exposed skin. What does McComas do with a burn? "Cold water and a painkiller" such as aspirin are the first order of business, McComas says. And then, "a glassblower with a bad burn goes straight to the hospital." (Don't give aspirin to children because of the risk of Reye's syndrome.)

Howard Fisher, program director of the New England Culinary Institute in Montpelier and Essex Junction, Vermont, is another burn veteran. His students can stand the heat of the kitchen, but when skin gets cooked along with the food, Fisher says, "we get it under cold water as fast as possible."

Cold is the best first-aid for burns, confirms David Sigelman, M.D., a pediatrician in Holyoke, Massachusetts. The cold doesn't have to come in the form of water either. "Immediately apply anything cold—ice, cold water, even a chilled soda can—and keep it there for 20 minutes," Dr. Sigelman says. Doctors say the cold reduces the swelling and pain of a burn.

Make a Jelly Sandwich

After your skin is fully cooled, you can keep it moist and comfortable with good old petroleum jelly, say burn-savvy healers. Timothy Bent, a farmer, fire fighter, and emergency

Are You Scorched Enough to Go In?

Anyone under the age of 1 or over the age of 60 should see a doctor for any kind of burn. Otherwise, most first-degree burns do not require a doctor's care, unless the area covered by the burn is more than the size of a silver dollar (or, on a child, the size of a quarter). If a burn develops any blisters—the chief sign of a second-degree burn—you should get medical help immediately. Second-degree burns involve damage to layers of skin below the surface cells and can occasionally cause scars. The most common causes are hot liquids and open flames. A second-degree burn usually takes two to three weeks to heal.

Even worse are third-degree burns, which penetrate through the entire skin, all the way down to the fat and muscle underneath. While first- and second-degree burns can be extremely painful, victims of third-degree burns usually don't feel the heat. Nerve tissue in the skin has been destroyed, preventing any pain signals from getting to the brain. All third-degree burns need close medical attention. Depending on their size, they may also require hospitalization, as do second-degree burns that cover more than 5 percent of the body.

First-degree burns (A) are the least serious. Blistering indicates a second-degree burn (B). Third-degree burns (C) extend down to the fat and muscle beneath the skin.

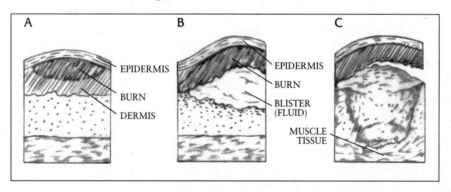

medical technician in Hanover, New Hampshire, turned to petroleum jelly after he got burned in a building blaze a few years back. "A hot ember went down into my glove," Bent recalls. "I got a burn on my hand a little smaller than a quarter. After washing with soap and water, I kept the burn lubricated with petroleum jelly and covered my hand with a large bandage."

Exactly right, says Charles Hammer, M.D., a dermatologist with the North Country Outreach Program of the Lahey Hitchcock Clinic in St. Johnsbury, Vermont. "Use cold water initially to reduce the thermal injury, then keep the burn moist and covered. Petroleum jelly with a nonstick gauze will reduce the pain significantly. Burns hurt if they are allowed to dry out. Keeping them moist will speed recovery and reduce scarring."

Skip the Higher-Priced Spread, Though

Although people have long put butter on minor burns to keep them moist, the practice is controversial in the medical community today. It's safer to use other salves, Dr. Sigelman says. "Butter is a good medium for bacteria to grow in," he points out. "Put butter on a burn, and you're asking for an infection."

Tell Burns Goodbye with Aloe

One of the best natural burn remedies is the "burn plant," aloe vera, according to Mark Quitadamo, M.D., a dermatologist at the Lahey Hitchcock Clinic in Bedford, New Hampshire. "Some people grow the plant indoors—it's a popular ornamental," Dr. Quitadamo says. "When you get burned, simply break open a stem and apply the sap directly to the burn." You can also buy processed aloe vera gel over the counter in drugstores. Look for products that contain at least 70 percent aloe. Aloe soothes burns by inhibiting the body's pain-producing chemical, bradykinin. The gel also can cut down on the formation of thromboxane, another natural chemical that keeps wounds from healing. By promoting the healing, aloe vera may prevent the scarring that often accompanies severe burns.

Ask Your Doctor about This Salve

Doctors often prescribe a soothing salve called Silvadene for patients who come in with burns, says Hugh P. Hermann, M.D., regional medical examiner for Windsor County, Vermont. "Silvadene by prescription is such a great remedy for first- and second-degree burns—it's used by clinics and hospitals across the country—that it is worth calling your doctor to see if you can obtain some to keep on hand."

BURSITIS
Battling the pain of joint maneuvers

Do you know what keeps your joints lubricated? If you've ever removed the ball bearings from a bicycle hub to clean and oil them, you can appreciate the marvel of your body's "ball bearings"—fluid-filled sacs called bursae (rhymes with "mercy"). You don't have to remove these sacs for oiling, because the sacs themselves—filled with synovial fluid produced by the body—act to reduce friction. The bursae smooth the way wherever tendons or muscle meet bones or where tendons rub against each other, such as the knees, hips, elbows, and shoulders.

Like any piece of equipment, however, a bursa can have mechanical difficulties. An overzealous tennis schedule or a hard fall while skiing can cause the little sac to become inflamed. The result is bursitis, an aching pain in the joint that gets worse when you work it. Bursitis also can be caused by a buildup of calcium, by rheumatoid arthritis, or, rarely, by a bacterial infection.

Depending on where your bursitis hits, you can get a pain with an interesting name. Weaver's bottom, an inflammation of the ischial bursa in the base of your derriere, comes from long bouts of sitting on a hard surface such as a bench. You can also get miner's elbow from working with your weight on your elbow. And the bursitis you can get from scrubbing floors is called housemaid's knee.

Bursitis caused by sports activity is often indistinguishable from the kind caused by gout or infection. And it can be hard to tell the difference between bursitis and tendinitis—an inflammation of the tendon itself. (The most common distinction is that with bursitis, you feel a dull ache; tendinitis generally causes a sharper pain.) So it's best, doctors say, to get medical attention for your joint pain. If it's run-of-the-mill (or mine or kitchen) bursitis, calm it down with these cures.

Get Some Heat in the Joint

"A bit of heat can often help bursitis," says Sarah Johansen, M.D., medical director of emergency services at New London Hospital in New London, New Hampshire. A heating

Get a Far-Ranging Shoulder

IF YOU have bursitis of the shoulder or you're recovering from an injury and want to regain your range of motion, try these exercises recommended by Sarah Johansen, M.D., medical director of emergency services at New London Hospital in New London, New Hampshire.

1. Bend over slightly so that your arms hang loose. Now gently pretend to paint circles on the floor. Make the circles as large as you can without causing pain.

2. While standing, paint imaginary circles on the wall. Keep your arms straight.

3. Stand at arm's length from the wall, perpendicular to it (your side, not your front, should be facing the wall). Extend one arm toward the wall. Using your fingertips and starting from just above your waist, slowly "crawl" your hand, spiderlike, up the wall to shoulder height. Turn and repeat on the other side with your other arm.

Paint an imaginary circle on the floor as large as you comfortably can (A). "Crawl" your fingers up a wall (B).

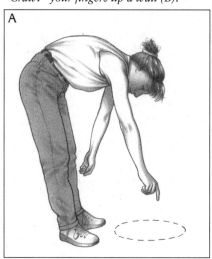

A

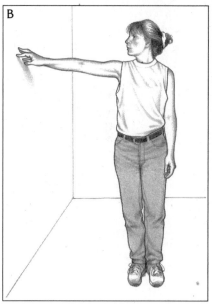

B

pad placed over the aching joint is a good way to get relief, she adds.

And Chill It, Too

Cold also works for bursitis, Dr. Johansen says. "Put some ice in a plastic bag and wrap it up in a towel. Then place the

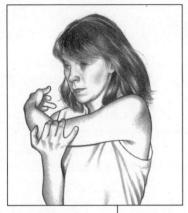

Stretch by pulling your elbow gently across your chest.

ice-filled towel on your sore joint." Hold it on the joint for about 15 minutes, she advises.

Then Stretch It

"Stretching can help relieve bursitis of the shoulder," says Lawrence H. Bernstein, M.D., medical director at Jewish Geriatric Services in Longmeadow, Massachusetts. "Stand up and gently grip your elbow. Now pull your elbow gently across your chest until it just begins to hurt. Ease off a bit and hold that position for 20 seconds. Repeat on the other side.'"

Cut the Pain

"Over-the-counter anti-inflammatory drugs can relieve the inflammation of bursitis," Dr. Johansen notes. "Best of all is ibuprofen."

Sling Your Shoulder

"The most common place to get bursitis is in your shoulder," Dr. Johansen says. "Along with other cures, you'll also want to give your shoulder plenty of rest. And the best way to rest your shoulder is with a sling. You don't need to buy a fancy one. Just take a large fabric square and fold it in half to make a triangle. Then tie two of the corners together. Put this loop over your neck and insert your elbow to keep the weight off your shoulder."

C

CABIN FEVER
*The inside dope
on being stuck indoors*

Your own home can start to feel like a prison during the cold, wet months. You find yourself snapping at your loved ones, wanting to sleep in late, and compulsively pigging out on snacks. You have a serious case of cabin fever.

If it's any consolation, doctors have given a fancy name to that blue, wintry, indoor feeling. "Cabin fever that comes on during the late fall and lasts through the winter is probably seasonal affective disorder, or SAD," says Peter Mason, M.D., a family doctor and chairman of ambulatory care at Alice Peck Day Memorial Hospital in Lebanon, New Hampshire. "We see a fair bit of SAD in our neck of the woods, and it can result in a fairly significant depression. When the days are long and sunny in summertime, everyone is smiling. When spring comes late and people are stuck indoors during a cold and wet April and May, I see some pretty unhappy-looking patients."

Spring does come eventually. But what do you do in the meantime? The hints below offer a breath of fresh air.

Lighten Up

Charles Ravaris, M.D., Ph.D., emeritus professor of psychiatry at Dartmouth Medical School in Hanover, New Hampshire, and an expert on seasonal depression, recommends installing fluorescent lighting in the rooms you tend to live in most. "The kitchen is a good place, because that's where you tend to spend the most waking time at home," he says. Fluorescent lighting gives you more of the light energy you need to help you with your cabin fever, Dr. Ravaris explains.

Evacuate

"You have to get yourself outside—there is no better cure for cabin fever than leaving the 'cabin,'" says Mary-Catherine Gennaro, D.O., a family osteopath in Warren, New Hampshire. "This takes real discipline if you live in a cold climate. Get yourself a good, rain-resistant jacket, warm down

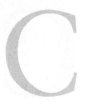

The Vacation That Wasn't

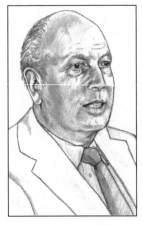

CABIN fever doesn't happen just in the winter. That cooped-up feeling can last right on through the spring and summer if you don't get outside.

During my years as a family doctor in the Lakes Region of New Hampshire, I treated a lot of cabin fever. Mothers with young children would come up here for the whole summer while their husbands stayed at their jobs in Boston or New York, joining their families just for the weekends.

A lot of mothers would end up in my office, complaining bitterly. "All I've got is a change of sinks," they'd say. They were relieved of all the conveniences of home but still had the responsibilities. They didn't have any physical problems but came to me just for support.

Everyone needs a vacation, but it should be a real one. You need a break from your routine. If child rearing is your main job, find a way to arrange baby-sitting, or get your spouse to take on the kid duties. If you work in the office all the time, get away from a telephone. A change in routine is one of the best ways to beat the summer version of cabin fever.

GERARD BOZUWA, M.D., *retired after 36 years as the sole family doctor for the town of Wakefield, New Hampshire.*

clothing, and some of that long underwear made of synthetic fabric such as polypropylene. That eliminates your excuses for staying indoors when it's cold and wet outside." Dr. Gennaro takes her own advice. "I put almost 1,400 miles on my bike in one year," she says. "I even biked after a big snowstorm we had in May. I would have gone crazy if I hadn't gotten out."

Find Company

"Join a group that does something outside together, such as walk or snowshoe," Dr. Gennaro says. "People are social creatures, and company relieves cabin fever."

Make Indoor Work

During the winter, focus on working creatively, says Francesca De Grandis, the Boston-born daughter of a Sicilian psychic and witch and a spiritual healer herself. "Staying indoors, people used to be too busy to feel cabin fever as much," she says. "Explore new arts and crafts. Get your children involved—young children can learn simple needlework on felt."

Dr. Gennaro agrees that staying busy helps. "I do knitting and bake bread," she says. "But do these things in addition to going outside."

CALLUSES AND CORNS

When the going gets tough on your skin, get going with these remedies

Weeks and years of hard use can cause your skin to toughen up in the places that take the most abuse. And that's not such a bad thing: The hardened skin that makes up a callus can serve as a kind of miniature body armor against rough treat-

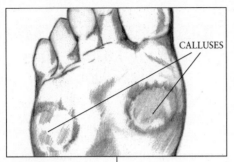

CALLUSES

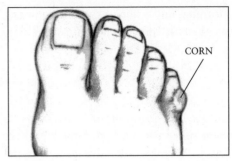

CORN

While calluses and corns are both hardened, dead skin, corns often have a painful core.

ment. But occasionally, the hard skin can build up enough to cause pain when you press on it.

If the rough spot has a hard, painful core, you probably have a corn. People with high foot arches tend to get corns from the pressure their feet exert on the toes. "Calluses and corns are really the same thing," says Laurence Bouchard, D.O., an osteopathic family physician in private practice in Narragansett, Rhode Island. "Both consist of dead skin building up in areas that get rubbed a lot." Calluses tend to appear on either hands or feet, while corns are generally limited to your long-suffering hooves. Not all corns are hard either; sometimes you can get a soft, painful kind of corn on the webbing between toes that rub together.

It's a Matter of Fitness

THE best way to prevent calluses and corns on your feet is to use the right shoes for the right occasions," says Ralph McCoy, a certified orthotic shoe technician and owner of the Shoetorium shoe store in Lebanon, New Hampshire.

"Don't run in anything but running shoes," McCoy says. "They have a wide, flexible toe box that expands when your foot lands, allowing your foot to flare out."

"If you walk regularly, buy walking shoes, not running shoes," McCoy continues. "The toe box in a walking shoe is a little firmer and gives more lateral support, which helps prevent the shifting that produces friction."

When it comes to dress shoes, the secret to comfort (and to avoiding calluses and corns) is a professional fit. "A toe box that's properly sized for you is key to preventing calluses and corns," McCoy notes. "I have refit people with new shoes, and

CALLUSES AND CORNS

If the rough stuff on your skin doesn't bother you, don't bother with getting rid of it, says Dr. Bouchard. But if your calluses or corns are making you sore, try these cures.

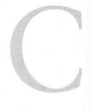

Get into a Tough Scrape

"Take a razor blade and carefully trim away the dead skin," Dr. Bouchard advises. "That will reduce the pressure and help prevent more skin from building up around your callus or corn." Always sterilize a blade before cutting skin by pouring rubbing alcohol over the blade, he cautions.

Arch Your Foot

"If you have calluses or corns on your foot, an over-the-counter arch support can help keep your foot in the proper position, so your shoe won't rub against the skin as much," Dr. Bouchard says. Arch supports by Dr. Scholl's and other makers can be found at any drugstore.

Fold a piece of moleskin and cut a semicircle (A) to make a callus-protecting hole (B). Then wrap the moleskin around the problem toe (C).

Try Fake Skin

A pad of felt moleskin or lamb's wool can help take pressure off a callus or corn on your foot. "Buy a piece of adhesive moleskin at your drugstore, fold it over, and cut a semicircle out of it," Dr. Bouchard advises. "Place the hole right over the callus."

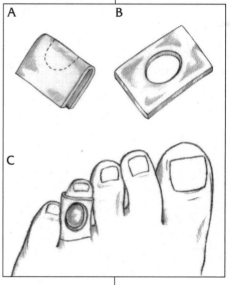

Get Wet

"Keep the callus or corn soft by using my wet-bandage cure," says Gerard Bozuwa, M.D., a retired family doctor in Wakefield, New Hampshire. "Get an adhesive bandage that is large enough to cover the callus or corn. Put it on dry so that it sticks. Then sprinkle the gauze part with a little water. Wet the gauze several times a day to keep it from drying out." Most bandages have little holes in them that allow water to seep through. "The wet bandage will give the callus the appearance and consistency of dishpan hands, making it all soft and wrinkly. Change the bandage every day, keeping the callus or corn wet for as many days as necessary. Sooner or later, it should fall off."

CAVITIES
Keeping the tooth, the whole tooth

If you don't defend yourself, the nasty stuff that accumulates on your teeth—the bits of food and bacteria that mix with saliva to form gluey plaque—can wage chemical warfare on your chompers. Bacteria go to work on the sugars and starches in plaque, creating a potent acid that can eat through the protective enamel of your teeth, forming a cavity. If left unchecked, the acid can enlarge the cavity, eating a hole right through to the dentin—the layer beneath the enamel and the last bastion before the sensitive pulp at the center of the tooth. The delicate tissue becomes infected, and you're likely to lose the tooth.

The trick is to avoid giving the enemy a foothold. "You can save a lot of frustration if you brush at least twice a day and floss every day," says Gregory L. Baker, D.D.S., an orthodontist in private practice in Woodstock, Vermont, and West Lebanon and New London, New Hampshire. "Get your teeth professionally cleaned twice a year. Proper cleaning will rid your teeth of the plaque that's at the root of a lot of dental evils."

Thanks to fluoridation of public water supplies and the widespread use of fluoride toothpastes, the incidence of cavities among children has declined significantly from earlier times. But caries, which is the term dentists use for tooth decay, remains the most common childhood disease that can't cure itself or be fixed with antibiotics. Moreover, if you have one cavity, you're likely to have more than one. A nationwide study by the National Institutes of Health showed that

In a healthy tooth (A), the enamel is intact. When acids from food and bacteria eat through the enamel (B), decay begins. If the root becomes infected (C), you can lose the tooth.

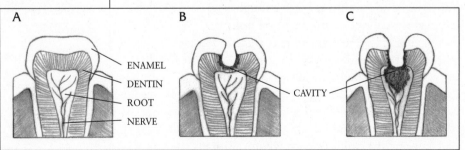

| A | B | C |

ENAMEL
DENTIN
ROOT
NERVE

CAVITY

cavities don't visit people equally: One-quarter of children ages 5 to 17 suffered from 80 percent of the tooth decay that the researchers found.

Here's how you can be among those who have fought off the cavity invasion.

Do the String Thing

"You could save so much frustration with your teeth if you just flossed once a day," Dr. Baker says. Flossing in every space between teeth is important. "Make sure you get at the

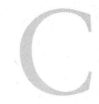

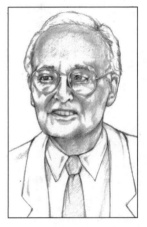

A WORD FROM DR. MARTIN

Look, Doc! No Holes!

Back in the early 1960s, a family vacationing in my town brought in a youngster with a bad mouth sore. While treating her, I was amazed to see that the girl didn't have a single cavity. I asked to see the mouths of her two brothers: Their mouths were perfect, too! I called my whole staff together to see those amazing teeth and congratulated the kids' parents on their astonishing luck.

What was the big deal, you ask? Those were the days before fluoride toothpaste. Especially for families without much money to spend on dentistry, dental care from a rural doctor or dentist sometimes amounted to simply pulling teeth. But the new toothpastes introduced in the 1960s changed things. People got the notion that if they took care of their teeth, they could actually keep them.

By the time I retired in 1993, kids' mouths were perfect more often than not. That lucky family went from being a freak of nature to the norm.

Fluoride is one of the great medical discoveries of the twentieth century. Use fluoride toothpaste; it's your best defense against cavities.

Brewster Martin, M.D., *a retired family doctor in Chelsea, Vermont (population 1,166), and cofounder of the Chelsea Family Health Center. He was named Vermont Doctor of the Year in 1991.*

---

sides of your molars in the way back," he says. "No brush can get in there."

Go Sour on Sweets

"Watch your diet if you really want to prevent cavities," Dr. Baker advises. "The sugar in chewy candy and dried fruit raises the acidity level in your mouth for as much as half an hour before your saliva returns to normal. Acidity deteriorates enamel, especially between the teeth." If you eat candy, brush your teeth immediately afterward, he says.

Ah, Chew

"Sugar-free gum can help stimulate the flow of saliva and reduce the acidity in your mouth," Dr. Baker says. "It also has a slight mechanical cleansing effect on the teeth." Research on gum chewers also shows that sugar-free gum cuts down on cavity-causing bacteria.

Try the Swish Technique

"If you aren't near a toothbrush after eating something, swish and swallow," Dr. Baker says. "Fill your mouth with water, swish it around several times, and swallow."

Learn Eve's Lesson

Swiss researchers have found that apple juice tends to soften the enamel of teeth, inviting cavities. Their study suggests that it's wise to brush your teeth after drinking the stuff.

Say "Cheese"

Researchers at Tufts University in Boston found that eating cheese can prevent cavities. You might consider switching snacks from candy bars to chunks of Cheddar.

CHAFING

Finding the right remedy when your skin rubs you the wrong way

If your thighs rub together when you walk, you probably know about chafing. The friction of skin against skin can make the area sore and red. Unless you take care of the problem, the rubbing can wear away skin and cause oozing. Moistened by sweat, the sore spot becomes an ideal home for microorganisms such as bacteria and yeast, and infection may result.

Thighs are not the only target of chafing. Any moist area where skin rubs against skin can become painful. "Chafing is very common in obese people," says Gerard Bozuwa, M.D., who is retired after 36 years as a family doctor in Wakefield, New Hampshire. "But you don't have to be obese to suffer from chafing. You can get chafed from horseback riding or from clothes that don't fit properly. And your skin can chafe in the groin, on the thighs, under the arms, under the breasts, and even between the toes."

The secret to preventing chafing, doctors say, is to keep problem areas clean, dry, and friction-free. Here are some methods recommended by New England country physicians.

Create a Desert Breeze

"Using a hair dryer on folds of skin or under heavy breasts is very effective in getting the skin thoroughly dry," says Mark Quitadamo, M.D., a dermatologist at the Lahey Hitchcock Clinic in Bedford, New Hampshire. Use a low setting to avoid an accidental burn.

Soak Up Sweat

Dr. Quitadamo recommends sprinkling Zeasorb powder on sensitive areas to absorb moisture and keep the skin dry. Zeasorb is available over the counter at drugstores.

Think Zinc

"Zinc oxide is an old-fashioned remedy that works well for chafing," Dr. Quitadamo says. "One of the principal ingredients in Gold Bond powder is zinc oxide." Zinc oxide, an antibacterial remedy that absorbs moisture, also can be found in Balmex baby powder and in Desitin ointment. All are available over the counter.

Use Lotion When in Motion

"I am a devotee of Eucerin, a lotion that consists of homogenized petrolatum, mineral oil, and water," Dr. Bozuwa says. "Put Eucerin on your skin wherever you tend to get chafed."

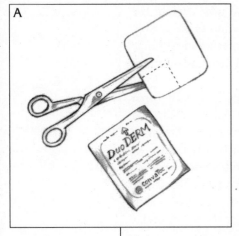

A

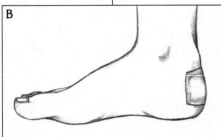

B

Duoderm is a stick-on layer of plastic. Cut a piece to the appropriate size (A) and apply to the chafed spot (B) to relieve friction.

You can buy Eucerin over the counter at drugstores.

Just One Word: Plastic

"One means of mechanically protecting the skin is called Duoderm," Dr. Bozuwa says. "It is like plastic wrap with a little adhesive on it." It's used mostly by joggers to protect their feet from blisters, but Dr. Bozuwa says that Duoderm works to prevent any kind of irritation caused by friction. "Just cut out a square of Duoderm and place it on the chafed area." You can buy Duoderm at drugstores and sporting goods stores.

Give Breasts Extra Support

"Women with large breasts may find that placing a piece of an old sheet or pillowcase under their breasts is helpful to wick away the moisture," Dr. Quitadamo says.

Destroy the Plant Life

"Sometimes chafing is accompanied by the growth of fungus," Dr. Bozuwa notes. "Whenever I diagnose it on a patient, as a simple family doctor I recommend an antifugal like Lotrimin. It is available over the counter at any drugstore."

Make the Bare Times Be Rare Times

"If you are so heavy that you chafe frequently, you should lose weight," Dr. Bozuwa says. "In the meantime, wear clothes to keep skin from rubbing against skin." Often obese people will be fine in colder weather when they wear pants, Dr. Bozuwa explains. "But when it is summer and they put on shorts, they run into trouble, because there is nothing to keep the thighs from rubbing against each other."

Maybe Ironing Isn't So Bad

In rare cases, a person who suffers from persistent dermatitis in the thighs or under the arms is allergic to the formaldahyde in permanent-press clothing. If you suspect an allergy, Dr. Quitadamo recommends that you ask your allergist or dermatologist for a patch test to see if formaldehyde is the culprit.

CHAPPED HANDS
Get a grip on the dryness

Dry air, both indoors and out, can suck the moisture right out of your hands and leave them red and scaly. What can you do to soften the blow?

Give Your Fists the Old One-Two

"Use two kinds of hand cream: sticky and not sticky," recommends Murray Hamlet, D.V.M., chief of the Research Support Division at the U.S. Army Research Institute of Environmental Medicine in Natick, Massachusetts. "Use the sticky kind at night, and wear gloves to seal in the moisture."

One of the stickier remedies is Bag Balm, a goopy, lanolin- and petrolatum-based salve that you can buy at feed stores and some drugstores. Made to heal cows' sore udders, Bag Balm gets high marks from farmers who use it on their hands. Dr. Hamlet says the sticky goo can be removed in the morning with baby oil. During the day, he recommends using nonsticky creams containing glycerin, such as unscented Neutrogena Hand Cream and Corn Huskers Lotion, available at most pharmacies. "You need to rotate your hand creams every two weeks through the winter," Dr. Hamlet says. "They lose maximum effect if used continually."

Ever See a Badger with Chapped Hands?

Stephen Comeau, a registered pharmacist at Spears Pharmacy in Enosburg Falls, Vermont, says he sells a lot of Bag

You Can Skip the Gold and Myrrh, Too

To GET rid of "chaps in hands," Thomas Palmer, a seventeenth-century Massachusetts doctor and clergyman, recommended giving your skin a mixture of oil of roses, white wax, frankincense, and hen's grease. Although we couldn't find any pharmacist (or wise man, for that matter) who would recommend frankincense, "just about any kind of oil will do," says Stephen Comeau, a registered pharmacist at Spears Pharmacy in Enosburg Falls, Vermont. "Most of the topical remedies you see today have the same stuff in them—oils, mostly."

Jorge Crespo, M.D., a dermatologist and former New Englander who now works with the Clark & Daughtrey Medical Group in Lakeland, Florida, confirms that oil is one of nature's best weapons against hand dryness.

Balm to dry-skinned customers. But he says a popular new remedy is Badger Cream, which contains olive oil, beeswax, castor bean oil, sweet birch, and aloe vera. You can buy Badger Cream (it's smooth enough for daytime use) at drugstores throughout the Northeast.

Go Heavy on the Metals

"Make sure you're getting enough trace minerals in your diet," Dr. Hamlet says. "They appear to strengthen the collagen, or protein molecules, in your skin." A healthy collagen layer helps keep moisture in. "Zinc is the most important, but you also need copper, cobalt, manganese, and sulfur. Make sure they're in any multivitamin you buy." Oysters, red meat, fish, poultry, whole grain bread, peas and beans, organ meats, and seeds are especially high in zinc.

Put Your Troubles in Oiled Water

"If your hands are just dry and not predisposed to eczema, try this really nice treatment," says Jorge Crespo, M.D., a dermatologist and former New Englander who now works with the Clark & Daughtrey Medical Group in Lakeland, Florida. Fill a small basin with lukewarm water. Add a bath oil such as Alpha Keri, which contains mineral oil. Keep your hands in the bowl for 10 to 15 minutes—long enough for them to soak up the oil and water. Pat your hands dry with a towel, then cover them with a thin layer of petroleum jelly to keep the moisture in. Put on a pair of thin cotton gloves before you go to bed. Repeat this routine two or three times a week.

CHAPPED LIPS
Removing cracks in the smackers

You'd think that after ages of evolution, your lips would be able to take care of themselves. But unlike skin, lips do not have oil glands to keep them moist. Nor do they protect themselves against the sun. Whereas your skin has a natural sun-fighting pigment called melanin, your lips do not. And even your skin would have problems if your tongue were right next to it. Saliva contains digestive enzymes that help dry out tissue. And so you get the classic vicious lip cycle: Licking your lips makes them drier, which makes you want to lick them again.

"Chapped lips are usually precipitated by one of three things," says Thomas Watt, M.D., a dermatologist in private practice in Bangor, Maine. "Lips get chapped from getting licked; from an irritant, such as sunburn or an allergic reaction to food, lipstick, or toothpaste; or from a fever."

The problem gets especially bad in the winter, according to Richard Baughman, M.D., a dermatologist who has established dermatology clinics throughout rural New Hampshire. "The skin on lips gets worse in the winter because the keratin—the skin's protein barrier—breaks down due to low temperatures and humidity," Dr. Baughman says.

Naturally, the best way to prevent chapped lips is to hold your tongue. "Easy for you to say," replies the lizard-lipped victim. Here are some more practical remedies.

> ### TIME TO SEE THE DOCTOR
> ### *Got to Go, Old Chap*
>
> THERE'S no need to panic prematurely, but if your lips are still chapped after you've been treating them yourself for two or three weeks with a good lip balm like Chap Stick's Sunscreen, it may be time for a visit to a dermatologist, says Thomas Watt, M.D., a dermatologist in Bangor, Maine. Badly chapped lips that last may be a sign of malignancy. And if your lips are persistently cracked, you may have a yeast or bacterial infection.

Do a Smear Campaign

To soothe chapped lips, Dr. Watt recommends a lip balm such as Chap Stick. "Go for the plain stuff," he says. "Avoid the balms that have phenols or camphor listed as ingredients on

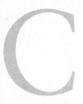C the label." At night, he says, "you can use petroleum jelly, which works just as well but can be messy during the daytime." Wet your lips with cool water before applying the jelly. And avoid flavored balms, Dr. Watt cautions. They just make lip licking more tempting.

Spread Tradition

A traditional remedy is Bag Balm, a lanolin- and petrolatum-based skin softener that dairy farmers use to keep cows' udders smooth and comfortable. Bag Balm has a growing number of human fans who use it as a lip balm. It's available at farm supply stores and vet supply stores, as well as some pharmacies and health food stores.

Before there was Bag Balm, country people used beeswax as a lip balm. It still works, too. Or you can do what many farmers have done for centuries: Rub your finger against the side of your nose to pick up some of its natural oils, then rub it against your lips.

Know Your Own Strength

Avoid irritating your lips with overly rigorous application, advises Beach Conger, M.D., a family physician in Hartland, Vermont, and author of *Bag Balm and Duct Tape: Tales of a Vermont Doctor*. The rubbing, even of helpful goo, can make your lips even more chapped. "It doesn't really matter what kind of emollient you use—petroleum jelly, vegetable shortening, lanolin, even bear grease; all of them work fine to keep the moisture in your lips. Just put it on gently and be careful not to rub it in."

Stay Moist Inside

"Keep drinking liquids if you have a problem with chapped lips," Dr. Conger advises. "Hydration will not prevent chapped lips, but dehydration will make it worse."

ANNALS OF MEDICINE

Lip Sufferers, Lend Me an Ear

WANT to save money on lip balms? Protect your lips with earwax, recommended Lydia Maria Child in her 1829 book *The Frugal Housewife*.

"Well, you wouldn't hurt yourself doing that—earwax has antibacterial qualities," says Beach Conger, M.D., a family physician in Hartland, Vermont. "But there are plenty of more palatable remedies around these days."

Earwax may have offered an added advantage during Victorian times: the prevention of unauthorized kissing.

CHARLEY HORSE
Ride that muscle pain
out of town

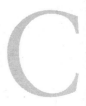

When a leg muscle suddenly cramps up in a squeezing pain, that's no ordinary steed you're riding. No, it's a horse of a different color—a charley horse.

Because a charley horse can strike at night as well as during the day, some people think the charley horse may have gotten its name from "Charley," the nickname given to night watchmen in seventeenth- and eighteenth-century London. The Charleys were the all-news networks of their day, calling out the neighborhood conditions every hour. Many a Londoner was aroused out of a sound sleep by a Charley calling from the street, "Two o'clock and all's well." Other people say nay to that theory, claiming that the cramp is named after a lame race horse named Charley.

Wherever the name came from, you'll know it when you've got it. If you lack minerals in your diet or you're dehydrated, you're more likely to get this sudden cramp, especially in your calf. "You can also get a charley horse from a bruise, such as the one you get when a baseball hits you hard in the leg," says Raymond Rocco Monto, M.D., an orthopedic surgeon at Martha's Vineyard Orthopedic Surgery and Sports Medicine in Oak Bluffs, Massachusetts. The pain can hit you later, especially after your leg has been still for a while, Dr. Monto says.

Here's how to break that painful steed.

Walk Your Horse
"Walk around slowly to keep the blood moving in your leg," Dr. Monto suggests. "The pain should go away gradually."

Have a Ginless Tonic
"Tonic water, which contains quinine, can help alleviate a charley horse," Dr. Monto says. In fact, doctors say that any kind of water is good to drink to prevent dehydration.

RICE Goes with the Grain
"Treat your charley horse with RICE—rest, ice, compression, and elevation," says Michael Ackland, M.D., an or-

thopedic surgeon in private practice in Hyannis, Massachusetts. "Don't try to go running with a charley horse. Apply a bag of ice to the painful spot for 20 minutes at a time until the pain diminishes. Then wrap the muscle with an elastic bandage and put your feet up." You can buy an elastic bandage at your drugstore.

Give It a Hand

"Self-massage is good for a charley horse," says Jon Didriksson, a massage therapist and former Olympic miler living in Belmont, Massachusetts. "Rub the affected muscle gently, then gradually increase the pressure until your rubbing hurts just a bit. Keep rubbing until your leg starts feeling better."

Offer Your Tummy a Treat

"Charley horses can stem from a lack of calcium in the diet," Dr. Monto says. "If you're getting a lot of cramps, I recommend calcium supplementation of 500 milligrams or more per day." A good source of calcium, according to Dr. Monto, is Tums, an antacid that is available over the counter in 500-, 750-, and 1,000-milligram tablets. Alternative calcium sources are milk and other dairy products.

CHICKENPOX
All-over relief when you're seeing spots

It's easy to see that chickenpox deserves its name—the itchy skin caused by the varicella virus can get your child scratching like a starved roaster hen. Actually, chickenpox got its name by being one of the less harmful childhood maladies. Folks used to say it was too mild to harm a chicken.

Chickenpox usually starts with a low fever and proceeds to the characteristic itchy blisters, which—to the relief of child and parent alike—scab over after a week or so and lose their itch. And that's about it. Once she's gone through the chickenpox ringer, your child will probably remain immune to the disease for life. The bad news is, although someone who's had chickenpox is unlikely to get *that* disease again, the virus can linger in the body's nervous system for years, popping up again as shingles later in life. Chickenpox can lead to other ailments as well. "You should see your doctor if the fever that accompanies chickenpox lasts for more than two or three days, if the ears become sore, or if the pox are full of pus and gook," says Patricia Edwards, M.D., a pediatrician in private practice in Concord, New Hampshire.

If you never had chickenpox yourself as a child, you're not out of the woods just because you're past childhood. You can get this highly contagious disease as an adult. But take heart: The remedies below can get you through the weeklong scratch as comfortably as possible.

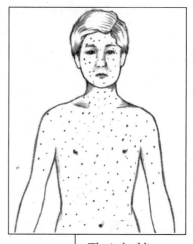

The itchy blisters of chickenpox scab over after a week or so.

Head for the Medicine Cabinet

"Chickenpox sores hurt and ache as much as they itch," says Carole Stashwick, M.D., a pediatrician at the Dartmouth-Hitchcock Medical Center in Lebanon, New Hampshire. "Older children especially will tell you the lesions are tingly or sore rather than itchy—much the same feeling that a cold sore on the lip has for an adult. Acetaminophen can help relieve the pain as well as reduce the fever that accompanies chickenpox."

Benadryl Works, Too

"You can give a child Benadryl liquid to help with the itching," says Everett Orbeton, M.D., a pediatrician who is retired after 44 years as a family doctor in Portland, Maine. "Available over the counter, Benadryl has a nice side effect: It makes the child sleepy, so he doesn't scratch as much."

Don't Substitute

If you don't have either acetaminophen or Benadryl on hand, don't reach for the aspirin, warns Peter Brassard, M.D., a family doctor in private practice on Block Island, Rhode Island. "Avoid aspirin at all costs," Dr. Brassard says. "Children who take aspirin are susceptible to Reye's syndrome, which can be deadly."

Use the Shower's Healing Power

"I like to have the child take a bath or a light shower," Dr. Stashwick says. "This is especially helpful if you have a shower with a handheld nozzle. Use warm, not hot, water—hot water can make the rash itch even more. Gently blot the skin with a clean towel until it's nearly dry but not entirely. Let the air dry the rest. Air drying is very soothing to irritated skin. Repeat this shower or bath routine several times a day during the worst of the chickenpox. This will help dry the scabs sooner and make them fall off without having to be scratched or rubbed off."

When Relief Is a Mush

John C. Robinson, M.D., a pediatrician in Quincy, Massachusetts, recommends soaking in oatmeal. "Aveeno, made with a special kind of oatmeal for irritated skin, is very soothing," he says. Aveeno is made of finely ground oats,

---

AN OUNCE OF PREVENTION
Now You Can Put a Pox on the Pox

CHICKENPOX no longer has to be a childhood rite of passage. A vaccine using a weak version of the varicella, or chickenpox, virus became available in doctors' offices in 1995.

"I was very skeptical of the varicella vaccine at first," admits Peter Brassard, M.D., a family doctor on Block Island, Rhode Island. "But I've spent a lot of time checking it out, and now I am very pro-vaccine." The vaccine does not guarantee immunity; a few people who have been vaccinated got the disease anyway. "But vaccinated people who contract chickenpox tend to have far fewer lesions and are less uncomfortable than those who aren't vaccinated before

getting the pox. And one vaccination seems to do the trick. The immunity from the vaccine shows no sign of waning over time."

According to John C. Robinson, M.D., a pediatrician in Quincy, Massachusetts, any woman contemplating pregnancy who did not have chickenpox as a child should ask her doctor for the vaccine. "Chickenpox can be dangerous for a pregnant woman in her last trimester," Dr. Robinson says. "A child born to a woman with chickenpox could have congenital varicella or encephalitis. Both of these are debilitating or even deadly diseases in a baby. However, the safety of using the vaccine *during* pregnancy is uncertain, so you need

called colloidal oatmeal, which form a coating on your skin. You can buy Aveeno at drugstores.

Armor with Hammer

"Use a quarter cup of baking soda in a bathtub filled with warm water," Dr. Edwards recommends. "Baking soda cleans your tub at the same time it soothes the child."

Dr. Orbeton says that you can also make a paste out of baking soda and water. "Just put a little water in the baking soda and put the paste right on the pox. It helps stop the itch."

Stick to PJs

"Dress the child in loose, light, cotton clothing, such as big pajamas or a nightgown," Dr. Stashwick says. "Skip the underpants or any binding elastic. You don't want anything rubbing against the sores."

Paint the Mouth

"If a child has chickenpox in the mouth," Dr. Edwards says, "you can numb the sores to allow eating and drinking by mixing equal portions of Benadryl and Maalox. Paint the mixture on the sores with a Q-Tip before giving the child something to eat or drink."

COLD HANDS AND FEET

What to do when Jack Frost has your digits' number

Are those really your hands and feet, or did someone strap blocks of ice onto your arms and legs? It doesn't take extreme cold to put a chill in your extremities, says Linda B. Dacey, M.D., an internist living in Hanover, New Hampshire.

"Blood circulates through smaller and smaller vessels the farther it gets from the center of your body," Dr. Dacey says. "By the time blood reaches your extremities, it goes through very small blood vessels. The vessels in your fingers and toes are not buried deep in fat and tissue, as are most other blood vessels in the body. Having less insulation, the vessels in your

C hands and feet get cold more easily. And when they get cold, the vessels constrict, supplying less warming blood to the region."

How can you give those chilly places a hand? The simplest way, experts say, is to make sure the rest of your body is toasty. "To keep your extremities warm, you need to keep all of you warm," Dr. Dacey notes. "Mittens and socks won't do much good if you aren't wearing a coat." Here are some other tips for warming your tips.

Put a Lid on It

"Up to to 55 percent of the body heat you lose goes out your head," says Murray Hamlet, D.V.M., chief of the Research Support Division at the U.S. Army Research Institute of Environmental Medicine in Natick, Massachusetts. "So wear a hat whenever the temperature outside dips even slightly. You'll be amazed what that does for your extremities."

And Don't Let Your Neck Get Naked

Besides the old hat trick, notes veteran mountain guide Nick Yardley of Shelburne, Vermont, "also remember that the blood to your head goes through your neck. So to keep that blood warm, wrap up your neck." Yardley recommends a neck gaiter—a doughnut-shaped scarf made of polyester pile material, available in sporting goods stores and catalogs.

Swallow Some Warmth

"Warming your trunk, or body core, can help your extremities, too—hence a hot drink can help your toes," Dr. Dacey notes.

Both hot and cold liquids are important, adds Yardley. "The liquid helps your circulation, bringing warm blood to the extremities," he says. "But leave coffee, tea, and most caffeinated sodas behind. Caffeine is a diuretic; you'll lose more fluids than you take in."

Lay on the Layers

To keep your whole body warm and bring the heat to hands and feet, you might do what the Eskimo do. George Wenzel, Ph.D., associate professor of geography at McGill University in Montreal, has spent seven winters studying the Eskimo (also called Inuit) on remote Baffin Island in northern

Are Your Hands Looking Too Patriotic?

IF YOUR hands or fingers turn a blotchy white, blue, or red when they're exposed to cold or vibrations, or when you're under emotional stress, you might have Raynaud's disease. As many as one in five people have this disease, a usually harmless ailment in which blood vessels in the hands occasionally constrict.

You can test yourself for Raynaud's disease by driving a car in the winter, according to Murray Hamlet, D.V.M., chief of the Research Support Division at the U.S. Army Research Institute of Environmental Medicine in Natick, Massachusetts. "Keep the heat off for a while and look at your fingers," Hamlet advises. "If you have Raynaud's, the cold, vibrations, and raised level of your hands should make your fingertips turn blue or white or sometimes red."

Although Raynaud's disease itself is no great cause for alarm, see a physician if you have the telltale signs, doctors say. Raynaud's may be a precursor to other problems with your connective tissues.

Canada. "All the clothing the Inuit wear is in layers," he reports.

Traditional Inuit use materials such as caribou, seal, and dog skins, which are rather hard to find in department stores. But Dr. Wenzel says people in less remote areas can still apply the same principle with clothing made of manmade fabrics and wool. Experts say that when you're going out into the cold for prolonged periods, you should avoid cotton, which tends to stay wet after you sweat and to lose its insulation as it gets damp.

Instead, wear long underwear made of a manmade fabric such as polypropylene or Capilene, which wicks moisture away from your skin. Over that first layer, put on pants and a shirt made of a heavier artificial fabric, such as polyester pile. Even if the temperature dips well below zero, a jacket or vest made of goose down as a third layer can keep you toasty. ("Make sure you have the opportunity to dry your down every couple of days," Dr. Wenzel notes. "Wet down is useless.") Top off your clothing with pants and a wind shell or parka made of coated nylon to keep out rain and snow and still allow your body's moisture to escape. Gore-Tex is one of the most popular of these weather-resistant fabrics.

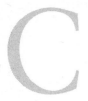

. "Layering creates air pockets between clothing that add insulation," Dr. Wenzel notes. "And if you're wearing more than one layer, you can keep putting on and taking off clothing as you warm up and cool down."

Wear Multiple Mittens

New Hampshire's Mount Washington, highest mountain in the Northeast, has clocked some of the worst weather in the world, including 200-mile-per-hour winds and winter temperatures that dip to –40°F—on a mild day. So how do the researchers who live in the weather observatory on the mountain's summit keep their hands warm? The key is in multiple layers of clothing, according to Michael Pelchat, summer manager of Mount Washington State Park and an emergency medicine instructor who teaches first-aid to the summit weather observers.

"Next to your skin, wear glove liners made of polypropylene," Pelchat says. "The gloves allow you to work with your fingers without exposing skin to the cold."

"Over the gloves, pull on mittens made of wool or polyester fleece, fabrics that wick moisture away to the outside," Pelchat adds. "For your outermost layer, top everything with a nylon mitten wind shell."

And where do you get this clothing without freezing your assets? "Army surplus stores have a good selection of inexpensive but functional cold-weather gear," Pelchat says. And all three kinds of hand protection are also available in outdoor-gear stores and catalogs.

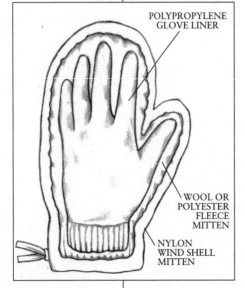

POLYPROPYLENE GLOVE LINER

WOOL OR POLYESTER FLEECE MITTEN

NYLON WIND SHELL MITTEN

When working or playing outdoors, layer on the protection with gloves and mittens of the right materials.

Double Up on Your Feet

At least two pairs of socks are essential if you go out into the cold, advises Dudley Weider, M.D., an otolaryngologist who lives in Hanover, New Hampshire. "First put on polypropylene socks, which you can buy at sporting goods stores. Then add wool socks, or socks made of an artificial moisture-wicking fabric. Some people have a middle layer of artificial fabric, along with an artificial or wool sock over that." Dr. Weider says that polypropylene and pile are ideal artificial fabrics for moisture wicking and insulation.

Stay Footloose

Dr. Weider warns against constricting your feet amid all that clothing. "Tight boots can restrict the flow of warming blood and actually make your feet colder." To solve that problem, he recommends "comfortable footwear at least two sizes too big. I got my pair of boots in Fairbanks, Alaska, over 30 years ago. They're two sizes too big, they still feel fine, and I'm still wearing them."

Bring Extra Heat

People whose hands and feet are especially sensitive to the cold should consider buying heat packs—plastic packets filled with charcoal or chemicals, says Pelchat. "Heat packs can be purchased at hardware stores and any sporting goods store that sells outdoor equipment. They're relatively inexpensive and last six to eight hours. Slide the packs between your glove liners and mittens. Some people might get burned by putting the packs next to their skin." You can use the packs in your boots by putting them between your layers of socks. "And there is a smaller size made to go on the toes—but your boots have to be large enough to hold the extra baggage."

Put Your Hands through Army Training

Dr. Hamlet developed this wintertime technique for soldiers in the U.S. Army. First, make sure the room where you're practicing is at a temperature that is comfortable for you—not too hot and not too cold. Sit for 5 minutes with your hands in an insulated container filled with hot tap water. Then wrap your hands in a towel and move to a near-freezing area—the porch or garage, for example. Now unwrap your hands and dunk them into a second hot-water container for

10 minutes. Go back indoors for another 2- to 5-minute dip. Repeat this routine 3 to 6 times every other day for a total of 50 times. "Our studies showed that after the immersion procedure, hands remained several degrees warmer when exposed to cool air," Dr. Hamlet says. The results can last 2 years or longer, he adds.

COLIC
If your child's wailing has you in tears, try these remedies

As many as one in five babies put their parents through the colicky ringer: crying, even screaming, that goes on for hours, especially during the afternoon and evening. Hard stomach. Legs drawn up. Hands clenched. Face beet red. Nothing the parents do seems to calm the poor child down. What makes these hollering sessions even worse is the absence of a good clue for the cause. Gas might be one. It could be an intolerance to some food or to something in Mom's milk. Maybe it's something no one thought of. Or maybe it isn't colic at all. Even the baby's doctor might be baffled.

There is one small bit of good news: The problem usually diminishes within three months. In the meantime, here are some remedies to try at home.

Give the Lass Molasses

"You can give a colicky baby molasses or dark corn syrup. Either one will help immediately by soothing the stomach," says Patricia Edwards, M.D., a pediatrician in private practice in Concord, New Hampshire. Mix 2 teaspoons molasses or dark corn syrup with ¼ cup warm water. "Put the mixture in a bottle and give it to the baby to suck." Dr. Edwards warns against giving a baby honey or light corn syrup. Either could contain botulinum, a bacterium that could kill an infant.

Stop for Gas

"Infants' Mylicon drops, which contain simethicone, help quiet a colicky baby by calming the innards," Dr. Edwards says, adding that simethicone absorbs some of the gas that causes discomfort. You can get Infants' Mylicon drops over the counter.

Don't Fill Up with Gas

"If the colicky baby is being breastfed, the mother should check her diet for foods that can cause gas," Dr. Edwards says. "Avoid too much milk, legumes such as beans and peas, spicy foods, onions, caffeine, and vegetables from the broccoli family—including broccoli, cauliflower, and brussels sprouts." Cabbage, onions, and chocolate also can make a breastfeeding baby colicky, according to researchers.

Stop Pumping Iron

"Get a baby with colic off formula that contains extra iron," advises Peter Brassard, M.D., a family doctor on Block Island, Rhode Island. "Instead, use a formula with little or no iron, because iron can be hard for a baby to digest. If possible, switch to breastfeeding. That's the best alternative of all."

Fight Noise with Noise

"The sound of a vacuum cleaner calms some colicky babies," Dr. Edwards says. "Some parents even tape-record the sound of the vacuum and play it for the fussy baby."

Or Try the Hard Rock

"Taking a colicky baby for a car ride is a classic cure," Dr. Edwards notes. "A lesser-known, but equally effective, trick is to place the baby in a baby carrier on top of a running washer or dryer. As with a car ride, the movement of the washer or dryer can calm a colicky baby." Dr. Edwards warns, however, that you should not leave the baby unattended. The vibrations could move the baby right off the machine.

TIME TO SEE THE DOCTOR

A Constant Crier Should See the Doc

SEE your pediatrician if your baby cries more than three hours a day, day after day," says Carole Stashwick, M.D., a pediatrician at the Dartmouth-Hitchcock Medical Center in Lebanon, New Hampshire. "The doctor will want to examine a colicky baby from time to time to be sure of the diagnosis and ensure the baby's growth and parental sanity. Parents who are angered or upset by the crying need to get some counseling rather than risk hurting the baby."

Peter Brassard, M.D., a family doctor on Block Island, Rhode Island, says it's also important to seek medical attention if your colicky baby runs a temperature. "Abdominal pain with a fever means a mandatory call to the doctor," he says.

Seek a Soak

"A warm bath will sometimes soothe a colicky baby," Dr. Edwards says.

Give Peace a Chance

Sometimes all a chronically crying baby needs is a bit of calm comfort, says Carole Stashwick, M.D., a pediatrician at the Dartmouth-Hitchcock Medical Center in Lebanon, New Hampshire. "In the evening, give the baby a bath and then do the feeding in a quiet room," Dr. Stashwick says. "You might try lying down to nurse the baby. After the little one falls asleep, you can leave."

COMMON COLDS

How to have an uncommonly comfortable time with your cold

It's called the common cold for good reason. Kids get 6 to 10 colds a year on average. Adults, whose immune systems are veterans of the cold wars, typically suffer from 2 to 4 a year. Colds and other respiratory tract infections cause the average grown-up to stay home from work almost seven days a year.

So if we can put a man on the moon, why can't we conquer the sniffles? Well, for one thing, we're fighting on many fronts. There are more than 200 cold viruses seeking a beachhead in your nose. When one of them establishes itself, you can expect to suffer for an average of two to six days, according to David Sigelman, M.D., a pediatrician with Holyoke Pediatric Associates in Holyoke, Massachusetts.

Most colds go away within a week, although some of the symptoms may bug you for up to several weeks. "The small viruses that cause colds stimulate

---

TIME TO SEE THE DOCTOR

Don't Mess with a Stuffed-Up Chest

A STUFFY nose is one thing, says Mary-Catherine Gennaro, D.O., a family osteopath in Warren, New Hampshire. But if you're feeling a tightness in your chest, get it checked by your doctor. "This may indicate bronchitis," she says, "especially if you're coughing up discolored sputum."

Also see a doctor if your chest congestion is accompanied by chest pain or swollen ankles—signs of possible heart disease.

---

the mucous glands in the nose and else-where in the upper respiratory system," says Hugh P. Hermann, M.D., a family doctor in Woodstock, Vermont. "The mucous glands create the characteristic clear discharge that lets you know you have a cold." You also may have some swelling in the linings of the nose, throat, and sinus areas. Fever isn't common in adults with colds, but a child could run a temperature of up to 102°F.

That old wives' tale about catching cold when you forget to wear your scarf doesn't seem to be true, by the way. According to medical research, being cold or wet doesn't make you more susceptible to the sniffles. (Modern-day stress, however, does appear to weaken the body's defenses against a cold.)

Although not all ancient wisdom about colds is true, some of the old cures still work. Here is a selection of the best—along with some more modern treatments.

Do the Fluids Thing

That old advice to drink plenty of fluids still holds, according to Dr. Sigelman. "Drinking a lot will help a little," he says. "It thins the mucus and makes you feel less stuffed up."

The Painkiller Thing, Too

Ibuprofen is best for aches and pains, Dr. Sigelman says. Avoid aspirin, which can cause Reye's syndrome in children.

And Don't Forget the Rest

"Get plenty of rest when you have a cold," says Brewster Martin, M.D., a retired family doctor in Chelsea, Vermont. "I don't recommend staying in bed all day. Just get adequate rest, with 8 hours of sleep and maybe a 20-minute nap in the afternoon. Get up and move around once in a while to keep the juices flowing."

Get the Right Drugs for the Job

THE ingredients in cold remedies can be quite a mouthful. What should you look for on the labels? The American Academy of Oto-laryngology–Head and Neck Surgery recommends the following generic ingredients for your particular symptoms.

- Stuffiness and nasal congestion: pseudoephedrine, phenylpropanolamine, phenylephrine, oxymetazoline
- Pain: ibuprofen, acetaminophen
- Runny nose: diphenhydramine, chlorpheniramine
- Cough: dextromethorphan

Get Unstuffed

"Decongestants are considered by doctors to be better than antihistamines," Dr. Sigelman says. "Antihistamines dry up secretions and make them harder to move out." Decongestants reduce the swelling in nasal passages to make it easier for you to breathe. You can buy decongestants over the counter in pill or liquid form. Follow the directions on the label.

ANNALS OF MEDICINE

Overstuffed Trunk? Play Elephant

Thomas Palmer, a seventeenth-century New England country doctor, prescribed the following technique to clear up a cold-stuffed head: "Fill your Mouth with water & then snuff up the juice of Primrose into your Nose."

"Who knows? It could work," says Mary-Catherine Gennaro, D.O., a family osteopath in Warren, New Hampshire. But a more tried-and-true solution is salt water. Dr. Gennaro recommends buying sodium chloride nasal spray, such as Ocean Spray (that's the saltwater remedy, not the cranberry juice) over the counter at the drugstore. "Snuff it up when you feel stuffy," she says. "It will help thin the mucus and keep nasal tissues moist."

Seek Citrus

"Warm lemonade is especially helpful for a cold," says Paul Lena, M.D., a retired physician of internal medicine in Concord, New Hampshire. "The vitamin C in lemonade is good for you, and the heat helps loosen secretions."

Get a Yen for the Hen

"There really is something to be said for hot chicken soup for a cold or the flu," Dr. Martin says. "Hot liquids are good for a cold in general. Plus the broth appears to stimulate the immune system."

Give "C" an A

"Vitamin C, in amounts totaling at least 1,000 milligrams daily, is helpful to prevent and alleviate colds and the flu," Dr. Hermann says. You can buy vitamin C in pill form over the counter at pharmacies. Or you can make sure your diet includes lots of foods high in vitamin C. Great providers are citrus fruits such as oranges and grapefruits, cabbage, dark green vegetables such as spinach and broccoli, cantaloupe, strawberries, peppers, tomatoes, potatoes, papayas, mangoes, and kiwifruit.

Get Sweaty

"For a pure cold without complications, a moderate, brief sauna is helpful in getting the blood to flow, stimulating the immune system, and easing your aches and pains," Dr. Hermann says. "Don't stay in for more than 20 minutes, and skip the traditional plunge into cold water or snow afterward. That could be hard on the system."

Lick It with Garlic

"Take garlic at the first hint of a cold or the flu," says Corinne Martin, a certified clinical herbalist in Bridgton, Maine. She recommends taking garlic pills, available at health food stores, or simply adding garlic to your meals. "Garlic is considered to be antibiotic and antibacterial," Martin says. "It kills germs in test tubes. More important, garlic goes specifically to the lungs, so it is good for fighting those things that attack the lungs." Martin says that upping your daily dose of garlic can help prevent colds.

Red Clover Is Lucky

"Red clover tea is very mild, easy to obtain, and good-tasting, so your kids will use it," Martin notes. "Have your child help you collect red clover in the summer. It stimulates the immune system, and it's a decongestant and expectorant, helping to clear up your stuffy head. Harvest red clover and dry it, then steep it in boiling water when your child has a cold or the flu. She'll enjoy using it, having helped make it." You also can buy red clover tea at many grocery stores and health food stores.

Purple Works, Too

Rosemary Gladstar, an herbalist in East Barre, Vermont, was taught the ancient use of herbs by her Armenian grandmother. Gladstar says that "the best possible remedy" for colds, the flu, or a suppressed immune system is tea made from purple coneflower, or echinacea. "Echinacea tea is effective against disease," she says. "It increases white blood cell count, which is part of the first line of defense of the body's immune system." Gladstar recommends drinking two or three cups of tea a day in cycles—five days on, two days off. "Prolonged use lowers echinacea's usefulness," she

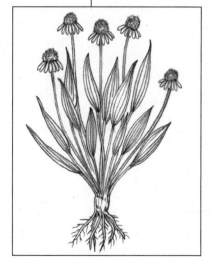

Purple coneflower, in the form of echinacea tea, is a traditional—and effective—cold remedy.

cautions. And don't take it at all if you're allergic to ragweed, a close relative of echinacea.

Take It to the Shower

"Treat yourself to a steaming hot shower," says Mary-Catherine Gennaro, D.O., a family osteopath in Warren, New Hampshire. "That will clear out your nasal passages better than anything."

CONCEPTION PROBLEMS
Ways to coax the stork to make a visit

A rule of thumb among medical experts is that you have a fertility problem if you've been trying unsuccessfully to conceive for one year. Before that, you may have an impatience problem, but there is little need to go to a specialist.

Even after a year, an unfilled nursery does not mean that you're infertile as a couple, according to Thomas J. O'Connor III, M.D., an obstetrician-gynecologist in private practice in Rockport, Maine. "It may be that just one of you is subfertile, or less likely to conceive readily," he says.

What's the best solution, once major physical problems have been ruled out? "Keep trying," Dr. O'Connor says. "Fifty percent of couples who did not conceive in the first year will conceive in the second. Half of those who still haven't conceived will succeed in the third year of trying." He adds that balky fertility is one disadvantage of being at the top of the food chain. "Unlike humans, voles and mice are brisk and efficient at reproducing. They have to have babies quickly before they are eaten. Our bodies don't have to work so fast."

So what can we do to become a little more rabbitlike, re-production-wise? All kinds of imaginative techniques have been tried over the years. As recently as the 1930s, the farm home of the famous Dionne quintuplets became a mecca for yearning couples. A workman was kept busy full-time digging up stones from the Dionne land for people to keep as fertility charms. People thought there must be *something* about that Dionne place to produce five kids at a pop!

Though they may be less charming, here are some remedies that are true as well as tried.

Boxer Yourself

If you are a man, to give you and your mate a good chance at conception, make sure that you have enough sperm by asking your doctor to have your sperm counted in the lab, Dr. O'Connor advises. And what should you do if your count is low? Switch to boxer shorts. "A man's brief-style underwear can bring his testes in close proximity to his body, causing sperm to heat up," he explains. Boxer shorts "allow him to hang loose, and sperm production can be enhanced at the lower temperature the boxers allow."

Don't Sweat It

Avoid saunas and hot tubs if you're a man trying to conceive a baby, says Hope Ricciotti, M.D., an obstetrician-gynecologist in Boston. "It takes 72 hours for your body to make new sperm. Don't kill most of them off with heat."

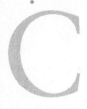

Space Your Passion

"Couples wishing to conceive should have intercourse at least every other day during the time of the month when the woman is fertile," says Eric A. Sailer, M.D., an obstetrician-gynecologist at the Dartmouth-Hitchcock Medical Center in Lebanon, New Hampshire. But don't overdo it. "If you have intercourse more than two or three times a day, the sperm count can go down."

Stay with an Old Standard

"The most fertile position is the standard missionary position, in which the man is on the top and the couple face each other during intercourse," Dr. O'Connor says. "If the woman is on top or on her hands and knees, the sperm can spill out."

Skip the Douche

"Don't douche after intercourse," Dr. O'Connor cautions. "That washes out the sperm."

Re-Honeymoon

"Stress can stop ovulation, the dropping of the egg into the womb that readies a woman for conception," Dr. Sailer

---

A WORD FROM DR. MARTIN

I'm Sour on This Remedy

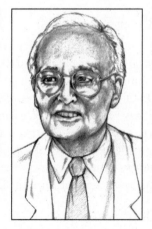

A LOT of Vermonters believe that a mixture of honey and vinegar is good for infertility. I never prescribed it, though. It won't hurt you, but there isn't a scintilla of evidence that it will help.

I had more than one patient say, "I've taken honey and vinegar every day for six months, and I'm still not pregnant!" I'd reply, "Well, did you go to bed with your husband?"

BREWSTER MARTIN, M.D., *a retired family doctor in Chelsea, Vermont (population 1,166), and cofounder of the Chelsea Family Health Center. He was named Vermont Doctor of the Year in 1991.*

notes. If you're having trouble getting pregnant, try to reduce the sources of stress in your life, he says.

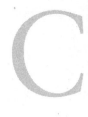

Catch Up on "Z"

"Take zinc if you're having trouble conceiving," Dr. Ricciotti advises. "Oysters are a great source of zinc. Their power in aiding fertility may be how they got their reputation as aphrodisiacs." A small zinc deficiency can make conception difficult, she explains.

Nix the Smoke and Drink

"Smoking and alcohol both impair conception," Dr. Ricciotti says. "Abstain from both if you're having fertility problems."

Try a Cough Cure

Cough syrup containing guaifenesin is an old-time remedy for women with fertility problems. Does it work? "In theory, it should," Dr. Ricciotti says. "Guaifenesin's function in the body is to thin secretions. It probably does the same thing to the mucus inside the woman, ensuring that the sperm have an easier time reaching the egg." Take the cough syrup several hours before intercourse.

Get a Kid with a Kit

Dr. Ricciotti strongly recommends buying an ovulation predictor kit if you're having trouble conceiving. Available inexpensively over the counter, the kit measures the level of the luteinizing hormone in the urine. This hormone tends to increase just prior to ovulation. When the kit registers the hormone change that shows you're fertile, "have intercourse the next day."

CONSTIPATION

Some moving advice
for when your innards come to a halt

Constipation—our forebears called it "costiveness"—comes in several varieties, according to Linda B. Dacey, M.D., an internist at the Dartmouth-Hitchcock Medical Center in Lebanon, New Hampshire. "Constipation means many

C things to many people—from trouble having a bowel movement, to uncomfortably hard stools, to straining to defecate, to abdominal discomfort prior to a bowel movement." Taken together, this mixture of discomforts accounts for more than 2 million visits to the doctor every year, and nearly three-quarters of a billion dollars spent on laxatives.

Lots of things slow down a body's digestive system and lead to constipation, according to Dr. Dacey. Medications such as antacids and antidepressants can be constipating. A lack of water and fiber in the diet, a lack of exercise, and an excess of iron are common causes. Obstacles in the digestive tract, such as tumors, also can trigger constipation. And so can a problem called colonic inertia, in which the colon fails to push waste products downward.

Doctors' advice? Don't overuse over-the-counter laxatives. That could make you even more constipated. Instead, add fiber to your diet. "Good sources of dietary fiber include fruits, vegetables, whole grains, or bran," says John Bancroft, M.D., a gastroenterologist in Portland, Maine.

If you're still stuck for a solution, try these remedies to get your system moving again.

Fiber Up Your Breakfast

One of the easiest means to get extra bulk in your diet is to eat a high-fiber cereal each morning—or sprinkle wheat bran on top of your usual choice. People whose diets contain 15 grams of fiber a day tend to have twice as many bowel movements per week as other people. When you add fiber to your diet, make sure you drink plenty of fluids to keep stools soft and moving.

Habit *Your* Way

"Keep to the same bathroom routine every day," Dr. Dacey advises. "Sit on the toilet for only a short period at the

TIME TO SEE THE DOCTOR

Is It More Than Constipation?

S EE a doctor if your constipation is accompanied by weight loss," says Linda B. Dacey, M.D., an internist at the Dartmouth-Hitchcock Medical Center in Lebanon, New Hampshire.

Other signs that a constipated person needs medical attention, according to Dr. Dacey, include the following:
- Vomiting
- A stomachache that gets progressively worse
- Stools that are becoming narrower in diameter
- Stools that have an unusual texture or color
- Sudden constipation for which you can't pinpoint the cause—such as a drastic change in your routine or diet

Even My Initials Are Regular

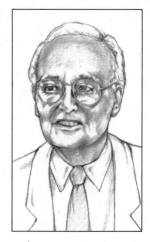

MY INITIALS are B.M., and I'm proud of them—despite a little episode involving them in medical school. During my last year as a med student, I was assigned to a hospital. Along with several other students, I followed a doctor on his rounds. He told us what medications to prescribe and allowed us in turn to put our own initials on the order chart—a little rite of passage toward becoming doctors ourselves.

For one patient with constipation, the doctor prescribed Milk of Magnesia, a useful remedy to this day (and available over the counter). I dutifully wrote down "30cc Milk of Magnesia. BM."

We happened to be working in a Catholic hospital run by nuns. At the end of the day, the mother superior came up to us and said, "Okay, who is the smart aleck who signed this order 'BM'?"

Ever since that time, I've derived a special little pleasure from signing laxative prescriptions with my initials.

BREWSTER MARTIN, M.D., *a retired family doctor in Chelsea, Vermont (population 1,166), and cofounder of the Chelsea Family Health Center. He was named Vermont Doctor of the Year in 1991.*

same time each day, whether you feel the urge or not. But don't wait around if you don't feel anything coming."

Keep Moving

"Exercise is another way to avoid constipation, because the moving around keeps things moving inside you," Dr. Dacey says. Research shows that people who exercise regularly tend to have fewer constipation problems than those who exercise rarely.

Do the Thermometer Trick

"For an infant having difficulty passing a hard stool," Dr. Bancroft says, "try taking the baby's rectal temperature with

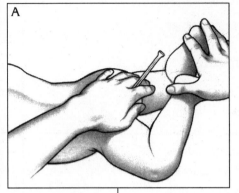

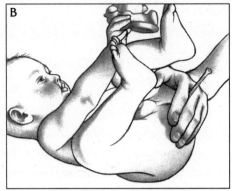

A rectal thermometer may help stimulate a baby's bowel movement. Insert the thermometer while the child is lying on his stomach (A). Or, if it's more comfortable for the baby, place him on his back and bend his knees (B).

a well-lubricated rectal thermometer. It may provide the necessary lubrication and rectal stimulation to help things along."

Gulp Some Grape

Rosemary Gladstar, an herbalist in East Barre, Vermont, and author of *Herbal Healing for Women*, suggests a daily glass or two of grape juice to combat chronic constipation. "Welch's is fairly concentrated, giving you good fruit fiber for constipation," Gladstar says.

Do a Power Lunch

IF YOU need a concentrated fiber supplement to maintain softer, more frequent bowel movements, try Power Pudding," says John Bancroft, M.D., a gastroenterologist in Portland, Maine. He recommends this recipe, passed on to him by T. R. Flygt, M.D., an internist in Baraboo, Wisconsin.

Power Pudding
3¼ cups cooked prunes
2 cups apple juice
2 cups prune juice
1 cup bran

Puree the ingredients and refrigerate the mixture.

Start with a two- or three-ounce serving three to seven days a week. "Adjust the amount and frequency to achieve a normal stool pattern," Dr. Bancroft says. He notes that some people gain weight eating this rich mixture, "and the large amount of sugar may cause difficulty for some diabetics." But for those who can handle the extra sugar, this can be good medicine. It has been proven especially effective with constipated elderly people who are housebound.

Prime the Pump

An enema can help to soften a hard stool that refuses to pass. "An enema can be prepared from equal measures of milk and molasses," Dr. Bancroft says. "You can use this mixture for a constipated child. Give 1 ounce per 10 pounds of body weight—in other words, a 30-pound child should be given 3 ounces." Up to 5 ounces of the formula is safe for a large child or adult. "Insert the enema into the rectum using an enema bag. Gravity is enough to let the mixture go in. Retain the mixture inside for 5 to 10 minutes, then go to the bathroom to expel it." Dr. Bancroft recommends that you consult your doctor if you feel the need for an enema more than twice a month.

COUGHING
Bark up the right tree with these remedies

You might not appreciate this fact while you're coughing in the middle of the night, but that hacking is your body's way of getting rid of stuff that doesn't belong there, such as dust from the air or the excess mucus that comes with a bad cold. Any irritation to your breathing passages—pet dander, pollen, smoke, airborne chemicals—will automatically trigger a cough in response. An infection in your chest caused by a virus or bacteria can inflame the respiratory system and cause a cough as well.

So there's a reason for that hacking. But too much of a good thing can simply add to your miseries. Doctors distinguish between a "productive" and an "unproductive" cough. "In a productive cough, you bring up the mucus along with some of what's causing the cough in the first place," says Mary-Catherine Gennaro, D.O., a family os-

---

ANNALS OF MEDICINE
That Old Black Magic Really Works

ONE of the oldest cough cures is licorice. "For a tickling Cough . . . I think there is not the like medicine. A charm by God's blessing," wrote Thomas Palmer, a seventeenth-century Massachusetts physician, who recommended combining licorice shavings and water. These days, herbalists recommend simply mixing a pinch of licorice powder (found at health food stores) in a cup of tea. A pinch is enough—taken in large doses, licorice can make you sick.

teopath in Warren, New Hampshire. "An unproductive cough is one where no mucus comes up." Asthma or post-nasal drip can cause an unproductive cough. Or sometimes a cold or the flu can cause your cough reflex to kick into overdrive, making you hack more than you need to.

That is why doctors have been trying to suppress coughs for centuries. Cotton Mather, the Puritan clergyman and part-time doctor, prescribed castile soap shavings, drunk in wine or beer, to get rid of a cough. Our doctors don't recommend that approach today, but they do offer some more palatable cures.

Grandmother's Cure Saved a Life

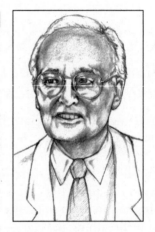

WHEN I was an intern in a country hospital 40 years ago, a pair of infant twins were brought in with the croup. They were less than a year old, and they were in rough shape, wheezing terribly. One of the little ones died during the night. The doctors on duty went out into the hallway to decide how to save the other baby—leaving me alone with the nurse.

I asked her for a dropper and a glass of water. Then I put a drop of water on the baby's tongue. A baby's instinct is to swallow, and that's what this one did. I immediately put another drop on the tongue, then another and another.

The doctors came back in and asked me what I was doing. "I'm doing what my grandmother would have done hours ago," I replied. She knew that you can't swallow and cough at the same time; that's the principle behind cough drops.

I stayed with that baby all night, until the worst of the crisis was over. Those little drops of water kept the baby from coughing to death.

BREWSTER MARTIN, M.D., *a retired family doctor in Chelsea, Vermont (population 1,166), and cofounder of the Chelsea Family Health Center. He was named Vermont Doctor of the Year in 1991.*

Use Sweet and Sour

"For the tickly kind of cough, mix equal amounts of honey and lemon juice," says Elizabeth Lowry, M.D., a pediatrician who is retired after 38 years of practice in Guilford, Connecticut. "Take a spoonful whenever you feel the cough coming on."

Just Drop It!

"Cough drops work because it is impossible to cough and swallow at the same time," says Brewster Martin, M.D., a retired family doctor in Chelsea, Vermont. "Sucking a cough drop will help relieve an irritating cough."

Buy Codeine

"Only cough medicines that use ingredients from the codeine family affect the cough center in the brain," Dr. Martin says. "If your cough comes from pneumonia or a chronic lung disease, the only thing that works is a codeine-derivative cough syrup." Many codeine or codeine-derivative medicines—such as Tylenol with Codeine, Triaminic Expectorant DH, and Actifed with Codeine cough syrup—are available with a prescription.

Take a Nightcap

"Mix yourself a hot toddy for a cough that won't let you sleep," Dr. Gennaro recommends. "Mix a jigger of whiskey and a jigger of water, then add lemon juice and sugar to taste. The alcohol will settle the cough and numb a sore throat, while the lemon will cut the mucus."

Bark at Yourself

"Slippery elm is excellent for coughs," says Rosemary Gladstar, an herbalist in East Barre, Vermont, and author of *Herbal Healing for Women*. A traditional cough treatment approved by the U.S. Food and Drug Administration,

TIME TO SEE THE DOCTOR

If a Cough Lasts, Report It

SEE your doctor if your cough doesn't go away within two weeks, if you're coughing up colored phlegm or what looks like coffee grounds, or if your coughing is accompanied by chest pain or a fever.

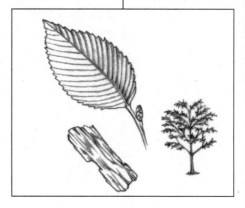

The powdered bark of the slippery elm tree is a cough cure approved by the FDA.

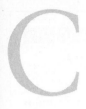

slippery elm bark is available in powder form at health food stores. Stir 1 to 3 teaspoons slippery elm into 1 cup water, boil for 15 minutes, and drink it down.

CRADLE CAP

Humble hints for when your baby has a less-than-regal crown

You marvel at the perfect skin of an adorable little baby until you take a glance at the top of his head, where a yellow, dry crust tops off an otherwise ideal picture. Cradle cap is a skin inflammation that's often found in babies—and sometimes in older children as well. "Cradle cap is just seborrhea, an inflammation caused by the excess secretion of sebum, a thick fluid from sebaceous glands in the skin," says Patricia Edwards, M.D., a pediatrician in private practice in Concord, New Hampshire.

The cap often shows up on an unwashed scalp, according to Everett Orbeton, M.D., a pediatrician who is retired after 44 years in private practice in Portland, Maine. "Some parents are afraid to wash a baby's head because of the soft spot up there, so the head doesn't get washed adequately."

Doctors say cradle cap is usually not harmful or even irritating to the baby, and it eventually goes away on its own. But if the cap gets too noticeable and modest bonnets just aren't your child's thing, take these baby steps toward a prize scalp.

Hit the Flakes

"Use dandruff shampoo on a baby with cradle cap," Dr. Edwards advises. "Get up a good lather on the scalp and rinse it right off the baby's head—don't let the shampoo sit." After rinsing, Dr. Edwards recommends using a toothbrush, a soft baby brush, or just your finger to loosen the flakes that remain on the scalp. "Repeat the shampooing once a day for a week and then as often as needed."

Don't Be Rash

Some babies' scalps react to strong shampoos. "Before using a shampoo on a baby's head, you can test an arm or a leg to

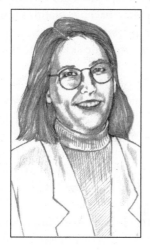
see if a rash develops within the hour," Dr. Edwards notes. Some babies are especially sensitive to the dandruff shampoos Selsun Blue and Head & Shoulders. "Neutrogena is a milder shampoo," she says. "You can also try T/Gel, available in most drugstores." Remember to keep shampoo away from your baby's eyes.

Oil's Well That Ends Well

"Use a good-quality vegetable oil on your baby's scalp," says Rosemary Gladstar, an herbalist in East Barre, Vermont. "I use olive or almond oil. And I add a drop or two of jojoba oil and vitamin E oil to each bottle of olive or almond oil." All of these products are available at health food stores. Warm the oil mixture slightly and rub just three or four drops into your baby's head. "You don't want to worsen the

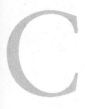

problem by making the head too oily," Gladstar cautions. The gentle oil massage stimulates the sebaceous glands in the skin, lubricates the scalp, and helps remove dead skin, she explains. "Use an oil massage daily until the skin clears up."

Tune Up for Grandma

"I am a massive fan of Cortaid for cradle cap," says Peter Brassard, M.D., a family doctor in private practice on Block Island, Rhode Island. Cortaid is an over-the-counter cream that contains the steroid hydrocortisone in a 1 percent concentration. "Kids will outgrow cradle cap anyway, but mothers will often bring their babies in to me because the grandmothers are coming," Dr. Brassard says. "I tune them up for Grandma with hydrocortisone in prescription form. But you can make your baby's cradle cap disappear by rubbing on the Cortaid two or three times a day for five days."

CRAMPING
*Cures for muscles
that put the squeeze on you*

Nothing puts a cramp in your style faster than a muscle that won't stop contracting. It can happen while you're moving about or while you're sitting still. You're minding your own business when—boom—you feel a deep pain in one or more of your muscles.

"A muscle cramp is an involuntary contraction of a muscle," says Gerard Bozuwa, M.D., a retired family doctor in Wakefield, New Hampshire. "It's caused by a chemical imbalance—an erroneous chemical signal from the nervous system to the muscle telling it to contract." Overuse of a muscle can throw the chemicals out of whack. That's why runners often get cramps in their calves and diarists get writer's cramp in their hands.

Some cramping is actually useful to your body, says Sarah Johansen, M.D.,

TIME TO SEE THE DOCTOR

That Gut Feeling Could Be Serious

SEE your doctor if your crampy feeling is in the lower right-hand part of your belly, says Sarah Johansen, M.D., medical director of emergency services at New London Hospital in New London, New Hampshire. "You could have appendicitis, which needs immediate surgery," she explains. Also get yourself checked out for any cramping that doesn't go away within 12 hours, she says.

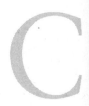

medical director of emergency services at New London Hospital in New London, New Hampshire. "When you're in labor, involuntary contractions of the uterus are what push the baby out." Women often get cramps during the middle of their menstrual cycles. "The pain of an egg being released from the ovary, usually felt in one or the other side of the lower abdomen, is called mittelschmerz," Dr. Johansen explains. "It's a natural, if uncomfortable, part of your cycle."

Regardless of where it hits, a muscle cramp generally goes away after an hour or so, says Dr. Bozuwa. "A muscle can't stay in spasm for very long. The muscle eventually runs out of the chemicals that signal it to contract."

But you may not feel like waiting around for a miscommunicating muscle to finish its message. Here are some sources of faster relief.

Heat a Cramp

"Apply heat, such as a moist, warm towel, directly to a muscle cramp," says Daniel Caloras, M.D., a family doctor in private practice in Charlestown, New Hampshire. "At the same time, take an over-the-counter anti-inflammatory drug such as aspirin or ibuprofen." If the person being treated is a child, do not give aspirin, which can cause Reye's syndrome in youngsters.

Take a Tonic

"The best cure for muscle cramps, including the leg cramps some people tend to get at night, is quinine," Dr. Bozuwa says. "Quinine is contained in tonic water. Sometimes if you drink a glass of it, your cramps will disappear quickly."

And Just Drink

"Stomach cramps are often the result of constipation," Dr. Johansen notes. "Drinking fluids and eating fiber are key to maintaining normal bowel movement and preventing cramps." While you're having stomach cramps, she says, sit

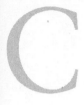

on the toilet with your feet propped up on a stool. "You should feel prompt relief. If your stools are hard and difficult to pass, use an over-the-counter stool softener such as Colace."

Skip the Caffeine

"Too much caffeine can lead to muscle cramps," says Tiffany Renaud, D.C., a chiropractor in South Burlington, Vermont. "Limit yourself to a maximum of two cups of coffee or tea a day."

Visualize Whirl Peace

"A whirlpool bath can do wonders for muscle cramps," says Randal Schaetzke, D.C., a chiropractor at the Wholistic Health Center in Quechee, Vermont.

CROSSED EYES
Straightening out skewed vision

Crossed eyes, a condition that doctors call strabismus, is not uncommon in babies under six months of age, according to Eugene J. Bernal, O.D., an optometrist in White River Junction, Vermont. One or both of your baby's eyes may turn in, out, up, or down, because nerves in the brain have not yet trained the eyes to see as a team. In most infants, however, the eyes eventually straighten out. "It is not considered normal for eyes to turn either inward or outward after half a year," Dr. Bernal says.

It's not always easy to tell if your baby's eyes are crossed. "Some parents worry that their baby is cross-eyed, when in fact the baby may simply have a broad nose bridge that makes the eyes look askew," Dr. Bernal notes. To make sure, buy a small penlight at a hardware store. "Shine the light in each eye. The point of reflection from the pupil of the eye should be in the same location in both eyes.

TIME TO SEE THE DOCTOR
Crossed Signals

A TUMOR in the eye or brain can cause eyes to cross inward or outward," says William Lavin, M.D., an ophthalmologist in private practice in Waterville, Maine. "Don't try any home treatments for crossed eyes until you've had them evaluated by an eye doctor."

"If your baby is one year old and still has crossed eyes, don't wait to see if they'll be outgrown," Dr. Bernal cautions. The brain tends to turn off a straying eye to prevent double vision, so if an eye is straying, it's also not seeing properly. "Early vision problems can be easily corrected, but if an eye is not used, its vision may be reduced permanently." Most adults with crossed eyes were born with the problem and never had it corrected.

If an illness or injury causes eyes to cross in adulthood, it's often too late for the brain to make adjustments. In that case, crossed eyes can lead to blurriness or double vision. But if your eyes tend to cross briefly after you take off your glasses, don't worry. That's probably just your vision readjusting.

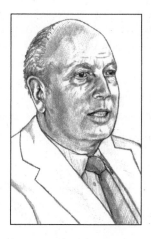

A WORD FROM DR. B.

My Father Got Me to See Straight

CROSSED eyes are the abnormality most missed by parents. A parent often doesn't recognize that his own child has crossed eyes—even when that parent is a doctor.

When my son, Paul, was several months old, my parents came over from Holland to see him. My father, an old navy man with no medical background, took one look at the baby and said, "His eyes are crossed."

Well, I wasn't about to take that from a layman, whether he was my father or not. "Of course they're not crossed," I said. "Paul is perfectly normal." I took him to an ophthalmologist—who recommended surgery. Two operations later, Paul's eyes were nearly normal.

Monthly checkups are a good idea during a child's first year. Ask your doctor to look for any serious eye problems. Don't leave it to your own all-knowing parenting.

GERARD BOZUWA, M.D., *retired after 36 years as the sole family doctor for the town of Wakefield, New Hampshire.*

C

And, by the way: Remember all those warnings about crossing your eyes when you were a kid? Yet another old grandmother's tale. "Your eyes won't stick if you cross them," says Henry Kriegstein, M.D., an ophthalmologist in private practice in Hingham, Plymouth, and Sandwich, Massachusetts.

If your eyes are crossed on their own, you need to see your doctor. Here are the sorts of things he'll advise you to do under his supervision.

Try Eye Aerobics

"Sometimes children have one eye that occasionally strays outward," says William Lavin, M.D., an ophthalmologist in private practice in Waterville, Maine. "This condition, known as intermittent exotropia, can be controlled with eye exercises." Once your doctor diagnoses your child's condition, you can try having the youngster do "pencil pushups." Have the child place a different-colored unsharpened pencil in each hand and hold the pencils at arm's length. While keeping one arm straight, the child should slowly bring the other pencil in toward his eye, concentrating his vision on that pencil. If he has the optical illusion of holding two pencils in one hand, that's actually a good sign: It means that both eyes are working the way they should, Dr. Lavin explains. Have your kid do this routine twice a day for five minutes at a time, alternating the hand that approaches the eye.

To do "pencil pushups," a child should hold both pencils extended at arm's length (A), then focus on one of the pencils while bringing it closer to the eyes (B).

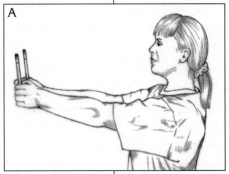

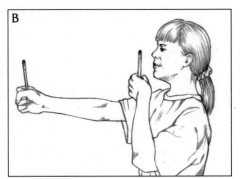

Do the Pirate Look

"A simple eye patch over the good eye can save the other eye," Dr. Kriegstein says. "The patch makes sure that the weaker eye is exercised. Ask your doctor if a patch is right for your child."

Get Specs

"In children, farsightedness can make crossed eyes worse," says Stephen Moore, M.D., an ophthalmologist in Great Barrington, Massachusetts. "This problem can be taken care of with prescription glasses."

CROUP
Coping with a child's strange cough

Croup is laryngitis with a vengeance. Whereas most adults and older children respond to this viral infection of the voice box by sounding hoarse, children under four can develop a nighttime cough that sounds like the mating call of a sea creature. Your child also might have a slight fever and be gasping for breath.

The reason: The air passages of a baby or preschooler are narrow, and the inflammation that accompanies a virus can cause the walls along the passages to swell. "It's the rule of

---

TIME TO SEE THE DOCTOR
Some Crouplike Coughs Are Not Croup

ALTHOUGH most cases of croup are fairly harmless, another disease that produces a croupy cough can be life threatening. Epiglottitis, an inflammation of the cartilage flap that covers the windpipe, affects all ages, not just babies. "Epiglottitis can close off the airway entirely," says Dudley Weider, M.D., an otolaryngologist at the Dartmouth-Hitchcock Medical Center in Lebanon, New Hampshire. "The disease requires immediate treatment in a hospital with antibiotics and relief to the airway."

The most obvious sign of epiglottitis is the person's position when he coughs. "A person with epiglottitis sits with the chin and neck thrust forward, trying to get air," Dr. Weider says. Other signs of the disease include a high fever, drooling, and difficulty swallowing. "Epiglottitis is usually caused by bacteria called *Hemophilus influenzae*," Dr. Weider says. "But it can also occur as an allergic reaction to nuts, shellfish, or a bee sting." The condition can be life threatening, he adds, so see a doctor if you suspect you may have this problem.

thumb," says John C. Robinson, M.D., a pediatrician in private practice in Quincy, Massachusetts. "A person's airway is about the diameter of his thumb. That means a baby's airway is pretty tiny—just the width of *his* thumb. The smaller the airway, the more turbulence there is as breath rushes through. The cartilage lining the airway in a baby is soft. Inflammation can increase the effort of breathing, causing the airway to collapse: The baby could end up with an airway the diameter of the lead in a pencil. The air going through that tiny passage is what makes the sound of croup."

It may be small consolation to a parent listening to the midnight howling, but croup becomes much less common as your child's windpipe grows. If croup keeps coming back frequently, ask your doctor to check for reflux. In some children, acid flowing up into the throat from the stomach seems to cause frequent bouts of croup.

In the meantime, here's how you can de-frog your child's croak.

Head into Some Steam

Drape sheets over the top and three sides of baby's crib, then direct steam from a humidifier in the open side to ease the symptoms of croup.

"When I was first in practice, the local hospital had a steam room," recalls Everett Orbeton, M.D., a pediatrician who is retired after 44 years as a family doctor in Portland, Maine. "Nurses wearing raincoats would hold croupy babies in the steam. You can do the same thing by running a hot shower. Hold the baby in the bathroom—not in the shower—with the door closed to keep the steam in."

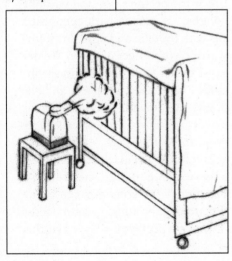

Make the Crib Tropical

"You can make a mist tent out of the baby's crib," notes Patricia Edwards, M.D., a pediatrician in private practice in Concord, New Hampshire. "Drape sheets over the top and three sides of the crib. Leave one side open and aim the nozzle of a steam humidifier into the open side."

Follow Steam with Cold

"Prescription steroids will take care of croup pretty quickly, but in the middle of the night, you can use home remedies," Dr. Edwards says. "After keeping your baby in a steamy bathroom for 15 minutes, bundle the baby up and take her out into the night air for another 15 minutes."

Place the Tummy Down

"When you put a croupy baby down in the crib, place him on his stomach," Dr. Orbeton says. "That lets the phlegm run out from the windpipe through the mouth, rather than down into the chest."

Give TLC ASAP

"Get up and hold your baby when you hear a croupy cough," Dr. Orbeton advises. "It is important to keep the child calm. If he panics, his windpipe will get even tighter."

CUTS AND SCRAPES
Say bye-bye to boo-boos

A scraped knee is one of the badges of a happy childhood. Small cuts and scrapes are part of an active life, and our skin is well-adapted for handling them—preventing infection with germ-fighting blood and growing new skin where it's needed. "Your skin is one of nature's most adaptable organs," says Owen Reynolds, M.D., a dermatologist in private practice in North Andover, Massachusetts. "The best remedies help your skin to do its thing."

Here are some ways to give your skin a little boost when it's broken.

Get Rinsed

"The sooner you clean a cut or scrape, the better," says Harry Rowe, M.D., a family doctor in Wells River, Vermont. "Use running water—a stream will do if you're out in the woods. Then apply

---

TIME TO SEE THE DOCTOR

Get Stitches for the Big Stuff

Any cut on your face that is more than half an inch in length should get medical attention," says Robert F. Wilson, M.D., a pediatrician who is retired from his family practice in Dover, New Hampshire. "You may need stitches to minimize scarring. Unless a cut won't stop bleeding, you usually don't have to worry about stitches if it's small."

Years Ago, Some Smart Guy Forgot to Take Out the Garbage

From Latin America to Europe, cures for cuts throughout the ages have included the use of molds to prevent infection. Brazilians gathered a fungus called *puf,* which grows wild, and applied it to cuts and minor abrasions. Europeans of old were big on mold. A tradition in their households was to sacrifice a loaf of bread, leaving it to mold on a rafter. When someone got a cut, the woman of the house would mix the mold with water and paste it on the wound.

They were on to something. Penicillin, the first of the wonder drugs, was discovered growing in—where else?—bread mold.

Here's another ancient wound-healing technique that's still used, though rarely: ants. In ancient India, surgeons closed up the wounds from their operations with large ants. The doctors would hold ants up to the incision, let the jaws shut, and then snap off the bodies. Voilà! Instant sutures. North American Indians apparently used leaf-cutting ants for the

an antiseptic. Hydrogen peroxide, available in any drugstore, is one of my favorites. You can apply it to any part of your body except the eyes, and it's very impressive to see the way it bubbles up on a wound."

Stay Wet

"Moist healing is enhanced healing," Dr. Reynolds says. "Keep a cut or scrape moist with petroleum jelly, Aquaphor, or Bag Balm, all available in drugstores and grocery stores. I'm very fond of Bag Balm myself." Made to soothe the udders of milk cows, Bag Balm can moisten human skin as well, he says. "If it's good enough for cows' teats, then it's good enough for you." Over-the-counter antibiotic ointments, such as Bacitracin, keep wounds moist while killing germs. A study by surgeons at the University of Oklahoma Health Sciences Center found that patients given antibiotic ointments had significantly fewer infections than those who were given petroleum jelly alone.

Air Your Trouble

"Most cuts heal better if left to the air, so it's best to leave them uncovered," says Patricia Edwards, M.D., a pediatrician in private practice in Concord, New Hampshire. "If your child is troubled by the sight of a cut, you can put an adhesive bandage on it," she says. "But don't leave it on for more than a day. Bandages can get pretty dirty."

Thank Charlotte

"To stop the bleeding from a cut or scrape, use a trick my husband learned on an Indian reservation," says Julia Foote, R.N., a retired nurse in Norwell, Massachusetts. "Put a spiderweb over the cut. Webs are relatively germ-free, and they make an ideal natural bandage."

"I haven't tried it myself, but I've read about it," says Daniel Caloras, M.D., a family doctor in private practice in Charlestown, New Hampshire. "You collect webs, ball them up, and place them over the cut. The webbing helps to coagulate the blood."

Leave the Cut

Foote grew up on a farm in Florence, Vermont, where her mother knew some natural remedies of her own. "When we got cut, my mother would pick a plantain leaf from out in the yard, wash it off, and place the entire leaf over the cut," Foote says. "She'd cover the whole thing with a bandage."

Dr. Caloras confirms this remedy: "Plantain leaves contain a natural antiseptic and are appropriate to use on any infection."

Get Kneady

"If you get a raised scar from a cut or scrape, try massaging it," Dr. Reynolds says. "Rub it for 10 minutes daily for a couple of months. That should help to remodel the scar tissue, flattening it out."

D

DANDRUFF

To *clear snowy shoulders,* catch the drift *of these remedies*

If it looks like the sky is falling every time you wear a dark suit, don't panic: Everybody gets dandruff to some degree or another. Your scalp sheds skin cells just as the rest of your skin does. And maybe the fact that your dandruff always seems to be worst during a first date or a job interview is just Murphy's Law—anything that can go wrong will go wrong.

Sometimes, though, your Chicken Little attitude is justified when dandruff comes down in excessive amounts, covering your shoulders. Doctors call this heavy precipitation scalp scaling. Any of several causes could be at the root of your problem. A common cause of scalp scaling is a yeast infection called seborrheic dermatitis. Often appearing during the pimple-prone teenage years, seborrheic dermatitis inflames your scalp and makes it shed skin cells in self-defense. The flakes you shed are greasy and yellowish. Your skin also may shed cells under your eyebrows, in your ear canal, or in the middle of your chest. Acne is a common accompanying misery.

Or your flakes could be the result of a fungus called *Tinea capitis*. "That's related to the fungus that causes athlete's foot," says Sarah Johansen, M.D., medical director of emergency services at New London Hospital in New London, New Hampshire. "It's like athlete's foot of the head."

Often the cause of dandruff is a simple dry scalp, owing to naturally dry skin or the overly enthusiastic use of harsh shampoos. Whatever the reason for the flakes, you can give them the brush-off with these remedies.

It's a Wash

"No matter how good the shampoo you're using is, you need to wash your hair at least every other day to control dandruff," says Charles Hammer, M.D., a dermatologist with the North Country Outreach Program of the Lahey Hitchcock Clinic in St. Johnsbury, Vermont.

Pick Two of Three

"There are three basic categories of over-the-counter dandruff shampoos," Dr. Hammer explains. "First, you have the tar shampoos, such as T/Gel, based on a special form of tar. Don't worry. Tar shampoos don't smell at all like road tar." A second category, Dr. Hammer says, has the chemical selenium sulfide as its active ingredient. Selsun Blue is in this group. The third kind of shampoo, which includes Head & Shoulders, is based on pyrithione zinc. "Buy shampoos in two of these three groups, and every two weeks switch back and forth between them," Dr. Hammer says. "That way, your dandruff is less likely to build up a tolerance or resistance to your shampoo."

> ### TIME TO SEE THE DOCTOR
> ## When You're More Than Just Flaky
>
> GET your head looked at if you have any of these symptoms.
> - A scalp that won't stop itching
> - Thick, scaly dandruff that resists dandruff shampoos
> - A yellowish crust on your scalp
> - Red patches of skin anywhere above the shoulders
> - No improvement in your condition after two months of using home remedies

Brew Your Hair

"Tea tree dandruff shampoo is great for dandruff," says Happy Griffiths, an herbalist at Enfield Shaker Museum in Enfield, New Hampshire. You can buy tea tree shampoo at health food stores.

Try the Strong Stuff

"If regular dandruff shampoos don't work, you might try an over-the-counter salicylic-acid-based lotion, such as Scalpicin," says Owen Reynolds, M.D., a dermatologist in

D private practice in North Andover, Massachusetts. "Rub it in according to the instructions on the label."

Switch Back

"Use antidandruff shampoos only until the dandruff is gone," advises Valerie Major, a licensed cosmetologist and manager of Beth's Salon in Woodstock, Vermont. "Return to your regular shampoo if you're not seeing flakes. Otherwise, the dandruff shampoo will eventually lose its effect and will be useless if the problem crops up again."

DARK CIRCLES UNDER THE EYES

Is your face being shadowed?
Try these cures

You're noticing dark patches under your eyes—discoloring that makes you look like a zombie. What is going on?

"A lot of things," says Charles Hammer, M.D., a dermatologist with the North Country Outreach Program of the Lahey Hitchcock Clinic in St. Johnsbury, Vermont. "In many cases, dark circles under the eyes are inherited. If your parents have them, you'll probably have them." Dr. Hammer says that some people are born with thinner than usual skin under their eyes, allowing blood vessels to show through as dark areas.

Especially pale skin can make the patches under your eyes look dark, too. And conditions that make you pale—such as a cold, menstruation, or just being pooped—can give you that raccoon effect. "Any swelling under the eyes can accentuate the skin folds, creating a dark shadow," Dr. Hammer says. "If you get shadowy creases under the eyes, that can be a sign of an allergy—they're called allergic shiners. You'll want to see your allergist for solutions."

TIME TO SEE THE DOCTOR

Problems Above and Below?

IF YOU develop dark circles under your eyes within a one-week period and your ankles become swollen at the same time, see your doctor," says Charles Hammer, M.D., a dermatologist with the North Country Outreach Program of the Lahey Hitchcock Clinic in St. Johnsbury, Vermont. "These symptoms could indicate heart trouble, kidney failure, or a liver problem."

For those plain old ugly dark patches, here are some ways to lighten up.

Bag the Late Night

"If you wake up one morning with dark circles under your eyes, chances are good that you're not getting enough sleep," says Robert Averill, M.D., a dermatologist in private practice in western Massachusetts and northern New Hampshire. "A lack of sleep causes swelling in the skin under the eyes. Get at least eight hours of rest every night."

Cover Up

"Use an over-the-counter cosmetic concealer," says Owen Reynolds, M.D., a dermatologist in private practice in North Andover, Massachusetts. "Women already know how to hide their dark circles with makeup, but men don't. Makeup works just as well to cover up men's dark circles."

Drink Juice

"Dark circles under a child's eyes, especially if it's a girl, may be a sign of a chronic bacterial infection of the urinary tract," says Laurence Bouchard, D.O., an osteopathic family physician in Narragansett, Rhode Island. "Have her drink a lot of cranberry juice and call the doctor."

Flub the Rub

"In springtime, I see children come in with vernal conjunctivitis—a springtime allergic irritation of the eyes," says Eugene J. Bernal, O.D., an optometrist in private practice in White River Junction, Vermont. "Their eyes itch so much that they dig their knuckles in and grind them. That bruises the area under the eyes." To minimize the problem, "discourage your kid from rubbing his eyes and fight the allergy with over-the-counter antihistamines and cold compresses for immediate effect."

Are You Looking through Rose-Colored Glasses?

"If dark circles under your eyes are a part of your natural coloring," Dr. Bernal says, "you may want to have an optician blend and tint the lenses of your glasses to match your skin color. This can cover up the circles or make them less noticeable."

DEHYDRATION
Catching a runaway thirst

You've spent several hours of a beautiful hot day weeding your garden, and now you've worked up a good healthy thirst, right?

If so, your timing is off, says John Bland, M.D., a rheumatologist in Cambridge, Vermont, and author of *Live Long, Die Fast: Playing the Aging Game to Win.* "By the time you feel thirsty, you are already dehydrated," he says. If you haven't anticipated that thirst, your postgardening glass of water may not prevent dehydration and its symptoms, which include dryness in the mouth, a run-down feeling, weakness, low blood pressure, and even fainting. Check your urine after a bout in the garden: You can tell your water level is going down if your urine is a dark yellow or has a powerful smell.

But summer activity isn't the only way you can drain yourself of fluids. Fever, an infection, diarrhea, and vomiting also cause dehydration. Dr. Bland notes that it's wise to be especially careful to drink plenty of fluids if you're over 40. As

Thirst Is Not Just a Summer Affair

You need to drink plenty of fluids before and during any outdoor activity, even in the winter, according to Michael Pelchat, an instructor of emergency medicine who has taught first-aid to the weather researchers on New Hampshire's Mount Washington. "Dehydration can be especially tricky in the winter," Pelchat says. "You often don't realize you're sweating when it's cold, because your sweat can evaporate quickly. And the dry air of winter can make you lose a lot of water through your breath."

A lack of fluid in your body can make your blood thick and sluggish, slowing its flow to your fingers, toes, and the tips of your ears and nose—prime targets for frostbite, Pelchat says. If the tiny veins in these parts aren't getting enough warm blood, your flesh is more likely to get nipped by the cold.

The best prevention, according to Pelchat, is to "drink at least half a pint of liquids for every quarter hour that you're outside in the winter. Besides helping to prevent frostbite, you'll probably find that your energy level is higher than if you're thirsty."

I'll Have My Water Straight Up, Please

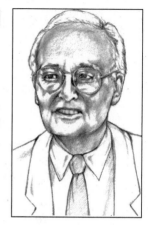

As a New Englander and a lover of the outdoors, I've learned the hard way that it's important to bring water with me whenever I'm away from a tap.

Years ago, when my children were still young, two of them spent a long day hiking with me on the Long Trail in Vermont. We climbed two mountains and got thirstier and thirstier. There were signs along the trail warning us against drinking the water in the streams, so we didn't drink any.

As soon as we got down from the mountains, we headed for a restaurant, where we asked for water. The waitress gave each of us a tiny glassful. "No," I said. "I want the whole pitcher." We each asked for a pitcher. It was all we could do to keep from grabbing them out of that poor waitress's hands. We must have looked as if we'd just come in from the desert.

A funny scene, but it could have been serious. Dehydration can cause headaches, vision problems, heart trouble, hypothermia, and, eventually, death—even in normally healthy people. Drink a few glasses of water before any outdoor activity, and bring water with you if you plan to be away from a reliable source of water for more than an hour. Make yourself drink a few gulps every 20 minutes.

BREWSTER MARTIN, M.D., *a retired family doctor in Chelsea, Vermont (population 1,166), and cofounder of the Chelsea Family Health Center. He was named Vermont Doctor of the Year in 1991.*

you get older, you tend to lose fluids more easily. The result can be serious. "Many older people arrive in emergency rooms near death—not for lack of proper medication or care, but for lack of water," he says. And how much water is enough? "Six to eight 8-ounce glasses of water a day are the minimum you need to be drinking for good health."

Here are some more tips for quenching that thirst.

Keep It Flowing

"Drink extra fluids at least an hour and a half before you begin a sweaty activity," says John C. Robinson, M.D., a pediatrician in private practice in Quincy, Massachusetts. "Then, during the activity, drink small amounts every 15 minutes or so. And keep drinking for an hour and a half after you stop." Dr. Robinson says he sees many cases of dehydration among young football players who practice in the August preseason. "All those hot pads cause a lot of sweating. Keep fluids beside the bench and encourage the kids to drink them."

Say No to Caffeine

"Avoid drinking anything with caffeine in it if you're trying to stay hydrated," says Sarah Johansen, M.D., medical director of emergency services at New London Hospital in New London, New Hampshire. "Caffeine, found in soda, coffee, and tea, makes you urinate, causing you to lose fluids." Stick to water, fruit juice, and sports drinks, she advises.

Brew Your Own

If water doesn't have enough taste for you, stay hydrated by mixing up an old-fashioned New England concoction. "Back before the days of Gatorade, farmers used to drink switchel when mowing hay," says Earl Proulx, longtime handyman at *Yankee* magazine and author of *Yankee Home Hints*. "My father used to make a batch on a hot day." The formula for switchel: Combine 1 gallon water, 2½ cups sugar, 1 cup dark molasses, ½ cup white or cider vinegar, and 2 teaspoons ground ginger. "Switchel is very sweet and has a strong, gingery taste," Proulx says. "My mother always complained that when it got hot, she couldn't keep ginger in the house."

DENTURE PROBLEMS
Keeping your chops in biting trim

One out of five Americans wears dentures of some type, and some 60 percent of them have problems with their biters, ranging from looseness to painful, swollen gums. Poor fit is the biggest reason for most of these complaints, according to Gregory L. Baker, D.D.S., an orthodontist in private practice in Woodstock, Vermont, and West Lebanon and New London, New Hampshire. "One way to tell if your dentures fit properly is to make an *F* sound," Dr. Baker says. "If you can't, your dentures need readjustment." The *F* sound, he explains, requires properly aligned teeth.

Here's what else you can do if you find yourself chomping at an uncomfortable bit.

Go Back for Alterations

Even dentures that initially fit perfectly will sometimes get out of whack. "The jaw changes over time, so the dentures need to be adjusted as well," Dr. Baker says. "If you find yourself needing adhesives to keep things in place, you should have your dentures refitted."

Ask about Implants

"New technology allows dentists to insert teeth right into the jawbone," Dr. Baker says. "Dentists call them implants, and they keep you from having to worry about adhesives and other means of keeping your dentures in place." Dr. Baker

---

ANNALS OF MEDICINE

George's Cherry Tree Didn't Go to His Mouth

THE ill-fitting dentures that vexed George Washington throughout his presidency and afterward really should have been made of cherry wood. That would have been poetic justice for his famous childhood crime of having hacked down an innocent cherry tree in its prime.

But Washington's choppers were not of cherry. In fact, they weren't made of wood at all. His first dentures, a set of lowers made by New York dentist John Greenwood in 1789, were made of ivory as well as a few genuine human teeth. Washington had just one lonely molar left, and Greenwood allowed it to stick up through a hole he left in the dentures. The dentist later made Washington a more expensive set of uppers and lowers out of gold, hippopotamus teeth, and hippo and elephant ivory.

This fancy dental work didn't make Washington any more comfortable, though. The dentures ruined his smile. These days, technology allows a better fit and regular adjustments—the keys to avoiding denture

---

notes that you should go to a dentist who places implants frequently. "That will assure you of the best care," he says. The downside of implants? "They're expensive."

Let Dentures Out at Night

"Removable dentures are like stars," Dr. Baker notes. "They should come out at night." Give your gums a rest when you go to bed.

Brush Up

"Brush your dentures with a toothbrush after every meal," Dr. Baker advises, "especially partial dentures, which can cause decay in the teeth that anchor the plate."

And Brush Cheap

"Use regular hand soap and warm water to scrub your dentures," says Gregory Colpitts, D.M.D., a dentist in private practice in Franklin, New Hampshire. "Over time, toothpaste will make your dentures less shiny." Dr. Colpitts says that it's a good idea to scrub your dentures both inside and out before you go to bed at night. "Then take another toothbrush—one that doesn't have soap all over it—and brush the roof of your mouth and your tongue."

DERMATITIS
Soothing cures for angry skin

Old-timers call this nasty skin rash eczema, but regardless of the name, it's hard to bear. In a reaction sparked by outside irritants or by internal allergies or illnesses, the skin becomes itchy, red, and swollen, creating oozing, crusty, and scaly patches. Some people can get dermatitis from stress. You also can get it from itchy clothing, extreme heat, cold, dryness, viruses, harsh detergents, gasoline, and overzealous washing—not to mention poison ivy, poison oak, and a host of other environmental hazards.

"Dermatitis is any irritation of the skin that doesn't go away," says Gerard Bozuwa, M.D., who is retired after 36 years of private practice as a family doctor in Wakefield, New Hampshire. "Your doctor will ask you whether anyone else in your family suffers from dermatitis or from other allergic problems, such as asthma and hay fever. If the answer is yes and your rash is behind the knees or inside the elbow, you probably have an allergic reaction. Alternatively, your dermatitis might be caused by an infection—bacteria, yeast, or fungus. Which remedy you use depends on what caused the problem in the first place."

Go to Cort

If your rash appears to be caused by an allergy, Dr. Bozuwa recommends applying the over-the-counter cream Cortaid with 0.5 percent hydrocortisone, the lowest concentration available. If two or three days of using Cortaid or any other remedy is unsuccessful, it's time to see your doctor.

Fend Off the Invasion

"Use over-the-counter antibacterial or antifungal remedies for an infection," Dr. Bozuwa says. Neosporin is a triple-antibiotic ointment that blasts a wide range of bacteria.

Work the Calamine

Charles Hammer, M.D., a dermatologist with the North Country Outreach Program of the Lahey Hitchcock Clinic in St. Johnsbury, Vermont, says good old calamine lotion is still one of the best anti-itch remedies. And you can pick it up at any pharmacy.

Hang Scratchy Clothes

"Some folks are irritated by wool clothing," Dr. Hammer says. "They should avoid wool or wear cotton against the skin."

Bar the Strong Soaps

"Some people with eczema have skin that acts like a defective sponge," says Mark Quitadamo, M.D., a dermatologist at the Lahey Hitchcock Clinic in Bedford, New Hampshire. "Anyone with sensitive skin should wash infrequently with lukewarm water and use a mild soap such as Dove, Basis, Camay, or Cetaphil, then lubricate with a face cream." Once a day is enough to cleanse the face, Dr. Quitadamo says; avoid repeated washings.

Maybe I Missed My Calling

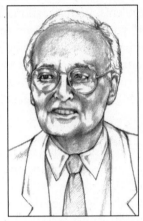

As a parishioner at our rural Vermont church, I love to wait tables during big functions. Once I helped out at a wedding reception. The groom's family was from Kentucky. One fellow on the groom's side kept drinking all the water in his glass. I filled it eight times, and he drained it every time: a pretty good sign of diabetes.

"You're an excellent waiter," the man said to me after dessert. "I own a restaurant chain in Kentucky, and if you ever want a job, look me up." And he gave me his card.

At that very moment, the groom's mother came up and introduced me as the family doctor. I thought that fellow would sink through the floor.

I never did find out if that guy had diabetes, but if you're making heavy water demands on waiters, you'd be smart to get yourself checked.

BREWSTER MARTIN, M.D., *a retired family doctor in Chelsea, Vermont (population 1,166), and cofounder of the Chelsea Family Health Center. He was named Vermont Doctor of the Year in 1991.*

Dress Like Your Aunt Mabel

"If your dermatitis is on your hands," Dr. Quitadamo says, "it is very good to lubricate your hands with hand cream or petroleum jelly, then cover them with cotton gloves to keep the lubrication on the skin and off everything else."

Cotton to Rubber

Some 7 to 10 percent of the U.S. population has allergic reactions to latex, the substance in rubber gloves found in doctors' offices and home kitchens. Studies show that children with spina bifida are especially susceptible to latex allergies, as are people who are allergic to bananas and avocados, which come from close relatives to rubber trees. If you are allergic to latex, buy cotton-lined rubber gloves.

Skip Sweet-Smelling Detergents

"People who find detergents irritating may find fragrance-free detergents helpful," Dr. Quitadamo says. "Cheer-Free, Tide Free, and All Free & Clear are detergents without fragrance."

Stick with Static Cling

"In a few, very rare cases, someone who is allergic to fiberglass will have a reaction to the fabric softener sheets used in clothes dryers," Dr. Quitadamo says. "These sheets can shed tiny pieces of fiberglass into the clothing and cause generalized itching." If you can't pinpoint any other cause for your problem and you find that the condition worsens after you do the laundry, try skipping the dryer sheets for a while.

Take a Quaker Bath

"Oatmeal is good for soothing irritated or itchy skin," Dr. Quitadamo says. Although you could sprinkle the breakfast stuff into your bath, he recommends an oatmeal product called Aveeno, specially made for bath use and available at drugstores and supermarkets.

Switch the Tube

If you have dermatitis around the mouth, try changing your brand of toothpaste. A study done by medical researchers in Finland found that half of the toothpastes in that country contained allergy-causing substances. The researchers traced 30 such substances in all. According to the study, cinnamon oil and peppermint are common irritants of sensitive mouths.

DIABETES
Dealing with sweet sorrow

Are you thirsty all the time and still find yourself making frequent trips to the bathroom? You might be one of the estimated 16 million Americans who have diabetes—a serious disease that requires a doctor's care. Diabetics can suffer from a variety of ailments, from hardening of the arteries to kidney disease to eye problems, in addition to the diabetes itself.

The Good News: You're Not Melting

ALTHOUGH people have known about diabetes for thousands of years, the disease has been poorly understood until recently. Observing diabetics' excessive urge to urinate, the ancient Romans believed that the flesh of their bodies was melting down and being funneled off into urine. *Diabetes,* in fact, comes from the Greek word meaning "funnel."

Even as late as the 1600s, physicians had little idea of what caused, or cured, the disease. "Snails burnt, and the Ashes taken, seldome fail of curing this Distemper," confidently asserted Cotton Mather, the famous Puritan minister and part-time doctor. As an alternative remedy, Mather recommended "Powder of a Burnt Toad, hung in a Bag, about the Neck."

Doctors now know that a diabetic's problem isn't melting flesh but simply too much sugar in the blood. Although you can do a lot of things for yourself at home (burning toads *not* being one of them), you should not attempt any cures without medical supervision.

If you have Type I, or insulin-dependent, diabetes, chances are you've already seen a doctor about it. Type I diabetics usually start showing symptoms as children. The common treatment is to add the hormone insulin to the bloodstream, which helps the body's cells take up sugar.

Type II diabetics usually don't show any signs of the disease until they're adults. In this form of diabetes, which is the more common variety, the body's sugar and insulin levels are out of whack. You may be producing excessive insulin because your body has developed a resistance to it. Or the insulin is not getting to the places where it's most needed to deal with your blood sugar. Either way, say doctors, obesity appears to be a culprit in the majority of Type II cases. The best way to treat it: Lose weight.

But before you try anything on your own, check with your doctor. "Diabetics must be under careful supervision," says Robert G. Page, M.D., a retired cardiologist living in Londonderry, Vermont. "You can't take care of yourself alone, or you risk coronary disease and other problems."

With your doctor's approval, though, you can use the methods below to reduce the risk of suffering from being too sweet.

Shed Pounds

"Losing weight is very important if you have diabetes," Dr. Page says. "In Type II diabetes (non-insulin-dependent diabetes mellitus), weight loss can actually make medication unnecessary in some cases." In young people with Type I diabetes (insulin-dependent diabetes mellitus), "weight reduction is a standard part of care. If young diabetics gain weight, they may require more insulin, and then they become resistant to it."

Get Starchy

Medical research shows that a diet high in carbohydrates—one that favors fruits, grains, and vegetables over red meat and fried foods—helps the body work with its natural insulin. "A low-fat, low-cholesterol, low-calorie diet is the single most effective home remedy for diabetes," says F. Daniel Golyan, M.D., a former New Englander who is now an electrophysiologist on Long Island.

Put Your Heart into It

A regular exercise program, such as a brisk daily walk or swim, is a good way to help make a weight loss diet work. Get approval for a workout routine from your doctor first, though. Diabetics are more likely than other people to have heart trouble, so it's good to be cautious before you get the heart pumping.

DIAPER RASH
Getting your baby's bottom problems behind him

As your youngster will be the first to tell you, diaper rash is a crying shame. What ends up in your baby's diaper is a chemical waste dump that's pretty unfriendly to tender infant skin. Dampness alone can cause a rash. Add uric acid and skin-eating fecal enzymes, and you have one raw baby bottom. "A lot of what we call diaper rash is actually an ammonia burn, caused by the ammonia from urine building up in a wet diaper," says Robert F. Wilson, M.D., a pediatrician who is retired from his practice in Dover, New Hampshire.

D

Fortunately, there are ways to make your baby's derriere smooth again.

Dispose of Your Problems

"Disposable diapers are treated to prevent ammonia formation," Dr. Wilson says. "If your baby suffers from frequent diaper rashes, try switching from cloth to disposable."

Embrace Change

"The key to clearing up diaper rash and preventing it from happening again is to change the baby's diapers often," says Kathryn A. Zug, M.D., a dermatologist at the Dartmouth-Hitchcock Medical Center in Lebanon, New Hampshire.

Teach the Alphabet

"For an ongoing case of diaper rash, use ointments that seal moisture out without irritating the skin further," Dr. Zug says. "An ointment containing vitamins A and D, available over the counter at drugstores, is among the most effective and cheap remedies."

Smear White Stuff

"Zinc oxide is great for preventing diaper rash," says Mark Quitadamo, M.D., a dermatologist at the Lahey Hitchcock Clinic in Bedford, New Hampshire. Zinc oxide is the ointment that prudent lifeguards put on their noses to prevent sunburn. It is available over the counter at drugstores.

Cream the Rash

"For a terrible rash, you can use over-the-counter hydrocortisone cream for a limited period—say, twice a day for a week," Dr. Zug says. "If it doesn't work after a few days, see your doctor. Your baby might have a secondary yeast infection that needs a prescription remedy to clear it up."

Birthday Suit Up

"Let your baby run naked for 20 minutes or so after you remove a wet diaper," says Brewster Martin, M.D., who is re-

---

TIME TO SEE THE DOCTOR

Are You Still Seeing Red?

ABOUT half of all diaper rashes clear up within a day. If your baby's bottom looks angry after three days, take the infant to a pediatrician or dermatologist. Sometimes a simple-looking rash can be a sign of something more serious, such as the skin disease psoriasis. Most baby skin diseases are treatable by physicians.

---

tired after running the Chelsea Family Health Center in Chelsea, Vermont, for 40 years. "Fresh air is the best way to dry up a bottom and kill the germs that can help cause diaper rash."

DIARRHEA

Ways to slow the runs to a walk

Our American ancestors called it the flux. The ancient Greeks came up with the word *diarrhoia,* which literally means "to flow through." You may have more choice words for the frequent trips to the bathroom to pass unformed stools.

No matter what you call it, diarrhea is simply excess water in your stool—caused either by increased fluids secreted in your digestive system or the body's failure to absorb the fluid in the stool. A viral or bacterial infection or a parasite can cause your digestive system to secrete extra fluid, leading to diarrhea. Bowel problems or lactose intolerance—found in people unable to digest milk sugar—can prevent your system from absorbing bowel water. Or you might have a speedy system in which your body's solid wastes move too rapidly to allow the absorption of water. Alcohol, caffeine, the excess magnesium found in most antacids, and some herbal

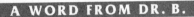

How I Got into Medicine

YOU might say that diarrhea made me a doctor. My childhood ambition was to be a sailor, not a doctor. I had originally planned to be an officer in the Dutch navy, like my father, who was a naval commander. He was sent back and forth between Holland and the Dutch East Indies—present-day Indonesia.

We happened to be living in the East Indies when the Japanese invaded in 1941. I was 15 years old. We were all sent to prison camps—including my father, who at the time was the commander of the Dutch naval air force. He tried to escape but was caught and spent the war in a prisoner of war camp in Manchuria. My mother and sister were sent to an internment camp. I was sent to a men's camp, an internment camp for men only.

Dysentery was a terrible problem in the camp. The disease caused unending diarrhea that sometimes resulted in such severe dehydration that it led to death. The commander of the 30 men in my ward asked for volunteers to work in the overcrowded infirmary. No one came forward. "If you are such terrible people that you won't help, then I don't want to be your commander," he said. What the commander said moved me. I couldn't help stepping forward.

I returned to Holland after the war determined to be a doctor. But for a while, it looked as if bureaucratic red tape was going to keep me from the first step: graduation from high school. Then Holland passed a law that allowed people who could prove they had studied in a POW camp to receive an "emergency diploma." While applying for the diploma, I ran into a guy I had nursed in the POW camp. He was the one giving out the diplomas. "I'll give you one if you promise to go into medicine," he said. I'd received training in the internment camp and was eligible for a diploma anyway. But my friend cut out a lot of the red tape and confusion that might have blocked me from the start. And so I went to medical school and became a doctor.

GERARD BOZUWA, M.D., *retired after 36 years as the sole family doctor for the town of Wakefield, New Hampshire.*

teas can cause an acceleration of what doctors call bowel motility.

Of all the causes of diarrhea, stomach viruses are the most common. You can get them from contaminated food or water or by touching a person who has the bug. Adults' bodies usually respond with diarrhea (in children, vomiting is a more common reaction to a virus). If you get a stomach bug, take heart: You should be feeling better within a week.

"Parents often worry that a child isn't eating during a bout of diarrhea," notes David Sigelman, M.D., a pediatrician with Holyoke Pediatric Associates in Holyoke, Massachusetts. "But eating little for a couple of days isn't very harmful." Dehydration—which can easily accompany diarrhea because of the loss of fluid in watery stools—is a greater concern. "The trouble arises when the child doesn't drink," Dr. Sigelman says.

So be sure to keep downing fluids. And slow that system down with these remedies.

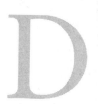

Slurp the Mother's Cure-All

An excellent way to replace electrolytes you lose in diarrhea—substances such as sodium and potassium, which allow the body to absorb water—is to sip some chicken soup. "Besides giving you electrolytes from salt, chicken soup is a reasonable source of calories and water," Dr. Sigelman says.

Don't Sweat over Gatorade

Doctors sometimes use the popular sports drink Gatorade to hydrate patients who have diarrhea. "Occasionally, this is an effective cure," Dr. Sigelman says. "But Gatorade is formulated to replace what the body loses from sweat, and sweat is very different from what is lost in diarrhea." You lose more electrolytes from diarrhea than you do from sweat. "Gatorade wouldn't be for infants, who don't have a reasonable store of electrolytes in their bodies," Dr. Sigelman says. "A baby would need Pedialyte or Rehydralyte to replace lost electrolytes." Pedialyte and Rehydralyte are liquids available over the counter at drugstores.

Go for the Pink

"Pepto-Bismol can help slow diarrhea," Dr. Sigelman says. Pepto-Bismol contains the mineral bismuth, which slows the passage of waste through the intestines. "It is especially useful in traveler's diarrhea. It's hard to get a kid to drink it, though."

But Bag the Red

Wine is a traditional cure for diarrhea. The Puritan minister Cotton Mather recommended a glass of wine for the "flux"—along with a few grains of rat's dung. These days, doctors say it's not a good idea to take wine for diarrhea. (You'll just get a funny look if you mention rat's dung.) "Wine is a diuretic—it makes you urinate," Dr. Sigelman says. "That means you lose more water if you drink wine, and you can't afford to lose water if you have diarrhea. So bag the wine."

And Skip the Coffee

"Caffeine is a gastrointestinal stimulant," Dr. Sigelman says. "It causes things to move along faster through your system. That's not something you want happening if you already have diarrhea." If your stools are loose, you might avoid your usual morning cup of coffee.

Give Your Baby Nature's Best

"Breastfeeding really works to restore an infant with diarrhea," Dr. Sigelman notes. What makes breast milk such a great diarrhea cure? "It is a source of fluid, has the right percentage of electrolytes and sugars, and contains a lot of antibodies, which are helpful in fighting the infection that caused the diarrhea in the first place. Nothing else can do all that."

Researchers at the University of California discovered that breastfeeding can actually help prevent diarrhea. In a study of American babies under the age of one, the researchers found that breastfed infants suffered from half the number of bouts of diarrhea as bottlefed babies.

Digest This Advice

"Avoid roughage when you have diarrhea," advises Elizabeth Lowry, M.D., who is retired after 38 years as a pediatrician in Guilford, Connecticut. "Cut out fruits, vegetables, and fruit juices. Always use something bland instead. Cream of Wheat is good to give someone with diarrhea."

Although fruit juices don't usually count as roughage, they contain high amounts of fructose, or fruit sugar. Some people have difficulty digesting large quantities of fructose, which can worsen their diarrhea. Honey, which also contains fructose, is another sugary food to avoid. And people who have diarrhea often have trouble digesting lactose, the sugar found in milk. Doctors say that you should avoid milk, ice cream, and other dairy foods for a week or more after you've had a bout of diarrhea.

Meet the BRAT

Maureen Williams, N.D., a naturopath in Hanover, New Hampshire, prescribes a BRAT diet: bananas, rice, applesauce, and toast. "This is a good, bland diet that is easy to digest," Dr. Williams says. "The rice should be really soupy. Cook the rice with twice the water that the recipe calls for."

Dr. Sigelman notes that all four foods are high in complex carbohydrates. "Carbs are reasonably easy to digest and reabsorb when the intestine is inflamed," he says. "Bananas, rice, pasta, bread, and crackers are all fine."

Take a Powder

"Sprinkle carob powder on your applesauce to help bind your stools," Dr. Williams says. "The carob powder will help slow the loss of fluid." You can buy carob powder at most health food stores.

DIZZINESS
What to do when you want to get off the spin cycle

Let's put a positive spin on your off-balance feeling: You have plenty of company. Dizziness is a common complaint—only backache sends more patients to the doctor. Most of the time, the problem is with your inner ears, the organs that tell you which end is up. But many other factors could throw you off balance, such as circulation problems, a head injury, a cold or the flu, allergies, or problems with your nervous system.

Before you or your doctor can pinpoint the cause, "you need to determine what you mean by dizziness," says Peter Mason, M.D., a family doctor in Lebanon, New Hampshire. "If the room seems to be spinning around, then you have vertigo, which is usually related to your inner ear balance system.

If you feel light-headed, as if you're going to pass out, then your problem may be low blood pressure, anemia, low blood sugar, internal bleeding, or an emotional response to trauma."

If your dizziness comes on suddenly, a virus is the likely cause, and your system should be stable in a week or so. But if your balance gets out of whack gradually and continues to get worse, you should see your doctor.

In the meantime, here's what you can do for yourself.

Lose the Booze

"If you are occasionally troubled by dizziness, avoid alcohol and stimulants such as diet pills and coffee," says Richard Nordgren, M.D., a pediatric neurologist at the Dartmouth-Hitchcock Medical Center in Lebanon, New Hampshire. "It doesn't take much to bring on dizziness. Don't make your problem worse."

Don't Disco

"Some dizziness is positional, meaning that you feel dizzy when you change position too quickly—getting up too fast or rolling over in bed," Dr. Nordgren says. "Until you and your doctor can pinpoint the problem, avoid sudden moves.

Stare at a fixed point, such as a spot on the wall, whenever you get out of bed or a chair."

Check the Salt

A hot summer day can make you dizzy by throwing your body's salt off balance, says Linda B. Dacey, M.D., an internist in Lebanon, New Hampshire. "I once had a patient approach me at the community lake, complaining of dizziness," she recalls. "I asked her what she'd been eating lately and decided her salt levels were low. So I sent her to the snack bar for a bag of potato chips. Soon after eating the chips, she was fine. Young women who have low blood pressure can get in trouble by avoiding salt, especially on hot days." See your doctor about maintaining the right balance of salt so that you can keep your balance.

Hit the Allergies

"Sometimes allergies play a role in causing dizziness," Dr. Nordgren says. "An allergy can plug up the middle ear, throwing you off balance. Try taking an over-the-counter antihistamine such as Benadryl. If that doesn't work, see an allergist."

DROWSINESS
Alert yourself
to these wide-awake remedies

If you find yourself getting sleepy every day, you may not be getting enough sleep—or the sleep you do get could be troubled by your breathing, says Michael Sateia, director of the Sleep Disorders Clinic at the Dartmouth-Hitchcock Medical Center in Lebanon, New Hampshire. "The cardinal causes of drowsiness are not getting enough sleep and sleep apnea," Dr. Sateia says. Obstructive sleep apnea, he explains, comes from a blockage in the upper airway, which causes breathing to stop for short periods. "If you snore at night and are sleepy during the day, you are a prime apnea candidate. See a doctor for diagnosis and treatment."

A rarer cause of drowsiness, Dr. Sateia says, is a hereditary neurological problem called narcolepsy. "Falling asleep routinely and suddenly during normal waking hours is one indication of narcolepsy," he says. "Again, see a doctor."

For those more occasional droopy-eyed moments, try these doctor-confirmed remedies.

Drop Weight

Drop the pounds, and you might drop off less during the day. "Overweight people tend to snore more at night, which disturbs sleep," Dr. Sateia explains.

Roll Over

You might gain more daytime energy by changing your normal sleeping position. "If you snore, try sleeping on your stomach," Dr. Sateia says.

Skip the Drugs

Avoid drinking alcohol at night. "It's a drug that disturbs the patterns of sleep, making you less rested the next day," Dr. Sateia notes. If you're having trouble getting to sleep, sleeping pills won't help in the long run. "You need to seek out the underlying cause of sleep problems and address them."

Get Some Sugar

You can perk up with a bit of fruit or candy, says Laurence Bouchard, D.O., an osteopathic family physician in private practice in Narragansett, Rhode Island. "Some people get drowsy from a lack of sugar in midmorning or midafternoon. If you're one of them, don't let yourself get too hungry between meals."

Are You Getting Your Full 40 Winks?

A GOOD cure for daytime drowsiness is to get lots of sleep at night, says Michael Sateia, M.D., director of the Sleep Disorders Clinic at the Dartmouth-Hitchcock Medical Center in Lebanon, New Hampshire. Well, sure. But how much is enough?

"*Enough* is defined as sleeping so that you wake feeling fully rested and alert through the entire day," Dr. Sateia says. "Ideally, you should wake naturally when you have had enough sleep. For most people, this means 7½ to 8 hours every night. Some people need 6 hours or less. On the other hand, some need 10 hours or more."

DRY EYES

Here are some cures that will bring you to tears

Those tears your eyes shed aren't just for emotion. They coat your orbs with a special film made of fat, water, and mucus. This film in turn lubricates your eyelids, provides needed nutrients to eye cells, fends off harmful bacteria, and cleans the surface of your eyes like a super window cleaner. Every time you blink, you refresh the tear film and spread it around.

Sometimes, though, your eyes just don't manufacture enough tears. Allergy and cold medicines can dry your eyes along with the rest of your head. A room with low humidity or a winter day on the ski slopes can make your eyes too dry for your tears to keep up. "Dry eyes are also common in post-menopausal women," says Eugene J. Bernal, O.D., an optometrist in private practice in White River Junction, Vermont.

It's enough to make you want to cry. Here's how to help those tears along.

Squirt the Air

"Dry eyes are particularly common in people who live in cold, dry climates," Dr. Bernal says. "If you're one of them, you need to alter your indoor environment." If you have a woodstove, place a pot of water on top and keep it full to release steam into the air. (Be careful not to let it boil dry; the pot doesn't have to boil to humidify a room.) "If you heat with more modern methods, keep a humidifier running at all times during the winter," Dr. Bernal says. "In some houses in New England, you'll commonly find that indoor humidity drops

TIME TO SEE THE DOCTOR

Don't Wink at Other Problems

GET medical attention if you have any of the following symptoms along with dryness.
- Red, bloodshot eyes despite the use of artificial tears
- Spots, blurriness, or other disturbances in your vision
- Eye pain

AN OUNCE OF PREVENTION

Shades Aren't Just for Sun

SUNGLASSES do more than protect your eyes against glare," says Eugene J. Bernal, O.D., an optometrist in private practice in White River Junction, Vermont. "They can also help reduce the amount of evaporation of your eye's moisture, especially on a windy day. Wear sunglasses when you're in the wind—even if it's cloudy."

5 to 10 percent during the winter. And the higher the humidity, the more comfortable your eyes will be."

Buy Some Tears

"Over-the-counter eyedrops are good for controlling the discomfort of dry eyes," Dr. Bernal says. How do you find the best artificial tears? "Look for products with the fewest ingredients. The simplest ones are less likely to produce an allergic reaction." He recommends Refresh, available at drugstores. Other effective artificial tears include Liquifilm Tears, Tears Plus, and Tears Naturale.

DYSPEPSIA
Smoothing out a rough ride inside

Dyspepsia is from the Greek for "bad digestion." In the days before refrigeration and modern hygiene, people had it in droves, with all kinds of folks suffering from the characteristic upset stomach and bloating.

People still get what doctors call non-ulcer dyspepsia, an illness that feels a whole lot like an ulcer—without the ulcer. For any of a variety of reasons—often mysterious ones—your insides periodically swell as gas builds up, and you can feel pain in the upper regions of your belly. The stomachaches come and go, often getting worse when you eat, though you can have them before meals as well.

If you feel bloated after a high-fat meal, particularly if you also experience discomfort behind the right lower side of your rib cage, you may have something else altogether: gall bladder disease, according to Peter Mason, M.D., a family doctor and medical director of the Alice Peck Day Community Health Center in Lebanon, New Hampshire. "See your doctor if you suspect gall bladder disease," Dr. Mason says.

Occasional digestive trouble can be treated at home. Here's how.

Don't Let Acid Reign

"Acid blockers work well to soothe dyspepsia," says Lawrence H. Bernstein, M.D., the medical director at Jewish Geriatric Services in Longmeadow, Massachusetts. "You can buy them over the counter at drugstores as Pepcid AC or Tagamet HB."

Spare Your Gut

"When you have dyspepsia, try to remember what you ate during the previous meal," Dr. Bernstein says. Common digestion pounders to avoid if you have dyspepsia are cabbage, citrus, tomatoes, spicy foods, alcohol, and caffeine.

Scrape Up This Cure

"If diarrhea is among your symptoms, try this old-time remedy," says Laurence Bouchard, D.O., an osteopathic family physician in Narragansett, Rhode Island. Peel an apple, he says. Then take a butter knife and scrape the inside of the peel. Throw away the peel and eat the scraped-off layer of fruit. "The inside of the peel contains pectin, a gelatin that helps absorb the water in your stool and stops diarrhea," Dr. Bouchard explains. "Pectin is one of the ingredients in the popular over-the-counter diarrhea medicine Kaopectate."

Balance Your Germs

"If you have dyspepsia, there may be an imbalance in your intestinal microorganisms," says Lawrence Bronstein, D.C., a chiropractor and certified nutrition specialist in Great Barrington, Massachusetts. "Try taking acidophilus, available over the counter at health food stores and some drugstores." You can also get acidophilus, a kind of "good" bacteria, in yogurt that contains live cultures. Look for acidophilus on the yogurt's label.

TIME TO SEE THE DOCTOR
Take in a Bad Ticker

A HEART attack can mimic heartburn or indigestion," says Laurie Duncan, M.D., an internist who moved from Cooperstown, New York, to Washington, D.C. "If your discomfort isn't easily relieved by antacids, get to a doctor quickly."

E

EARACHE

The best pain-popping nostrums you'll hear

Earaches often stem from infections in the middle ear or the outer ear canal. The pain frequently goes with a bad cold, which is one reason that kids—who get colds more than adults do—also succumb to more ear infections. "The only symptom a child with a middle ear infection may have is a plugged-up feeling," says Robert Fagelson, M.D., an otolaryngologist in private practice in Brattleboro, Vermont. Dr. Fagelson notes that babies are born with fully grown inner ears. ("The only other parts of the body that are full-size at birth are the eyeballs," he says.) Trouble is, the rest of the ears are still baby-size for the first several years, creating bottlenecks for fluid. "An inner ear infection in a child may occur in a matter of hours," Dr. Fagelson says. "I can examine a child's ear and it looks fine, then three hours later it can have a bad infection."

As your child gets older, his immune system and ears mature, and his body can handle the bacteria and viruses that cause infections. But germs aren't the only cause of ear pain. You can get a doozy of an ache if a virus causes swelling and mucus to gum up your eustachian tubes—the tiny channels that equalize the

---

TIME TO SEE THE DOCTOR

If the Ache Keeps On Aching

SEE your doctor if your earache lasts for more three days, says Elizabeth Lowry, M.D., who is retired after 38 years as a pediatrician in Guilford, Connecticut.

---

pressure in your nasal passages and inner ears. An object that gets stuck in your ear—a bug, for instance—also can trigger pain.

Your outer ear canal can start smarting if leftover moisture from a swimming pool or a smack upside the head causes an inflammation in the passageway. You can tell if you have an inflamed outer ear canal if a tug on your earlobe makes the pain worse.

If the pain lasts for more than a few hours, head for the doctor. Antibiotics can clear up bacterial infections, which are the most common causes of earaches. In the meantime, here are some tips for making your suffering ears more comfortable.

Do a Three-in-One in One

"You can treat an earache by warming up a little ordinary olive oil or mineral oil and putting a few drops into the sore ear with a dropper," says Elizabeth Lowry, M.D., who is retired after 38 years as a pediatrician in Guilford, Connecticut. "Do this while the child is lying down with the affected ear face up. Then hold a warm heating pad against the ear while the child is still lying down. You can also administer acetaminophen. Avoid giving aspirin to children because of the risk of Reye's syndrome."

Pacify a troubled canal zone with a few drops of warm olive oil (A). Then cover the ear with a toasty heating pad (B).

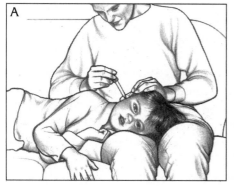

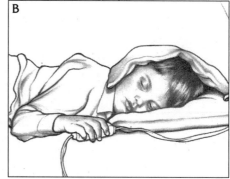

Dr. Fagelson notes that the heating pad heats up the mineral or olive oil in your child's ear. "It's the heat that provides relief," he says. "But don't put in oil if there's any drainage from the ear. That could indicate a hole in the eardrum."

Go After the Congestion

"Consider taking a decongestant to relieve the pressure of an earache," Dr. Fagelson advises. Try to find a decongestant that comes without an antihistamine, he adds. The antihistamine could thicken the liquid in your ears and keep it from draining.

EAR NOISES
How to cope with that all-too-familiar ring

The ringing, buzzing, swishing, hissing, whistling, chirping, or roaring noises you hear in your head are called tinnitus— a hearing disorder shared by almost 36 million Americans. Doctors aren't sure exactly what causes these noises, except that the nerves inside sufferers' ears appear to have gone haywire, sending signals of sounds that aren't really there. Sometimes tinnitus comes and goes suddenly, after a single loud noise or a few hours of deafening sounds—a rock concert, say. Expose your poor ears to too much of this abuse, and the ear noises could become permanent.

Tinnitus also can come from too much wax in your ears, hearing loss, a hole in the eardrum, high blood pressure, drugs such as antibiotics or aspirin, allergies, an ear infection, a jaw that's out of joint, even stress. Some people who have ear noises accompanied by bouts of severe dizziness suffer from Ménière's disease, which seems to stem from problems with fluid in the ears.

Age is a big factor in tinnitus. People ages 50 to 70 are the biggest sufferers. Some causes—such as impacted earwax or an ear infection—can be cleared up in a doctor's office. "But most cases of tinnitus just have to be tolerated," says Robert Fagelson, M.D., an otolaryngologist in Brattleboro, Vermont. If you can't get rid of the sounds, here are some ways you can at least make them more bearable.

If the Shoe Fits, Don't Wear It

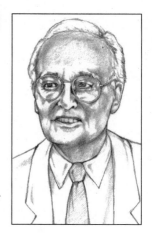

A<small>N OLD</small> doctor once told me that the best thing for tinnitus was to buy shoes that were too small for your feet. Then your feet will hurt so much you'll forget about the ringing in your ears. In most cases of tinnitus, distraction is the only remedy.

B<small>REWSTER</small> M<small>ARTIN</small>, M.D., *a retired family doctor in Chelsea, Vermont (population 1,166), and cofounder of the Chelsea Family Health Center. He was named Vermont Doctor of the Year in 1991.*

Get at the Wax

How can you tell if your ear noises are caused by wax buildup? "If fluid or wax is blocking the ears, you'll hear a low-pitched hum," Dr. Fagelson says. "You won't be able to hear sounds in the low frequencies, such as the bass fiddle in an orchestra. Remove the wax with an over-the-counter wax remover. If you have fluid in your ear, see a doctor."

Watch the Aspirin

"Sometimes a person who isn't feeling well will get an accidental aspirin overdose," says Peter Brassard, M.D., a family doctor on Block Island, Rhode Island. "The person takes a few aspirin, doesn't feel well, takes more, sleeps, wakes, still doesn't feel well, and takes more aspirin. That much aspirin can cause ear noises such as ringing or buzzing. They should go away within the week, but it's best to avoid taking too much of a good thing in the first place."

Avoid the Noisemakers

"Caffeine, salt, smoking, alcohol, and stress all exacerbate ear noises," Dr. Fagelson says. "Avoid them."

Take Magnesium

"Taking supplemental magnesium can sometimes help prevent ringing in the ears," says Maureen Williams, N.D., a naturopath in private practice in Hanover, New Hampshire.

"Magnesium capsules, available in most health food stores and many drugstores, are inexpensive and easily absorbed by your body. In military studies, soldiers who took magnesium supplements suffered less ringing in their ears and less long-term hearing damage after being exposed to loud noises."

Seek Peace

"Relaxing helps to open the blood vessels that contract when you are tense," Dr. Williams says. "When the vessels are constricted, the blood supply to the tiny hair follicles in the inner ear is restricted, and cells can be damaged." Research also shows that people who are relaxed are less likely to notice their tinnitus.

Treat Ménière's Disease

If your doctor diagnoses you with Ménière's disease, he may prescribe drugs to fight dizziness—a symptom that's particularly dangerous if you drive or operate heavy machinery. Your doctor also may tell you to quit caffeine, smoking, excessive dietary salt, and alcohol, which tend to aggravate both Ménière's disease and tinnitus.

EARWAX
Ways to make sure that excess wax is on the wane

A humble bodily product, earwax is nonetheless part of a system that really does work remarkably well—most of the time. "Earwax is a natural protection that coats the skin of the outer ear canal," explains Robert Fagelson, M.D., an otolaryngologist in Brattleboro, Vermont. Secreted by special glands in the canal, the wax traps dirt and germs. "The skin in your ears starts growing just outside the eardrum and then migrates forward, taking with it the wax," he says. Once outside the ear canal, the wax dries up and falls out of the ear or gets removed by proper cleaning. "It's nature's own way of self-cleaning."

Sometimes this nifty system gets bollixed up, either from a zealously used cotton swab pushing the wax back in or from overly productive wax-making glands. A wax buildup can make your ears feel stuffy and full and can even block your hearing. Leave it too long, and irritation can result. You'll want to get at the wax before that happens by following these hints.

Skip the Hog

"That which is thick filth gathered in the Ears is curable," wrote Thomas Palmer, a seventeenth-century Puritan minister who did double duty as a Massachusetts physician. And how do you cure a gunked-up ear? One of his recommendations: "Ox gaul & she goat Urine . . . mixt together drop oft into the patients ear." Doctors these days prefer hydrogen peroxide, available over the counter at drugstores. "A few drops of hydrogen peroxide in the ear two times a day for several days should clear up an earwax problem," Dr. Fagelson says.

Not only is this remedy superior to ox gall (and another of Reverend Palmer's favorite cures, a solution of child's urine), but Dr. Fagelson also prefers hydrogen peroxide to other, more modern methods. "Over-the-counter medications for wax removal may contain irritating chemicals," he says. "And the ear syringe provided to squirt the medicine can puncture the eardrum. Instead, use hydrogen peroxide and an eyedropper. Leave the peroxide in your ear until it stops bubbling, then allow it to drain. That should bubble the wax away."

Go Soft on Your Wax

"If your earwax is hard, use a mixture of half hydrogen peroxide and half glycerin to soften the wax," Dr. Fagelson says. Glycerin is available over the counter at most drugstores. "If earwax is a chronic problem," he says, "you can use this 50-50 mixture two or three times a week on a regular basis."

EYESTRAIN

These cures are definitely a sight for sore eyes

That all-night study session, or the double feature you sat through, or the tiny print in the thriller you read on the plane can take a toll on weary eyes. Our lifestyles often have a collision with our vision, including the problem your mother warned you about most: inadequate lighting. "The most common cause of eyestrain is doing work near improper lighting," says Eugene J. Bernal, O.D., an optometrist in private practice in White River Junction, Vermont.

Although a poor reading light can result in pooped peepers, a low-watt bulb will not "ruin your eyes," as Mom said. "Dim light does absolutely no harm," says Henry Kriegstein, M.D., an ophthalmologist in private practice in Hingham, Plymouth, and Sandwich, Massachusetts. "A long reading session may tire your eyes and even give you a headache, but it won't cause any physical damage to your vision. That's because eyestrain is really just tired muscles, not damaged eyes."

Dr. Kriegstein notes sadly that a doctor told the great seventeenth-century writer Samuel Pepys to stop his nighttime practice of keeping a diary. "Pepys followed his doctor's orders, putting a halt to the greatest diary ever written," Dr. Kriegstein says. "The awful thing was, no medical reason existed for Pepys to stop. That doctor did a great injustice to posterity."

Most forms of eyestrain are no more harmful than what Pepys experienced, but they can be annoying. Here are some ways to keep eye problems out of your own diary.

Carefully Monitor Your Computing

"The biggest mistake people make in the office is placing their computer screens incorrectly," Dr. Bernal says. "Position the top of the monitor at eye level, so that the middle of the screen itself is

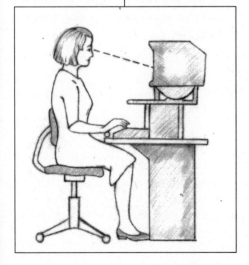

Screen out problems. Position the top of the computer monitor at eye level, so you look down slightly to see the middle of the screen.

slightly below eye level. And make sure you've placed the monitor so that there is no reflection on the screen from a window or light."

Dress for the Screen

"If you are having trouble with glare from your computer screen, try wearing a dark-colored shirt instead of a white

An Instant Cure for Blindness

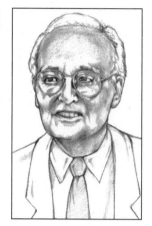

I ONCE came home to find a message on my answering machine from the sister of a patient of mine. "Julian's gone blind," said the voice on the machine. "Please come over."

I found Julian lying in bed looking about as unhappy as you would expect a man who's lost his sight to be. He was an elderly man who was almost blind without his glasses, but up until that point he had been able to see fairly well with his specs on. This decline in his sight was not good.

"When did you start having problems?" I asked Julian.

"It's been getting worse and worse over the past couple of weeks," he said. "Now I can't see anything except blurs, and my glasses don't help at all."

I noticed his glasses on the bedside table. They were filthy—completely coated with dirt and grease. I took them to the bathroom and washed them thoroughly. Then I handed them back to Julian, whose face broke out in a relieved smile. He could see again!

Julian is an extreme example, but you can do your eyes a favor if you get into the habit of cleaning your glasses every day with water and lens cleaner. You can polish them with special cloths bought from your optometrist or eyeglasses store, but a clean old linen towel or a piece of clean flannel works just as well.

BREWSTER MARTIN, M.D., *a retired family doctor in Chelsea, Vermont (population 1,166), and cofounder of the Chelsea Family Health Center. He was named Vermont Doctor of the Year in 1991.*

one," Dr. Bernal suggests. A light color tends to show up as a reflection on the screen, reducing the contrast and causing eyestrain. A dark shirt remains invisible on the screen.

Sit Back

"A good rule of thumb is to sit back from the television a distance seven times the diagonal measurement of the screen," Dr. Bernal says. "If you're too close, your eyes strain to capture the flickering images."

Light Up

"A single light to read by in a dark room isn't a good idea if you tend to suffer from eyestrain," Dr. Bernal says. "You should have general light as well as specific task lighting, such as a reading lamp. If you have fluorescent lighting, it's a good idea to mix it with incandescent light—the kind that regular bulbs produce."

Act Your Age

"A nearly universal sign of aging is presbyopia, the condition in which your eyes cannot focus on things up close," Dr. Kriegstein says. "Although it won't harm your eyes to go without reading glasses, the extra boost to your vision could prevent eyestrain." You can probably get by with an inexpensive pair of glasses from a drugstore, he adds, unless one eye focuses differently from the other. In that case, you'll need prescription glasses.

Swap the Specs

"If you are 50 years old and your reading glasses are more than 5 years old, you probably need a new pair," Dr. Bernal says. "Your eyes change over time, to the point where they have to strain to focus through old glasses. That's very tiring on the eyes."

Don't Rub the Wrong Way

"There is some evidence that people who rub their eyes frequently and hard may cause their corneas to become misshapen," Dr. Kriegstein says. "This condition, called keratoconus, causes blurred vision. So when your eyes are tired, don't rub them—or at least rub them gently."

F

FAINTING
Bright cures for blackouts

Although fainting is far from pleasant and a rough landing can cause other problems, such as bruises, most of the time the underlying cause is not serious, says Keith Michl, M.D., an internist in Manchester Center, Vermont.

What causes a swoon—or syncope, as doctors call it? "Fainting can happen when you're not getting enough oxygen to your brain," Dr. Michl says. "This makes you pass out for just a brief time, usually only a few seconds."

There are lots of ways to starve your brain of oxygen. One is the sudden drop in blood pressure when you stand up suddenly—in church, say. Overexertion can cause your body to use up more oxygen than it can take in, causing your brain to shut down suddenly. A phone call telling you of a death in the family or your winning lottery ticket can affect the nerves that control your blood pressure, cutting off oxygen to your brain. Coughing, stretching, and even urinating can interfere with the oxygen flow and cause a sudden blackout. And a drop in blood sugar, caused by skipping a meal or, more seriously, by diabetes, can make you faint.

One fainting episode is probably nothing to worry about, Dr. Michl says, although two within a period of as many days should send you to the doctor. As long as your blackouts remain less frequent than that, you can deal with them on your own. Here's how.

Get Your Head Down

"If you feel that you're going to faint—that feeling of the room closing in on you—put your head between your knees," says Peter Mason, M.D., a family doctor in Lebanon, New Hampshire. "Sit down quickly and put your head below the level of your heart. That way, gravity can pull more blood to the brain and make you feel less faint."

To help this process even more, Dr. Mason recommends having a friend place a hand against the back of your neck. "Try to push up against your friend's hand," he says. "You'll feel your face flush as more blood rushes to your head. You should feel better quickly."

Adjust Your Pills

"Among the most common causes of fainting are medicines for depression and for Parkinson's disease," says Richard Nordgren, M.D., a pediatric neurologist at the Dartmouth-Hitchcock Medical Center in Lebanon, New Hampshire. "Check with your doctor if you are on these medications and are blacking out frequently. He may be able to adjust the dosages to alleviate the problem."

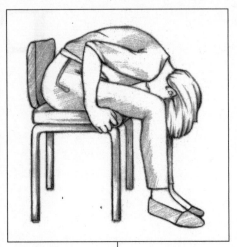

If you feel faint, grab a chair and sit down. Then put your head below the level of your heart.

TIME TO SEE THE DOCTOR

Does a Workout Cause a Blackout?

"IF YOU frequently faint during exercise, I would urge you to get to a doctor," advises Richard Nordgren, M.D., a pediatric neurologist at the Dartmouth-Hitchcock Medical Center in Lebanon, New Hampshire. "You could have a serious medical problem." Nordgren points out that even top athletes sometimes have undiagnosed heart trouble.

Other reasons to visit your doctor after fainting include the following:

- You feel faint whenever you change position, such as sitting up in bed.
- You've injured your head recently.
- You faint when you turn your head suddenly.
- You have a history of heart trouble.
- You've been having periods of forgetfulness.

Go Slow

If you feel faint when you get out of bed suddenly or when you stand up after kneeling in church, you may have a common and usually harmless problem called orthostatic hypotension, a temporary drop in blood flow to your brain, Dr. Mason says. "If you are bothered frequently by this problem, get into the habit of dangling your legs over the edge of the bed before you stand," he advises. "In church, rise slowly from a kneeling to a standing position." He recalls sewing stitches into a man who fainted after getting out of bed too suddenly. "He fell against a bookcase and almost sliced his ear off. He would have saved himself a lot of grief if he'd just taken his time."

Swallow a Gator

"Unless you have high blood pressure or congestive heart failure, you probably don't need to restrict your salt intake," says Thomas Roy, M.D., a cardiologist who moved from New Hampshire to Minocqua, Wisconsin. "Maintaining your fluid intake, especially during exercise or hot weather, is important to your body's functioning. An electrolyte-balanced drink such as Gatorade is a good idea."

Squeeze Some Fruit

"Some people are hypoglycemic, meaning their blood sugar levels get too low," says Laurence Bouchard, D.O., an osteopathic family physician in Narragansett, Rhode Island. "If you find yourself feeling faint at midmorning or midafternoon, drink some fruit juice immediately. Then go see a doctor. You could have a chronic blood sugar problem."

FATIGUE
Solving your personal energy crisis

If your inner batteries are low, you should try to figure out what drained them in the first place. "You can be fatigued for any number of reasons," says Laurie Duncan, M.D., an internist who moved from Cooperstown, New York, to Washington, D.C. "Illness, stress, anxiety, a poor diet, or a lack of adequate exercise and recreation all can drag you down."

So can more serious illnesses. "If you have fatigue that you can't put your finger on, check your appetite and see if your weight has dropped," Dr. Duncan notes. "Have your bowel-moving habits changed? Are there any lumps in your neck or groin or under your arms? Do you find yourself urinating more?" If you answered yes to any of these questions—or if your dragginess just won't go away—see your doctor, she says.

Some poor souls suffer from chronic fatigue syndrome, a mysterious illness that is the focus of intensive medical research. The disease appears to be a complex combination of physical and psychological problems. These tend to fade over a year or two in children but have proven frustratingly stubborn in adults. Nonetheless, doctors are coming up with increasing numbers of cures for chronic fatigue, so it's worth placing yourself under a doctor's care.

On the other hand, if that pooped feeling is only an occasional thing, you can perk yourself up with these remedies.

Snooze a Little Longer

"Many Americans have a sleep deficit of an hour or more per night," Dr. Duncan says. Most people need a minimum of 7 hours, and some need as many as 9. "Turn the TV off by 10 o'clock," she advises. Kids need even more sleep. A study of elementary school children in New Hyde Park, New York, showed that one of the biggest causes of fatigue among those youngsters was their refusal to go to bed on time. Kids between the ages of 2 and 12 need anywhere from 10 to 12 hours of sleep each night.

Variety Is . . . A Source of Fatigue

"Set the same time for going to sleep and waking up every day, even on weekends," Dr. Duncan advises. People who vary their sleeping habits tend to feel more fatigue than those who follow a regular sleep schedule.

Set Low Daily Goals

People who try to do too many things at once during the day tend to suffer more from fatigue, according to medical researchers. Set a limited number of achievable goals each day, and do one task at a time.

Check the Pressure

"Your blood pressure medication could be the cause of your fatigue," says Laurence Bouchard, D.O., an osteopathic family physician in private practice in Narragansett, Rhode Island. "If your doctor has given you a prescription for high blood pressure, tell him about your fatigue. He may want to change your prescription or dosage."

Hit the Iron

If you think you're anemic because of your monthly period, see your physician. "A woman should not be anemic from menstruation unless it's prolonged or excessive—in which case you should see a doctor," Dr. Bouchard explains. Once

---

A WORD FROM DR. LARRY

House Calls Are Good Exercise

I SPENT many years visiting patients in their homes in Connecticut. If the weather was good, I'd occasionally use my bicycle for transportation. Some patients were a little taken aback at seeing a doctor wearing tennis shorts, but biking to make house calls was a great form of exercise. Once the call was over, I'd keep going for a ride in a nearby state park.

People tell me they don't have time for exercise. One way to find the time is to build exercise into some part of your regular routine. Take the stairs instead of the elevator. Park at the far end of parking lots. Walk to a distant bus stop. Or do what I did: Bike to work.

LAWRENCE H. BERNSTEIN, M.D., *a family doctor who made house calls in Storrs, Connecticut, for 22 years. He now works at Jewish Geriatric Services in Longmeadow, Massachusetts.*

---

a physician gives you the okay, you can take over-the-counter Slow FE, "a very slow acting form of iron that shouldn't give you diarrhea or constipation. Take it in the recommended dosage two or three times a week." You can buy Slow FE at your drugstore.

Cran Can Make It Better

"In a young girl, fatigue may be a sign of a chronic infection in the urinary tract," Dr. Bouchard says. "Have her drink plenty of cranberry juice and get her checked by a doctor."

Gulp Down

"If you feel draggy after a day at the beach or a long run, you could be dehydrated," Dr. Bouchard says. "Drink plenty of fluids, and keep drinking the next day. The effects of dehydration can last a long time."

Pump Up

"Lack of exercise can cause fatigue," Dr. Bouchard says. "The less you do, the less you want to do. Try a brisk walk for 20 minutes or more three times a week, and increase your other physical activities."

Jolt Yourself

"Guarana tea, available at health food stores, is a powerful stimulant," says Rosemary Gladstar, an herbalist in East Barre, Vermont, and author of *Herbal Healing for Women*. "Guarana contains more caffeine than coffee, but it lacks the other harmful alkaloids that coffee has."

FEVER

How to chill out when your body gets tropical

"Fever is a symptom, not a disease," says Stephen Blair, M.D., a pediatrician in private practice in Claremont, New Hampshire. "Your body's immune system functions better at a higher temperature." Here's how it works: An invasion of bacteria or a flu virus causes the white blood cells to release a certain chemical. That chemical signals the brain to raise the body's temperature. The hotter internal climate makes it harder for the invaders to grow, which in turn allows time for the body's defenses to track them down and kill them.

Don't worry if you're running a slight temperature. In fact, there is no "normal" level, doctors say. The standard of 98.6°F is just an average. Your body tends to be at its coolest when you first wake up, and it usually rises a couple of degrees during the day until its peak in the late afternoon—which is when fevers tend to rage.

Despite the folk wisdom, your brain isn't in much danger of cooking during a fever. Most healthy people can get through a relatively high fever without any long-term effects.

What's more, a fairly high temperature might signal a relatively benign disease, while a relatively low reading could disguise a nasty ailment. "The seriousness of the illness is not in proportion to the temperature on the thermometer," says Robert F. Wilson, M.D., a pediatrician who is retired from his practice in Dover, New Hampshire. "A child with appendicitis might not have much of a fever, while a kid with roseola—a fairly mild childhood illness—may have a fever of 106°F."

Still, a temperature over 101°F in a newborn under 2 months old or in an adult over age 60 is reason for a quick call to the doctor, according to Lawrence H. Bernstein, M.D., a former family doctor who is the medical director at Jewish Geriatric Services in Longmeadow, Massachusetts. In a child other than an infant, a fever above 102°F deserves a consultation. And any adult should see a doctor for a temperature that exceeds 103°F. "I try to allow lower-grade fevers to run their course," Dr. Bernstein says.

Here's what you can do to deal with the accompanying discomfort of a fever after consulting your doctor.

Soak a Child

"You can soothe a small child who has a high fever with a lukewarm bath and acetaminophen," Dr. Blair says. "Avoid giving a child aspirin. It could result in Reye's syndrome, which can be deadly."

Sponge Yourself

"Try taking a cool, wet sponge or washcloth and wiping your arms, chest, and face," says Laurie Duncan, M.D., an internist who moved from Cooperstown, New York, to Washington, D.C. "You can also take a tepid bath. Get out immediately if you feel a chill coming on."

Down the Fever

"A fever increases the body's use of fluids," Dr. Duncan says. "Make sure the feverish person gets lots of fluids. If there is vomiting with a fever, give an oral rehydration solution to restore the body's fluids and electrolytes." You can buy such a solution at a drugstore.

Rest at Home

"If a child is sick for two or three days and then is feeling better, wait an extra day before sending the kid to school," Dr. Blair says. "At the tail end of a virus, your child probably isn't contagious but needs a day to recuperate."

FINGERNAIL INFECTIONS

Curing the ragged edge of your digits

It's as if your fingernail takes on a life of its own, starting with a light-colored spot that spreads. Your nail gets lifted up and becomes an ugly-looking, thick, brittle slab.

That crazy nail effect is probably caused by a fungus, says Charles Hammer, M.D., a dermatologist with the North Country Outreach Program of the Lahey Hitchcock Clinic in St. Johnsbury, Vermont. "Most nail infections are fungal, although a fungus can invite bacteria to infect the site."

The most common fingernail fungus is a yeast called candida. "The people who get it most tend to have their hands in water for long periods—such as restaurant dishwashers, meat packers, and factory workers who deal with solvents, water, coolants, or detergents," Dr. Hammer says. But you can't be sure that candida is the culprit. Any of a variety of microscopic nail biters can be responsible, and Dr. Hammer says the only way to know which one is attacking you is to have a doctor take a sample and get it examined in a laboratory. "The best cures are prescription medicines geared specifically to your infection."

Until you and your doctor figure out what the cause is, here's what you can do at home for a fingernail infection.

Nail the Infection

"Liquid Clotrimazole, available over the counter at drugstores, can help fight a nail infection," Dr. Hammer says.

"But it only works if you can limit the amount of time your hands are wet during the day."

Get Pickled

While constant soaking in water or detergent encourages infections, you can actually fight them by soaking your hands in Epsom salts, says Daniel Caloras, M.D., a family doctor in private practice in Charlestown, New Hampshire. In a bowl, dissolve 2 cups Epsom salts in 2 cups warm water (around 100°F). "Soak your nails at least twice a day for 10 minutes at a time until the infection goes away," Dr. Caloras advises.

Anoint the Area

"Apply over-the-counter Bacitracin ointment to the infected site if your doctor gives the okay," says Hugh P. Hermann, M.D., a family doctor in private practice in Woodstock, Vermont. "Bacitracin works only on bacterial infections, so you need to get any infection checked out by a doctor."

FISHHOOK CAUGHT IN SKIN

What to do when you catch yourself in a less-than-all-star cast

"My Uncle Russ—we called him Uncle Skinhead because he was bald—was an outdoorsman of the first order," says Thomas Lord, dean of students at Dublin School in Dublin, New Hampshire. "He owned a hardware store in Camden, Maine, which gave him plenty of time for fishing. I was eight years old the first time he took me out on the water. I thought I'd won the lottery.

"Well, I hooked a fish right off the bat, but it got away. I felt a little ashamed about losing the fish, and to make up for it, I made a heroic cast. I just cocked that rod way back and swung as hard as I could. Nothing happened. I turned around, and there it was—my fly was stuck right in Uncle Skinhead's ear. I thought he was really hurt, and I felt just awful about it. But my uncle just reached up to his ear and yanked the fly right out.

"It didn't seem to faze him at all. But he never took me fishing again."

Richard Hamel, an Orvis fly-fishing guide throughout the United States, says that plenty of other fishing companions have suffered Uncle Skinhead's fate. Accidents in fly-fishing are more common than in other forms of fishing, such as bait and spin casting, Hamel says, because in freshwater fly-fishing, the fisherman must whip a 30- to 60-foot line and its hook back and forth several times before completing the cast.

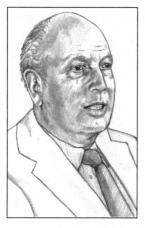

A Matter of Lure and Order

R IGHT over my desk in my home office is my place of honor for fishing lures—maybe 80 or so. I fished them myself—out of the skin of people who had caught themselves. Now that I'm retired, I keep the display as a souvenir of my patients.

The town where I live is surrounded by seven lakes, so we have our share of fishing accidents. Often, early on Sunday mornings in the summer, my doorbell would ring. There would be a father and son who had been out fishing, and one or the other was hooked. Usually it was the father, caught by his son's overenthusiastic or poorly aimed cast. The hook would be embedded in the ear, the hand, or the back of the head; one man had a hook right next to the eye. I'd give a shot of Novocain, remove the hook, and keep the lure for my collection. The exhibit would let the patient know he was not the only one.

Some of those lures I acquired over the years are quite expensive, and the fishermen would try to reclaim them. I'd just smile and say, "Ah, no, this goes in my place of honor."

From what I've seen of hooked fathers, I'd suggest that an inexperienced fisherman be placed in the back of the boat. That way the back cast is less likely to do damage.

GERARD BOZUWA, M.D., *retired after 36 years as the sole family doctor for the town of Wakefield, New Hampshire.*

F"Nine out of ten flies that catch humans get caught in the face, ear, or back of the head," Hamel says. "The fly comes fast past the head when you cast, and since most people don't fish naked, a miscast that hits elsewhere is likely just to get caught in clothing."

Saltwater fly-fishing is even riskier, Hamel says. "The line is 60 to 120 feet long. You have a lot of power, a weighted line, the wind, and the arc of the rod, so that fly can go deep into your skin."

If your fly gets caught in a sensitive spot, such as the area around an eye, Hamel says, "don't touch it. Get it to a doctor." Otherwise, here are some techniques you can use to extract the hook and treat the wound—ways that are somewhat less painful than the Uncle Skinhead method.

If you get hooked, press on. Push the barb farther in the same way it's already headed (A) until it breaks the skin again (B). Then cut the barb off and back the shaft out (C).

Put the Hook in Reverse

"The easiest way to remove a fishhook is to push the barb on through the skin, cut the barb off with wire cutters, and back the hook out," says Peter Brassard, M.D., a family doctor on Block Island, Rhode Island. "That works 95 percent of the time."

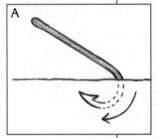
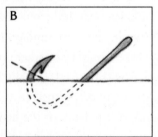
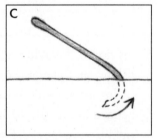

Or Give It the Old Heave-Ho

As an emergency room physician at the Northwestern Medical Center in St. Albans, Vermont, John Dunn, M.D., has seen his share of human catches. "I do a lot of fishhook removals, particularly during the big fishing derbies on Lake Champlain," Dr. Dunn says. "Once, two people came in hooked together on the same lure. One had gotten himself caught trying to get the hook off the other guy. I removed the lure one person at a time."

Besides the old push-the-hook-through-and-cut-the-barb-off technique, Dr. Dunn says another way to remove a fishhook is the "string method." Take some stout twine and loop

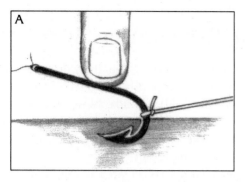

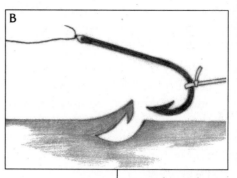

it over the hook so that it encircles the bend in the wire. Then push the shaft of the hook downward toward the skin. "This stretches the hole in the skin and disengages the barb." Finally, give a quick snap up on the string to pull the hook out. "Usually there is minimal damage. But you need to be very fast and very confident."

A quicker and more violent approach is the string method. Tie the string to the shaft just above the surface of the skin. Push the shaft of the hook down (A) and then pull up sharply on the string (B).

FLAT FEET
Fetching advice for lying-down dogs

Take a look at your footprints next time you walk barefoot on the beach: If you see the complete outline of your foot, you probably have flat feet, according to Lawrence H. Bernstein, M.D., a former family doctor who is the medical director at Jewish Geriatric Services in Longmeadow, Massachusetts. A foot with a working arch leaves a crescent-shaped indentation in the sand, he says.

If yours doesn't, you have flat feet. Now what? "If your feet don't bother you, don't worry about them," Dr. Bern-

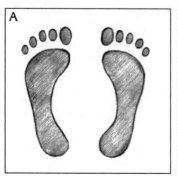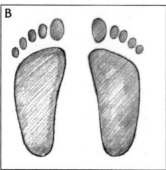

Untroubled soles (A) make the mark of normal arches in the sand. Flat feet (B) leave a broader impression.

Try These Exercises to Rebuild Your Arch

IF FLAT feet cause you pain and difficulty walking, you can stretch and rebuild your foot muscles with these two routines, according to Mary-Catherine Gennaro, D.O., a family osteopath in Warren, New Hampshire.

First, stand facing a wall that's two to three feet away from you. Place one foot in front of the other. Keep both feet flat on the floor, with most of your weight on your back foot. Now place your hands on the wall and lean into it. You should feel a stretch in both calves and feet. Hold for 20 to 30 seconds. Now reverse your feet and repeat the stretch.

Next, sit on the floor with your feet straight out. Take a belt and place it across the arch of one foot. Hold the belt with both hands and lean back gently.

"These exercises work well to help restore arches in the feet of people who can't move around easily," Dr. Gennaro says.

---

stein says. "When I was a young medical resident, the teaching doctor showed off pictures of his children with all their sports trophies. Then he showed pictures of their feet, which were perfectly flat. The kids didn't seem to be bothered at all by the lack of arches."

That could change after the kids pass the age of 40. Flat feet can cause aching in the bottom of the feet and in the calves, knees, hips, and back. And some people start out with perfectly good feet that lose their arches later in life, causing the same pains in the same areas.

Here's how to deal with the problem in no time flat.

Shop Archly

"If your feet are a little flat, be sure to purchase shoes with good arch supports," says Stephen Blair, M.D., a pediatrician in private practice in Claremont, New Hampshire. "Shoes made for walking and running often work fine. Avoid high heels and other dress shoes that don't contain an arch inside."

Save Your Arches and Your Dollars

"Buy a shoe insert from your drugstore or shoe store," says Laurence Bouchard, D.O., an osteopathic family physician in Narragansett, Rhode Island. "You don't have to pay $200 to get an arch support that works. Try Dr. Scholl's."

Follow Custom

There's no better shoe than one that's made especially for you, says Nicholas Vachon, D.P.M., a podiatrist in private practice in Ellsworth, Maine. "Benefoot, for example, works with podiatrists to custom-fit shoes for individuals. Your podiatrist can make a mold of your foot and send it directly to Benefoot."

Get a Heel

"I recommend Thomas heels, which are sold in shoe stores," says Robert F. Wilson, M.D., who is retired from his pediatric practice in Dover, New Hampshire. "They are special kinds of lifts added to the heels of Oxford-type shoes. They have one-eighth-inch wedges built into the heels on the inside edge, giving the shoes a very slight lift. Also, the heels extend farther forward on the inside than on the outside, helping to support flat feet."

FLATULENCE

*Air-purifying aids for those times
when life is too much of a gas*

Are you filling up with fiber? Belting down beans and broccoli? Good for you! Your loved ones and colleagues might not be quite as thrilled with your healthful eating habits, though. A good diet often means gas. After a fine meal, you may find those who are close to you needing some space.

"Flatulence—gas passed via the rectum—is usually dietary in origin," says Linda B. Dacey, M.D., an internist at the Dartmouth-Hitchcock Medical Center in Lebanon, New Hampshire. "The gas is the result of partially undigested food. Common culprits are dried beans, dairy products, and cruciferous vegetables such as cauliflower and broccoli— food items that tend to be good for you." The indigestible food gets attacked by bacteria that live in your gut. These microscopic creatures in turn release by-products such as hydrogen, carbon dioxide, and methane—a smelly, gaseous mixture that doctors call flatus.

Stress also can affect your digestion, increasing the amount of gas that needs to escape. Some people become incapaci-

F tated by large amounts of gas trapped in their bodies after abdominal surgery. And flatulence is sometimes a symptom of a serious disease. But "most of the time, it isn't a medical problem, just a social one," Dr. Dacey says. As Massachusetts doctor Thomas Palmer put it in a seventeenth-century medical guide, "wind issuing out gently & voluntarily is the best & holsomest sign" of health. But not of air quality. Here's how you can keep your personal atmosphere a little better smelling.

Expel Correctly

"If intestinal gas is bothering you," says Lawrence H. Bernstein, M.D., a former family doctor who is the medical director at Jewish Geriatric Services in Longmeadow, Massachusetts, "lie on your back and pull your knees to your chest. In that position, you will expel the gas."

Rock It Out

A rocking chair can be a comfort when you're feeling bloated. The rocking helps your body remove the gas, while the motion can relieve stress.

Get Seedy

"Chew anise, fennel, or celery seeds to relieve flatulence," says Corinne Martin, a certified clinical herbalist in Bridgton, Maine. As an alternative to chewing on seeds, you can relieve your flatulence by boiling half a teaspoon of seeds in a cup of water, letting the seeds sink to the bottom of the cup, and drinking the tea after it cools a bit.

Carry Caraway

Caraway seeds also work to control flatulence, according to Julia Foote, R.N., a retired nurse in Norwell, Massachusetts. Boil them up and drink the tea when you feel gassy, she says.

When Wind Isn't Your Only Problem

F LATULENCE or gas can be indicative of a more serious problem," says Laurie Duncan, M.D., an internist who moved from Cooperstown, New York, to Washington, D.C. See your doctor if your gas is accompanied by any of these other signs of illness.

- You notice a change in your bowel habits.
- Your gas is particularly malodorous.
- You also are constipated or have diarrhea.
- Your gas problems last for more than three days.
- Your weight drops as your flatulence increases.
- You have the worst stomachache you've ever had.

Beano Is Keeno

Beano, a product containing the enzyme alpha-galactosidase, can prevent flatulence before it starts. Just put eight drops on a meal that tends to give you gas—baked beans, say—and you can reduce your chances of getting windy. Medical researchers at the University of California in San Diego found that people who took Beano before a meal suffered from flatulence significantly less than those who were given fake drops. Beano is available over the counter at many grocery stores and drugstores.

Cook without Gas

"A friend of mine prepares beans in a way that seems to reduce their gassiness," says Laurie Duncan, M.D., an internist who moved from Cooperstown, New York, to Washington, D.C. "She covers the beans with cold water, brings the beans to a boil for five minutes, drains the water, rinses the beans, and reboils them before following the recipe as she normally would."

FLU
Loosening the grasp of "La Grippe"

People used to think you could blame the flu on the position of the stars. Hence the name *influenza,* which is Italian for "an influence"—as in, influenced by the heavens. Before English doctors picked up the name in the eighteenth century, people called the flu everything from the "jolly rant" to the "new acquaintance" to "La Grippe."

You may have your own terms for the flu, less suitable for polite company. She's a nasty ailment, La Grippe, with her relentless combination of fever, chills, muscle aches, headache, stuffiness, and cough. "Here in Vermont, when people say they have the flu, they can mean anything from a bad cold to a stomach bug," says Hugh P. Hermann, M.D., a family doctor in Woodstock, Vermont. "But *flu* as a medical term means a serious viral infection. In the very young or the very old, the flu can open the door to a more serious bacterial pneumonia."

F Vaccines are available to stave off the flu from year to year, and doctors recommend them for children and the elderly. But if you're already in the grip of La Grippe, here's how you can make yourself more comfortable during her typical three- to seven-day grasp.

Use the Triple Flu Threat

"Adequate fluids, adequate rest, and aspirin or aceta- minophen are still the best combination to fight the flu," says Brewster Martin, M.D., a retired family physician who ran the Chelsea Family Health Center in Chelsea, Vermont, for 40 years. "Drink at least two quarts of fluid daily, and sleep at least eight hours a night." Remember, don't give aspirin to children because of the risk of Reye's syndrome.

Decongestants, Not Antihistamines

"The current theory is that deconges- tants are more helpful than antihista- mines," says David Sigelman, M.D., a pediatrician with Holyoke Pediatric As- sociates in Holyoke, Massachusetts. "Antihistamines dry up secretions and make them harder to move out," he says. "Decongestants are far better, but neither will cure you. They just deal with the symptoms."

Stay Liquid

"Drink lots of fluids," says Paul Lena, M.D., a retired physi- cian of internal medicine in Concord, New Hampshire. "Lemon juice and water make a good remedy. Warm lemonade is even better. Any of these thins the mucus and makes you feel less congested."

Drink to Your Health

Rosemary Gladstar, an herbalist in East Barre, Vermont, and author of *Herbal Healing for Women,* recommends echi- nacea tea as a surefire flu remedy. Echinacea, or purple cone- flower, helps stimulate the immune system. But don't drink

---

> **TIME TO SEE THE DOCTOR**
>
> ## *Is Your Cough Colorful?*
>
> IF YOU have a fever for more than three days, or if you have a severe cough or one that produces thick, greenish yellow mucus, see a doc- tor," says Paul Lena, M.D., a retired physician of internal medicine in Concord, New Hampshire. What carried off most of the people who died in the great influenza epidemic of 1918 wasn't the flu but bronchial pneumonia, Dr. Lena adds.

echinacea tea if you're allergic to ragweed, she cautions. The plants are close relatives.

Chew on a Clove

"Take garlic when you're the only healthy person around, and it will lessen your chances of getting the flu," says Corinne Martin, a certified clinical herbalist in Bridgton, Maine. "Take garlic capsules, available at health food stores, or just eat more garlic with your meals."

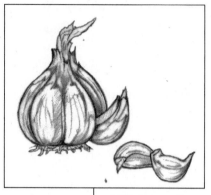

Garlic is a traditional means of keeping the flu at bay.

FOOD CRAVINGS

Crazed for a candy bar?
Acquire a taste for these remedies

You're going about your daily business when the craving hits: chocolate. You don't just want it; you *need* it. You find yourself headed for the candy machine as if you're under hypnosis. Have you been brainwashed by the candy industry? Is the Chocolate Industrial Complex sending radio waves to your head?

Most likely, your food cravings have more to do with your innards than with some diabolical plot. Women tend to get cravings more than men do, and the usual yen is for something sweet—especially chocolate. "Women get food cravings especially just before their periods start," says Marcia Herrin, Ed.D., M.P.H., R.D., coordinator of the Nutrition Education Program at Dartmouth College and adjunct professor of community and family medicine at Dartmouth Medical School in Hanover, New Hampshire. Dr. Herrin offers a simple explanation for premenstrual cravings: You're hungry. "Your body needs more calories at this time of the month, and you really should eat more," she says. "And there's no more efficient way to obtain calories than to eat a chocolate bar."

That raving hunger for something sweet can hit at other times of the month, too. People who are depressed often report food cravings, according to medical researchers. Some scientists think that a disruption in the transmission of signals

F from the brain to the rest of the body can cause a hunger for carbohydrates. And a craving for certain foods can be caused by a nutritional problem. "The first thing a nutritionist checks for if a patient comes in complaining of a food craving is whether the person is being deprived of an essential type of food, such as protein," Dr. Herrin explains. Diabetics, whose blood sugar levels tend to vary widely, often get sudden cravings for sugar.

See a nutritionist if you have constant, unexplained cravings that aren't patterned around your menstrual cycle, Dr. Herrin advises. Otherwise, to stop that occasional hypnotic march to the candy machine, try these remedies.

Fish the Cupboards for Tuna

"Sometimes a craving for a particular food can be caused by a dietary lack of a completely different kind of food," Dr. Herrin says. For example, you may feel the need for sweets when your body lacks protein. "Try eating tuna when your sweet tooth can't be satisfied."

Don't Go Cold Turkey

"Don't entirely deny yourself a food you crave," Dr. Herrin says. "If you try to give up chocolate completely, that may only make you crave it more, causing you to overindulge. Let yourself have one chocolate bar a day if you want to be in control of your candy habit. That'll give you something to look forward to, and it will make you less likely to go overboard when you treat yourself."

Go Sweet on Bitters

"Your craving for sweets may actually be caused by a dietary lack of bitters," says Rosemary Gladstar, an herbalist in East Barre, Vermont, and author of *Herbal Healing for Women*. "The American diet is lacking in bitter tastes." To make up for that lack, Gladstar suggests adding dandelion greens and chicory greens to your salads. You can buy these greens at many grocery stores or pick them yourself.

A more convenient way to add bitterness to your life, says Gladstar, is to buy a bottle of liquid Swedish bitters at a health food store. "Just put a drop of bitters on your tongue a couple of times a day. That will help reduce your craving for chocolate and other sweets."

FOOD SENSITIVITIES
What to do when your chow causes a row

Your body is a wonderful food processor—for most foods. Sometimes, though, it thinks you've swallowed an alien invader, and it mistakenly marshals its resources in defense. When your natural defenders meet the "enemy" food, the resulting chemical clash can raise some distinct discomforts. "The hallmarks of an allergic reaction to food are itching; swelling of the mouth, lips, and throat; asthma; and hives," says Wilfred Beaucher, M.D., an internist, allergist, and immunologist in Chelmsford, Massachusetts, and Nashua, New Hampshire. "Some people may even pass out because of a food allergy."

Reactions to foods can be life threatening on occasion. "Peanuts, strawberries, and shellfish can kill people who are allergic to them," notes Lawrence H. Bernstein, M.D., a former family doctor who is the medical director at Jewish Geriatric Services in Longmeadow, Massachusetts. Dr. Bernstein notes that these serious allergies are rare. More common are mild reactions to milk products, wheat, eggs, corn, or chocolate.

Some foods cause reactions that are more mysterious in origin. Monosodium glutamate, a flavor enhancer often found in Chinese food, can cause Chinese restaurant syndrome in some people—an uncomfortable but mercifully temporary ailment in which you sweat and your heart beats as if you've just climbed the Great Wall, explains John Dunn, M.D., an emergency room physician at the Northwestern Medical Center in St. Albans, Vermont.

AN OUNCE OF PREVENTION
Mother's Flows Best

ONE of the best ways to keep a child free from food allergies is to breastfeed from birth," says Stephen Blair, M.D., a pediatrician in private practice in Claremont, New Hampshire. "Babies who are breastfed until at least six to eight months of age are far less likely to have allergies. Hold off on solid foods until the baby is four months old. Then start in on rice cereal. I know some grandmothers who push turkey and mashed potatoes on four-month-olds, but I try to ward them off."

When a meal bites back at you, here's what you can do to soothe your tummy.

Don't Be Cowed by Milk

If milk products give you indigestion, you don't have to skip the milk and ice cream altogether. "If your body is intolerant of milk products, it probably means you have a deficiency of the enzyme that breaks down the sugar in milk," Dr. Bernstein says. "The undigested sugar can cause cramps and diarrhea." He recommends Lactaid, an enzyme product that helps break down milk sugar. Lactaid, which you down before drinking milk, is available over the counter at drugstores

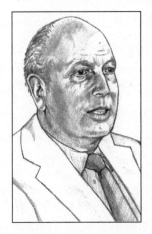

A WORD FROM DR. B.

The Attack of the Pound-and-a-Quarter Lobster

MY WIFE, Titia, and I live in New Hampshire, but very close to the Maine coast. In Holland, where I grew up, lobster is a very rare delicacy, eaten only at weddings and 25th anniversaries. So you can understand why Titia and I used to go frequently to Maine to eat lobster.

The only trouble is, I'm allergic to the creatures. I would eat some lobster and then immediately break out in hives. An antihistamine would clear things up, but I was skating on pretty thin ice with shellfish. Once we were driving back from Maine after a great lobster dinner when my throat suddenly began to close up. I told my wife to get me to a hospital, fast. I managed to croak to the nurse there that I needed an immediate shot of adrenaline. That's the last time I ate a lobster.

I miss it terribly, but you don't play with a food allergy like that. The best way to stay healthy is to avoid foods that cause serious allergic reactions in you.

GERARD BOZUWA, M.D., *retired after 36 years as the sole family doctor for the town of Wakefield, New Hampshire.*

in drops or pills. Or you can buy the problem and the solution in a single container: H. P. Hood makes milk with Lactaid already in it.

Learn to Read

"If you're sensitive to certain foods, learn to read the labels on packaged items," says Sandra McCormack, A.R.N.P., a nurse-practitioner with Allergy Associates of New Hampshire in Portsmouth. "Many prepared foods contain lots of ingredients, and some of them might cause reactions in you."

Don't Blame the Fish

If you're allergic to shellfish, it may be an allergy to iodine, and not fish, that makes you sick, according to Dr. Dunn. "Before you have an x-ray done of your blood vessels or undergo a CAT scan, make sure you mention your shellfish allergy," he says. "The dye used in these procedures contains iodine, which can be dangerous to you."

FOOT AND HEEL PROBLEMS
Give pain the boot
with these high-stepping healers

Did you know that a quarter of the bones in your body are down there in your feet? Add 100 or so ligaments and 19 muscles, and then pound this assembly with more than twice your body weight—the force your feet must bear during walking—and you can understand why your dogs can feel a little dogged now and then.

A jarring gait can cause a stress fracture on the heel bone, or a bruise on the bottom of the foot. Ill-fitting shoes can cause a whole passel of problems, from bunions and corns to an inflamed Achilles tendon, the cord leading up from the back of your heel. Obesity or walking problems can lead to plantar fasciitis, an inflammation of the bottom of the foot. And runners are all too familiar with heel spurs.

Diabetics tend to have some of the worst foot problems, according to Nicholas Vachon, D.P.M., a podiatrist in pri-

Fvate practice in Ellsworth, Maine. "Diabetics have a general decreased ability to fight infection, especially in their extremities, because their blood doesn't circulate easily," he says. "The feet are the most severely affected parts because they're the farthest away from the heart." A simple blister in a diabetic can easily turn into a nasty infection with dramatic loss of tissue, Dr. Vachon says. The best prevention is the same as for everyone else, he adds: good foot care.

Here are some home remedies to get you back in stride.

Stop Standing and Start Soaking

"I would tell my patients to soak a sore foot in warm water with Epsom salts for an hour twice a day for a few days," says Brewster Martin, M.D., a retired family doctor in Chelsea, Vermont. "Soaking helps with pain and infection, but to tell you the truth, the biggest benefit is from taking the weight off the foot during the soaks. The single best thing you can do for foot problems, other than to get the right shoes, is to put your feet up for a few hours."

Raise Your Heel

"If you have heel pain, try buying a heel wedge made of hard rubber—you can get them at a sporting goods store," says Lawrence H. Bernstein, M.D., a former family doctor who is the medical director at Jewish Geriatric Services in Longmeadow, Massachusetts. Just insert the rubber wedge into the heel part inside your shoe.

Turn Down the Heat

"You can deal with some inflammations in your foot by taking an over-the-counter anti-inflammatory medicine such as ibuprofen or aspirin," Dr. Vachon says. Don't give aspirin to children, though, because it can cause Reye's syndrome.

Head for the Freezer

"Take a bag of ice and apply it directly to the sore part of your foot for 10 to 15 minutes daily to reduce inflammation," recommends Donald Helms, D.P.M., a podiatrist at

---

If the Shoe Fits, Congratulations

I F YOUR shoes rub you the wrong way, consider our forebears. Up until the 1840s, a pair of shoes had no right and left; they were both the same.

The Man Who Loved His Shoes

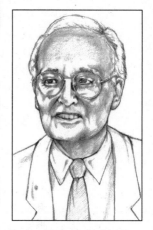

THE worst feet I ever saw were on an old farmer. Every one of his toenails was black or missing altogether. He told me he wore the same shoes every day all day until they wore out.

When I suggested that he change his socks every day, he wouldn't believe me. "Change my socks? Now, Doc, why would I want to do a thing like that?"

The reason is that you want to keep your feet clean and dry. Fungi love dirt and moisture. I wouldn't have wanted to live with that farmer's feet.

BREWSTER MARTIN, M.D., *a retired family doctor in Chelsea, Vermont (population 1,166), and cofounder of the Chelsea Family Health Center. He was named Vermont Doctor of the Year in 1991.*

the Dartmouth-Hitchcock Medical Center in Lebanon, New Hampshire.

Bridge over Your Troubles

"Gentle stretching exercises that focus on your Achilles tendon and calf can help with foot and heel problems," Dr. Helms says. Here's one stretch that can ease both foot and heel: Start out on your hands and knees and then raise yourself up, forming a bridge with your body while keeping your heels on the floor. Hold this position for 20 seconds.

FOOT ODOR
Wish your feet would take a walk without you? Try these remedies

If your feet sweat a lot, they may smell just fine. If they stink, though, the problem is not the sweat but bacteria on your feet, which happen to love the warm, moist environment you provide within your shoes. "People whose feet sweat a lot have a tendency to grow lots of bacteria," says Charles Hammer, M.D., a dermatologist with the North Country Outreach Program of the Lahey Hitchcock Clinic in St. Johnsbury, Vermont. "Just as bacteria cause underarm odor, the same microscopic creatures can make feet smell."

In other words, it's a jungle down there. Here's how to civilize things.

Sock It to 'Em

"Be not slovenly, wear Socks, often shifting [changing] 'em," said the famous Puritan Cotton Mather way back in colonial times. That's still good advice, says Robert F. Wilson, M.D., a pediatrician who is retired from his practice in Dover, New Hampshire. "Change your socks frequently," he says. "Kids seem to wear sneakers without socks. That's a great way to work up a powerful smell down there."

Sweeten with Sour

"Try soaking your feet in some diluted vinegar," Dr. Hammer advises. "Mix a couple of teaspoons of cider vinegar in half a gallon of water. It should sweeten things up."

Try a Pit Stop

"Use an underarm deodorant on your feet," Dr. Hammer says. "It works the same way it works under your arms."

Get at the Germs

"Wash your feet with antibacterial soap, such as Lever 2000, once or twice a day to kill the smell-causing bacteria," Dr. Hammer recommends.

Remove the Innards

"Buy shoes with removable insoles," suggests Ralph McCoy, a certified orthotic shoe technician and owner of the Shoe-torium in Lebanon, New Hampshire. "Take out the insoles after each wearing so they can dry out and get some air."

TIME TO SEE THE DOCTOR

Beat the Fungus

SOME foul foot odors are caused by a fungal infection," says Harry Rowe, M.D., a family doctor in Wells River, Vermont. "See your doctor if the smell is accompanied by itching."

FOOT ODOR

FOOT STEPPED ON BY A COW OR HORSE

Cures to get you galloping again

"A horse or cow stepping on a foot is a pretty common occurrence in the country," says Alcott Smith, D.V.M., a veterinarian in Hanover, New Hampshire. "The more protection you have on your feet, the better. Most people have on leather or rubber boots when they work around cows or horses."

Dr. Smith says that horses rarely just stand there after they step on a person's foot. "They usually step on you as they are changing positions." Cows, however, might be perfectly content to stand stock-still on top of your foot, "especially when you are milking them." The first order of business, Dr. Smith advises, is to get the cow off your foot—no easy task with upwards of 1,400 pounds of beef anchoring one of your limbs. "To get the cow off, you have to lean into her and shove her off. You may have to give her a whack to get her off balance enough so that she'll shift position."

Dr. Smith notes that a large animal can cause serious damage. Most of the time, the unlucky farmer limps off with nothing more than a bruise, but "the trauma can cause a break in the metatarsal bone of the foot. You also can get periostitis, an inflammation of the outermost layer of the bone. It's sometimes referred to as bruising of the bone. If you think you have a serious injury like that, get yourself to a doctor."

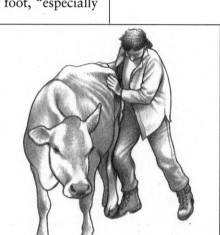

The proper way to reposition a misplaced bovine foot: Lean and shove.

Horses are a bit easier than cows to remove. "If a horse stands on your foot, ask the horse to step forward," says Susie Tann, R.N., an elementary school nurse in Bradford, Vermont, who breeds registered Percheron draft horses. "I say the horse's name and make a little kissing sound."

Toni Prince, who owns the Prince and the Pauper Riding Stables in Norwich, Vermont, trains young riders to react quickly when a horse comes to rest on one of their feet. "We train our children to, one, yell, and, two, take the palm of the hand and push on the horse's shoulder as hard as they can," Prince says. "I have the kids practice it."

Once you have removed the offending animal, here's how you can deal with your throbbing foot.

Use Instant RICE

"The best cure for a foot that's been stepped on hasn't changed in more than 100 years," says Lawrence H. Bernstein, M.D., a former family doctor who is the medical director at Jewish Geriatric Services in Longmeadow, Massachusetts. "Give your foot RICE—rest, ice, compression, and elevation." Stay off your sore foot for a few days. Put ice on it as soon as possible and keep the ice on for up to

---

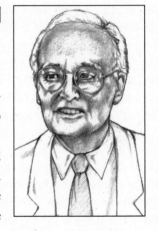

15 minutes at a time. Wrap your foot with an elastic bandage, available at drugstores and sporting goods stores, and keep it up when you sit down.

Get Help from St. John

Rosemary Gladstar, an herbalist in East Barre, Vermont, and author of *Herbal Healing for Women,* once spent four months riding the Pacific Crest Trail in California, Oregon, and Washington with her two-year-old son. Her cure for a swollen, horse-bruised foot: "Soak it in cold water and put Saint-John's-wort oil on it." Saint-John's-wort is a woody perennial. Its leaves and flowers have been crushed and mixed with oil as a wound remedy for hundreds of years. You can buy Saint-John's-wort oil at herbal stores.

TIME TO SEE THE DOCTOR
Do the Wiggle Test

IF A horse has stepped on your foot, wiggle your toes," says Lawrence H. Bernstein, M.D., a former family doctor who is the medical director at Jewish Geriatric Services in Longmeadow, Massachusetts. "If you feel a sharp pain when you wiggle your toes, you'll need an x-ray to see if a foot bone is broken."

FOREIGN OBJECT IN EYE

Removing a tiny object that looms large

As the Bible tells us, the smallest speck can seem like a log. "Most foreign bodies in the eye are microscopic," says Henry Kriegstein, M.D., an ophthalmologist in private practice in Hingham, Plymouth, and Sandwich, Massachusetts. "Half the time they are under the eyelid. Insect wings or legs can cause problems. So can sand or bits of metal." Foreign objects in the eye are a common problem in people who cut their own firewood. "They think it is a bit of sawdust," Dr. Kriegstein says, "but it is almost always a tiny piece of the saw."

However small those bits may be, they can cause big problems if left unattended. "If a foreign body stays in the eye, it can cause an infection of the cornea, the outside lens of the eye," Dr. Kriegstein says. "Corneal infections usually cause scars, and if they're in the center of your field of vision, the scars may interfere with your eyesight."

Always Ask for Credentials

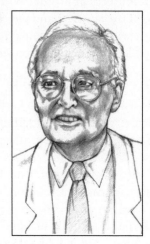

I HAD been practicing as a family doctor for 30 years when a couple brought in their 6-year-old son with something in his eye. I carefully explained to all three of them the procedure for removing a foreign object from the eye.

Just as I began, though, the little boy grabbed my arm. "Wait a minute," he said. "Can I ask you a question? Is this the first time you've ever done this?"

I assured him it wasn't and removed the object. Afterward, I told the parents that the boy would go far. It never hurts to ask a doctor whether he has done a procedure before.

BREWSTER MARTIN, M.D., *a retired family doctor in Chelsea, Vermont (population 1,166), and cofounder of the Chelsea Family Health Center. He was named Vermont Doctor of the Year in 1991.*

Some obstacles may be relatively painless. "A chip of metal can make a sharp cut in the eye that really doesn't hurt very much," Dr. Kriegstein says. "But if your vision is cloudy the next day, see a doctor immediately."

By contrast, a pain in the eye may not be caused by an object at all. "An infection or ulcer in the cornea may make you feel as though there's something in your eye," Dr. Kriegstein notes. "If you have problems with persistent pain or obscured vision, see a doctor."

To keep obstacles out of the eye, your best bet is to wear protective glasses or goggles, "especially if you are hammering metal with metal," Dr. Kriegstein says. "Striking a piece of metal with another piece—such as when you pound a nail or a sheet of metal—can make fragments fly off and cause a high-velocity injury to the eye."

People once believed that holding a magic stone to your eye could draw off a foreign object. Here are more down-to-earth cures that country doctors see clear to recommend.

Make a Stream

"If the particle is in the white part of your eye, you may try to remove it by washing it out with a gentle rinse from your bathroom tap," says Eugene J. Bernal, O.D., an optometrist in private practice in White River Junction, Vermont. "If the foreign body is in the colored part of the eye, try removing it with a good stream of water. If you can still see or feel it, get to an eye doctor." Avoid trying to wash out an object that's on the edge of your eye, Dr. Bernal cautions. "The water could drive the object farther in."

Try Cupping

"Try to remove the object with an eyecup," recommends Robert F. Wilson, M.D., a pediatrician who is retired from his practice in Dover, New Hampshire. You can buy an eyecup at your drugstore. "Fill it with warm water and hold it against the eye with your head tilted back to wash the object out," Dr. Wilson says. "If that doesn't work, you can try to remove the object with a wet Q-Tip."

Put in More

"The best way to remove a foreign object from the eye is to irrigate it with eyedrops," says Stephen Moore, M.D., an ophthalmologist in Great Barrington, Massachusetts. "A saline rinse like Dacriose is very helpful." Dr. Moore notes that your eye may feel irritated even after the object is gone. "That's because the cornea may be scratched. Wait 24 hours. If your eye is still bothering you, see a doctor."

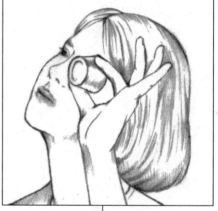

To remove an object, try getting a close look at an eyecup.

FORGETFULNESS

Reminders for—what was it?
Oh, yes—remembering

Ask Mary-Catherine Gennaro, D.O., the best way to deal with forgetfulness, and the Warren, New Hampshire, family osteopath laughs. "I forgot my husband's name on our first

F

date. To compensate for memory gaps, you need a sense of humor."

You may find that your own memory isn't as good as you, um, remember it to be. "By the time you are in your forties, you may start forgetting words, place names, even your spouse's name," says Peter Mason, M.D., a family doctor and medical director of the Alice Peck Day Community Health Center in Lebanon, New Hampshire. "It's common to have a word for something drop out of your head just when you need it, only to remember it suddenly in the middle of the night or the next day."

If you eventually remember what you've forgotten, you don't have to worry about Alzheimer's disease or other forms of senility. "You probably just have what doctors call benign senescent forgetfulness," Dr. Mason says. "It's a normal, if annoying, part of aging." Alzheimer's, however, is a progressive deterioration of the brain cells that leads to forgetting things permanently—often without any awareness on the part of the person doing the forgetting.

But the fact that your memory loss probably isn't serious doesn't mean you have to forget about it. Here are some ways to improve your recall.

Simplify

"Among my patients who aren't elderly, the ones who complain the most about memory loss are women with hectic schedules and more than one child," Dr. Gennaro says. "They are packing three or four lives into one. It's hard to remember the name of your child's teacher if you aren't even sure where you're supposed to be and when." The answer: "Use your memory loss as a barometer of busyness," she says. "Cut out the nighttime meetings and say no to driving your kids to some activities." Dr. Gennaro also suggests making a daily list of obligations, putting the most important first. "Then just cross out the bottom third. That'll give you less to remember." This is

---

TIME TO SEE THE DOCTOR

If It's Not Just Your Spouse's Birthday You're Forgetting

IF YOU suddenly find yourself unable to pinpoint where you are or you're confused about what month or year it is, talk to your doctor.

Also see your doctor if your memory loss is accompanied by dizziness, headaches, balance problems, or a lack of coordination in your hands or feet, says Peter Mason, M.D., a family doctor and medical director of the Alice Peck Day Community Health Center in Lebanon, New Hampshire. "These could be signs of a tumor or a stroke—a loss of blood to the brain cells," he says.

more easily said than done, she admits. "You just have to protect yourself by saying no to demands on your time."

Alarmed? Snooze

"If you find yourself forgetting things during especially busy times, it could be that you're not getting enough sleep," Dr. Gennaro says. "If you're like most people, you need at least

F

My Cosmopolitan Aunt

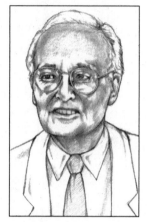

THE best kind of long-term memory is the kind that gets saved through the generations. I had an aunt who came to live with us in Pittsfield, Vermont, when I was a boy. Electricity hadn't come to Pittsfield yet, and that was a bit of a comedown for my great-great-aunt, who had moved from the relative metropolis of Lebanon, New Hampshire.

My aunt clearly thought that my family was rather uncouth. Whenever we got too loud and boisterous, her nose would go up and her voice would ring out, "In Lebanon, we had streetlights!" It was her way of reminding us that there was a better, more gracious world out there than what we had to offer.

She said it often enough that it became a family expression. Long after my aunt went to her well-lighted reward, someone would always break the tension of a family argument by saying, "In Lebanon, we had streetlights!"

One recent Thanksgiving, I was sitting down to dinner with my family. The talk became loud, and the conversation got a little out of control. Suddenly, one of my youngest grandchildren, a little boy of six, sang out, "In Lebanon, we had streetlights!"

My aunt was saved from the worst forgetfulness of all, that of family tradition. Through generational memory, she had achieved a kind of immortality—one that, in all likelihood, she would not entirely have appreciated.

BREWSTER MARTIN, M.D., *a retired family doctor in Chelsea, Vermont (population 1,166), and cofounder of the Chelsea Family Health Center. He was named Vermont Doctor of the Year in 1991.*

---

seven or eight hours of sleep a night. A lack of sleep can mess up your memory."

Air Your Brain Out

"Get regular aerobic exercise, such as walking, jogging, swimming, or biking, at least three times a week," Dr. Gennaro advises. "Exercise increases the amount of oxygen going to your brain, which helps your memory." On the other hand, she says, cigarettes are death to memory—literally. "Smoking cuts off oxygen to the brain. You'll save your memory if you quit the habit."

Play to Your Strengths

"Some people are better at storing visual memories, while others are better at verbal memory storage," says Kathleen Kovner-Kline, M.D., a child psychiatrist at the Dartmouth-Hitchcock Medical Center in Lebanon, New Hampshire. "Learn to compensate for gaps in your memory," she advises. "For example, if you find yourself losing your keys a lot, put a key rack by the door and get in the habit of hanging your keys there—that plays to your visual memory. For verbal memory, give yourself verbal prompts such as 'Keys by the door, coat in the closet.'"

Now, What Was That String For?

"The old-time memory techniques still work," says Gerard Bozuwa, M.D., who is retired from his practice as a family doctor in Wakefield, New Hampshire. "Tie a knot in your handkerchief to remember to buy flowers for your wife. Or tie a string on your finger to remember to pick up milk on the way home from work." Dr. Bozuwa has a friend who spins her engagement ring so that the diamond faces backward when she wants to remember something.

FROSTBITE
What to do when your skin starts to freeze

Frostbite is one aspect of winter that shouldn't be taken lightly. When your skin is exposed to below-freezing weather, the liquids within the tissue can literally begin to freeze. The affected parts of your skin turn pale and numb. People with frostbite often feel no pain as they're being nipped, although some people start to itch or to feel as if their skin is crawling. "Frostbite can creep up on you without your feeling a thing," says Michael Pelchat, an emergency medical technician who teaches first-aid to researchers atop Mount Washington in New Hampshire. "You can get frostbite in seconds if it is 40 degrees below zero with 100-mile-per-hour winds. You can also get frostbitten in half an hour—about the length of a ski run—if your skin is exposed to temperatures barely below freezing."

Early signs of frostbite can tell you when to head indoors, according to Pat Teter, R.N., a nurse who works at the first-aid station at Okemo Mountain Ski Area in Ludlow, Vermont. "Watch for tingling or pain in your hands or feet," she says. Try to get in before those sensations turn to numbness. "Also look for color changes in skin. Gray, white, yellow, or waxy-looking skin means it is past time to go in. Get yourself inside and rewarm the affected area. If you continue to have problems, contact your health care provider."

Here are some ways to keep frostbite from chomping too deep.

Watch Your Feet

"The most common places to get frostbitten are the fingers, toes, tip of the nose, and, most commonly, the prominence of the cheekbones," says Dudley Weider, M.D., an otolaryngologist in Lebanon, New Hampshire, who has spent much of his time adventuring north of the Arctic Circle. "If frostbite goes too far on your nose, you'll get a permanent brown spot and look funny. And without proper footwear, frostbitten toes and feet will bring you to your knees."

Dr. Weider recommends wearing at least two pairs of socks. First, don an inner layer made of polypropylene, a manmade fabric that wicks moisture away from the skin and keeps your feet dry. Over the inner layer, put on an outer

---

| TIME TO SEE THE DOCTOR |

Don't Rub

THE damage from frostbite can't be reversed, says dermatologist Richard Baughman, M.D., who lives in Etna, New Hampshire. "Once it's done, it's done." But you can keep it from getting worse. "Don't rub it. If it's in your feet, don't try to walk on it. You can do far more damage that way." The trauma to flesh from the frostbite's ice crystals biting into tissue can magnify the harm. "If you're seriously frostbitten, get yourself medical care as soon as possible."

F

layer of heavier polypropylene or heavy wool socks. Boots or shoes should be large enough to wear over the two pairs of socks without restricting circulation. Tight shoes can make your feet colder and more susceptible to frostbite.

Commit a BUBU

"That stands for big, ugly, bulky, and unrestricted clothing," Pelchat says. "It's the best kind of clothing to prevent frostbite. Buy clothes a size or two bigger than you'd normally buy them. Big clothing traps more of your own body's warm air."

Avoid stylish ski clothing, which tends to be made of fabric that's too thin to be warm enough. "When you're out in the cold, ugly is beautiful," Pelchat says.

"Your outdoor clothing also should be made of bulky material," Pelchat adds. "Thick or down-filled fabrics offer good loft and insulation." Finally, "cold-weather clothes should be nonconstricting. They should allow good freedom of movement, which allows warming blood to flow to the extremities."

Heat Your Head

"Treat your head the way you do your water heater," Pelchat advises. "Cover it up to keep heat from escaping, and it will keep your feet from freezing."

Hats made of polyester fleece material or wool are best. "They should cover the ears as well as the back of the neck," Pelchat says. "The hat should be windproof or wind-resistant and be of a material that breathes, allowing the moisture from your head and neck out into the air."

Tape Your Cheeks

If you wear glasses with a metal frame, frostbite can form anywhere the frame touches your cheeks, says Murray Hamlet, D.V.M., chief of the Research Support Division at the U.S. Army Research Institute of Environmental Medicine in Natick, Massachusetts. "Before going out, put a little piece of adhesive tape on each cheek where the bottom of the frame rests."

Glasses of all kinds also tend to push your ears out, making them more exposed to the cold. "So be sure to wear a hat that comes all the way down over the ears," Dr. Hamlet cautions.

Beware the Gas Station

"You can get instant frostbite if you spill superchilled gasoline on your hands," Pelchat notes. Gasoline is often stored above ground for refueling snowmobiles or snowblowers. The fuel retains cold temperatures for several hours, so if it was –40°F last night, the gasoline will still be –40°F this morning. "Don't take off your gloves when you're getting gas," Pelchat advises, "even if it's just at the self-service pump."

F

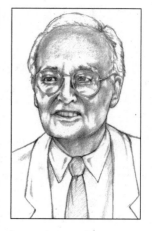

A WORD FROM DR. MARTIN

My Town Looks Better in Mud Season, Though

DURING the mid-1980s, the *Today* show did a segment on small-town America. Three towns were featured: one in Ohio, one in Colorado, and my own town of Chelsea, Vermont. The point of the story was to contrast a booming town with one that had boomed and gone bust and one that hadn't changed in 100 years. Chelsea was the one that hadn't changed. It's still as small as ever, and it looks exactly like pictures taken a century ago, except that many of the roads are paved. And, heck, when the snow comes in the winter, you can't tell they're paved.

The town hasn't changed in that time, but medicine has. Country doctors today are trained as rigorously as their city colleagues. But because they work in much smaller communities, country doctors often see their patients outside the office—in the local coffee shop, in the grocery store, at town meetings. That's holistic medicine at its best: knowing the whole patient.

And that's a principle you can apply at home: Consider yourself as the whole patient. When you think about how to treat yourself for an ache or pain, factor in diet, lifestyle, and daily stresses and strains.

BREWSTER MARTIN, M.D., *a retired family doctor in Chelsea, Vermont (population 1,166), and cofounder of the Chelsea Family Health Center. He was named Vermont Doctor of the Year in 1991.*

Skip the Booze

"Drinking alcohol does three things to you when you're out in the cold," says Thomas Watt, M.D., a dermatologist in private practice in Bangor, Maine. "First, it dulls the senses. It makes you think less straight, and can cause you to do foolish things that can lead to frostbite.

"Second, alcohol can cause flushing of the skin. You lose heat as the heated blood from the body's core rushes to the surface. This, too, can lead to frostbite.

"Third, although alcohol makes you *feel* warm, there is no evidence that it actually warms you. It deceives you, making you feel as though you don't need to bundle up even when you're in danger of frostbite."

Dr. Watt's advice: Save the sauce until you're back inside.

Protect Down Under

"The tip of a man's penis can literally freeze if he's not careful," Dr. Weider says. "It happens to runners. To keep the penis warm in bitter weather, a man should wear long underwear made of polypropylene." The Lifa (pronounced LEE-fuh) Company makes a particular style with a nylon panel in front, Dr. Weider says. "We call it Fig Lifa."

Cup Your Face

"Frost nip, which is what we call early frostbite, will show up first on the face and extremities," says Pelchat, who recommends using the "buddy system" to keep track of faces for early signs of frost nip. "You might see an area about the size of a quarter blanched white on your friend's face," he says. If your buddy sees it on *your* face, you can quickly re-warm the spot by cupping your hands over your face and blowing into your hands. "Then cover the area with a neck gaiter or another kind of scarf and get inside as quickly as you can." A neck gaiter, by the way, is a doughnut-shaped scarf that can be pulled up to protect more than half of the face from cold.

Use Your Pits

"If you feel your hands starting to tingle, put them in your armpits to warm them," Dr. Watt advises.

Avoid Premature Thawing

"Some of the biggest damage from frostbite can come from thawing the area before the person can be taken to a warm place," Pelchat warns. "The danger is that the thawed area can refreeze. The ice crystals that form from refrozen flesh are double the size of the original frostbite crystals when they reform. These larger crystals literally cut into your tissue and can do much more damage than the original frostbite." Until you can get to a warm place and get some medical attention, Pelchat recommends covering frostbitten areas without trying to warm them up much above freezing. "Clothing or your own hand will do," he says.

Once Bitten, Be Twice Shy

"If you have been frostbitten once, you are more likely to be frostbitten in the same place again," Dr. Hamlet warns. "The frostbitten area is more sensitive to the cold, so you need to cover up or go in someplace warm sooner."

G

GALLSTONES

Cures for fat
that turns hard on you

Although it's not the sort of stuff you'd want to describe at the dinner table, bile is a pretty important bodily substance. Your liver produces this thick, gooey liquid, which sits in your gallbladder waiting for your next meal. In the old days, doctors thought bile—which they called "yellow bile"—was one of the four essential "humors" in the body, along with blood, "black bile," and phlegm. If you were sick, that meant one of your humors was out of balance with the others.

These days, doctors credit bile with a more prosaic but still important function: to help digest the fat in your food. "The gallbladder is a small sac situated under the liver," explains Keith Michl, M.D., an internist in private practice in Manchester Center, Vermont. "The liver produces bile, and the gallbladder stores and concentrates it. When you digest, hormones in the intestine cause the gallbladder to contract and expel its bile into the gut, where it helps to digest fat."

Sometimes the bile can gum up the works by forming a gallstone made of cholesterol or other substances that have become crystallized. These "stones" can be as small as a grain of sand or as large as a robin's egg. "You may not feel any symptoms from a gallstone," Dr. Michl says. But

When one or more stones get stuck in the duct that passes bile, it can be a gut-wrenching experience.

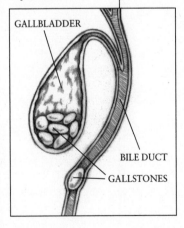

GALLBLADDER

BILE DUCT

GALLSTONES

some gallstones move around, and one or more can get stuck in the duct that passes the bile. The result is usually a pain in the upper-right-hand part of your abdomen or between your shoulder blades. "The pain comes when the gallbladder pumps to try to push out the stone," Dr. Michl says. "You also might feel feverish or sick to your stomach."

Poorly functioning gallbladders tend to run in families. Too much fat and cholesterol in your diet can also cause gallstones to form, and middle-aged, overweight women are especially susceptible. But if your doctor has found stones that aren't causing pain, don't be alarmed. "If stones are causing you no symptoms, you can leave them alone," Dr. Michl says. Although more than half a million Americans undergo gallbladder surgery every year, Dr. Michl says some of that surgery is probably unnecessary. "If the stones aren't bothering you and a surgeon wants to operate, get a second opinion."

In the meantime, here's what you can do to lower the chances of an attack.

Diet Slowly

Since being overweight puts you at risk for forming gallstones, it stands to reason that a good way to give your beleaguered gallbladder a break is to lose weight. And, in fact, studies show that people who shed pounds are much less likely to be attacked by their gallbladders. But if you do choose to get your weight down, be patient. A crash diet can actually increase your chances of getting gallstones.

Even worse is the "yo-yo" diet on which a person loses weight only to gain it back again. "I would see people who lost a great deal of weight, then gained it back, then lost it, and then regained it all over again," says Brewster Martin, M.D., a retired family doctor in Chelsea, Vermont. These people seem more likely to have gallbladder attacks, Dr. Martin says. So what's a safe way to diet? Lose one to two pounds per week, researchers say. And change your eating habits so the pounds stay off.

Find Friendly Fat

"Eat good fats," says Lawrence Bronstein, D.C., a chiropractor and certified nutrition specialist in Great Barrington,

G

G

Massachusetts. "Researchers suspect that omega-3 fatty acids, like those found in fish, can help prevent gallstones. You also may try taking a flaxseed oil supplement, available over the counter at health food stores." And what are the bad fats to avoid? "Trans fatty acids, like those found in margarine and deep-fried foods, especially those found in fast-food restaurants," which tend to fry much of the food on the menu.

Abstain from Pain

If you suffer from gallstones, ask your doctor about taking regular doses of nonsteroidal anti-inflammatory drugs (NSAIDs)—a fancy term for over-the-counter painkillers such as aspirin and ibuprofen. Researchers at Virginia Commonwealth University found that people who used NSAIDs regularly had less thick mucus in their gallbladder bile. People with concentrated mucus are more likely to develop new gallstones.

Help Your Digestion

To aid gallbladder function and digestion, "you may benefit from supplemental bile salts," Dr. Bronstein says. "Some general digestive enzymes—including protease, amylase, lipase, celluase, maltase, and sucrase—can help relieve the burden on your stomach and gallbladder function, making stone formation less likely." All these supplements are available over the counter at drugstores or health food stores.

GENITAL IRRITATION
Treatments for low-down problems

Oh, your poor genitals. The warm, moist darkness they dwell in can harbor bacterial, fungal, or—primarily in women— yeast infections. You also can get pimples when the hair follicles in your genitals are clogged. And then there are genital warts, which are just like warts on the rest of your body, except that these are transmitted sexually.

It wouldn't be so bad if your genitals weren't so darn sensitive. Here's how you can give them some tender loving care.

Use the Jock Cure

"The single most common cause of genital irritation in men is jock itch," says Stephen Rous, M.D., chief of urology at the Veterans Administration Medical Center in White River Junction, Vermont. "It's an infection by the fungus *Tinea cruris*. The dark, damp environment of your genitals is ideal for fungal infections. Any antifungal medicine will help. Ask your doctor for a prescription for Mycostatin."

Or Try a Woman's Cure

"In women, genital irritation can mean yeast infection," says Hope Ricciotti, an obstetrician-gynecologist at the Beth Israel Deaconess Medical Center in Boston. "Women often get yeast infections when they take antibiotics. Yeast is a normal inhabitant of the body. When the antibiotics kill off normal bacteria that keep yeast in check, the yeast tends to overgrow." The cure, she says, is the same as for men's jock itch: "Use an antifungal medicine. Monistat, for example, available over the counter, works very well. And be sure to get antifungals when you have to take antibiotics."

Swallow Bacteria

"Plain yogurt with active cultures, either eaten or applied directly to your genitals, will help keep vaginal flora in balance, helping relieve vaginal irritation," Dr. Ricciotti says. Leave the yogurt on for two minutes, then bathe, she suggests. "Not all yogurts have active cultures," Dr. Ricciotti adds. "Look on the label for acidophilus."

Take Tub Time

"Males and females suffering from genital irritation can get relief by bathing in a tub of cool water with half a cup of

TIME TO SEE THE DOCTOR
Watch for Strange Signs

SEE a doctor when you find any distinctive or unusual lesions on your penis," says Stephen Rous, M.D., chief of urology at the Veterans Administration Medical Center in White River Junction, Vermont. "Also go in if you have a genital scab that won't heal, a raised lesion, or a blister." You might have an infection or genital herpes—a sexually transmitted disease.

If you find tiny pimplelike growths on your genitals that form in a pattern of clusters like a cauliflower, seek medical help. "You may have genital warts, a sexually transmitted disease that is quite contagious," Dr. Rous says. Your doctor can treat you with prescription drugs. In the meantime, avoid unprotected sex. "The incubation period of the disease varies greatly," Dr. Rous notes. "It can last as long as 6 to 12 months, during which you're still contagious."

Avoiding Babies Can Be Irritating

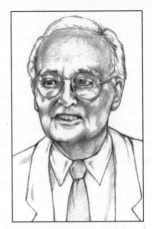

WHEN I first started practicing in rural Vermont in the 1950s, condoms were a common form of birth control. But most people used the rhythm method, which meant avoiding sex for a couple of days before the woman thought she was going to ovulate. As a result, people had a lot of kids.

The diaphragm came onto the market just as I became a doctor. It works great, but the spermicidal gel you're supposed to use with it can irritate some people's genitals. Stop using the gel, and the irritation will probably go away. But make sure you switch to another reliable birth control method, unless you like lots of kids.

BREWSTER MARTIN, M.D., *a retired family doctor in Chelsea, Vermont (population 1,166), and cofounder of the Chelsea Family Health Center. He was named Vermont Doctor of the Year in 1991.*

baking soda mixed in," says Paul Lena, M.D., a retired physician of internal medicine in Concord, New Hampshire. "Aveeno works, too." Aveeno is a brand of colloidal oatmeal, specially formulated to coat the skin. It is available at pharmacies. Follow the directions on the label.

Use Steroids

"Topical application of corticosteroids such as Cortaid, available over the counter, is very helpful for genital irritation," Dr. Lena says.

Ditch the Douche

"Some older women in particular are obsessed with douching," says Brewster Martin, M.D., a retired family doctor in Chelsea, Vermont. Dr. Martin explains that douching can upset the natural balance of yeast and bacteria in your genitals and cause irritation or yeast infections. "I had one patient who douched every single day, as her mother before her had," he says. "She couldn't understand why her vagina and labia were raw. She would have been much healthier if she'd never douched at all. Douching isn't a good habit."

Don't Be Crabby

"An insect like crabs can infest the pubic hair of men and women," Dr. Rous notes. "They look like dark freckles against your skin. They can cause itching and discomfort and are passed from person to person by direct physical contact. One application of Kwell, an over-the-counter shampoo, should take care of them."

Switch Devices

"Some people are allergic to the lubricants that coat most condoms," Dr. Rous says. "Other people have an allergy to the latex of the condom itself. First try switching condoms if they seem to be causing irritation. If you still have a problem, consider changing your method of birth control."

Check Your Meds

"An allergy to a drug, such as a decongestant, can cause a rashlike lesion on a particular part of your body—including the genitals," Dr. Rous says. "The strange thing is, a reaction that raises a lesion will tend to form that rash in the exact same part of your body every time you take that drug. Ask your doctor about switching medications."

GOUT

Stop feeling poorly
from the "rich man's disease"

There was a time when gout, a painful form of arthritis, was a kind of status symbol. A diet of red meat washed down with port can bring on the disease, so anybody who could afford to eat expensively could complain, with a certain amount of satisfaction, of agony in the first joint of the big toe or other joints in the foot or knee (and sometimes in the wrist or elbow).

G If you suffer from gout, you have some prestigious predecessors. The Old Testament's King Asa had gout, and "his disease was exceeding great." The pain drove sixteenth-century Spanish king Charles I to abdicate. His gouty son Philip II ruled from bed. At least 14 of the 86 Byzantine emperors had gout and other forms of arthritis. Benjamin Franklin wrote a dialogue between himself and "Madam Gout" in which the disease argued that it had saved the old philosopher from an even worse diet. By causing pain every time Franklin ate overly rich food or drank alcohol, the disease argued, "the gout, in such a subject as you are, is no disease, but a remedy."

Madam Gout had a point: Doctors now know that a major cause of gout is a diet rich in purines, which are often found in fatty foods such as organ meats, sardines, and anchovies. Yeast is also packed with purines, which is why heavy beer drinkers are gout-prone.

But you can be a teetotaling vegetarian and still have the disease. The major cause of gout is heredity. A genetic defect can cause uric acid to be concentrated in the body, leading to the formation of painful acid crystals in the fluid sur-

No Wonder Folks Hoped the Frogs' Eggs Would Work

IN THE days when the common diet (for people who could afford it) involved lots of organ meats and beer, gout was a common disease among the upper classes. The search for escapes from the piercing joint pain led to some desperate measures. From ancient times to the nineteenth century, people anxious to avoid gout sometimes abstained from sex, which was assumed to be one of the causes. Some doctors even went so far as to prescribe castration.

The ancient Greeks thought that another sure but unwelcome cure was dysentery. One medieval remedy called for a roast goose stuffed with chopped kittens.

Thomas Palmer, a country doctor in seventeenth-century New England, prescribed wool compresses soaked in hot "Frogge Water," which consisted of frogs' egg masses that had been aged for a few weeks. Modern doctors aren't fishing farm ponds for frogs' eggs, but they do endorse one old-time cure for gout: avoiding organ meats and beer.

rounding the joints. Men over the age of 40 are most likely to get gout, although women who have gone through menopause are also somewhat susceptible. Besides diet and genes, other triggers that can bring on a painful gout attack include dehydration, excessive use of aspirin, crash dieting, serious injury, and stress.

But you don't have to lose your own personal argument with Madam Gout. Here's how you can give the nasty old ailment the boot.

Eat Green

"If you get attacks of gout, avoid alcohol and rich organ meats such as liver and kidneys," says Gary Venman-Clay, M.D., a family doctor in private practice in Bellows Falls, Vermont.

Get Flushed

"Drink lots of liquids, such as water and cranberry juice, to help flush your system," says Laurence Bouchard, D.O., an osteopathic family physician in private practice in Narragansett, Rhode Island. "The more hydrated you are, the lower the concentration of gout-causing uric acid in your body."

Pop a Pill

"Take an anti-inflammatory such as ibuprofen for the pain of gout," Dr. Venman-Clay recommends. Avoid aspirin, which has been implicated in bouts of gout. Ibuprofen is safer.

Check Your Water Level

"If you have gout and you're taking medicine for your high blood pressure, ask your doctor about your medication," says Raymond Rocco Monto, M.D., an orthopedic surgeon at Martha's Vineyard Orthopedic Surgery and Sports Medicine in Oak Bluffs, Massachusetts. "Some diuretics, which are also called water pills, can make gout worse by increasing the concentration of uric acid in the blood," he says. "If you're taking a diuretic, regularly review the need for the medication—as well as the question of whether you should also be taking an over-the-counter potassium supplement—with your doctor."

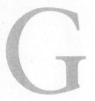

GRAYING HAIR
Rather not look quite so distinguished? Try these remedies

Are you getting snowy up on top? Look on the bright side: Your hair isn't going gray, it's going *clear*. "I call gray hair clear hair because it has no color," says Thaedra Thompson, a licensed cosmetologist and former New Englander who is a stylist at the Salon Montanna in Albuquerque, New Mexico. "As you age, your hair loses its pigment, turning transparent. It gets the appearance of grayness."

The bad news is, there is nothing you can do to restore that youthful color permanently. "If you don't want gray hair, then don't grow older," says Robert Averill, M.D., a dermatologist in private practice in western Massachusetts and northern New Hampshire.

If your hair turns white suddenly, that's probably another optical illusion. Stress or fright can cause your darker hairs to fall out, exposing the colorless ones. Chances are, your hairs—including the dark ones—will grow back, and you'll seem to regain some of that lost youth.

If your hair is getting frosty more gradually, here's how you can turn back the clock.

Kick the Butts

Smoke and graying hair don't make a very attractive combination, says Lorie Warren, a barber at Jack's Barber Shop in Ellsworth, Maine. "Smoking turns white hair yellow," she says. "I can tell by looking at someone if he's a smoker."

Prep the Gray

"Gray hair is resistant to color," Thompson says. "You have to soften it first with hydrogen peroxide and then use color if you want to cover all the gray." Hydrogen peroxide is available at drugstores, and it is usually included with hair-coloring products. Follow the directions on the label. Thompson says you should ask your hairdresser to recommend the proper color. "You have to be careful with over-the-counter hair-coloring products, because it is hard to tell from the box what color you'll wind up with."

How I Became the Doc Who Dyed

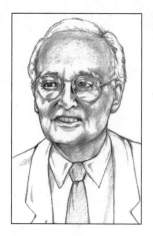

MY HAIR turned snow white when I was in my thirties. Even though I was about the same age as my partner in our community health center, people would always ask to see "the older doctor"—meaning me. I was taking 90 percent of the calls. Finally, my nurse suggested I dye my hair. I did just that, and my partner ended up getting more of the calls. (He still looks younger, though.)

You might think that dying your gray hair is vain. But sometimes you have to do it for professional reasons.

BREWSTER MARTIN, M.D., *a retired family doctor in Chelsea, Vermont (population 1,166), and cofounder of the Chelsea Family Health Center. He was named Vermont Doctor of the Year in 1991.*

Turn on the Highlights

Thompson recommends highlighting your hair—putting in subtle streaks of color—to beat back the aging look. "The point is to blend the gray with your natural color," she says. "It looks natural, and the highlighted color is reflected in the clear gray hairs." You can buy dark-colored highlighter in your supermarket or take your gray hair to a cosmetologist for some toning up.

Set a Condition

If you're nervous about doing anything long-lasting to your hair, use temporary dyes called color conditioners, says Debbie Irish, a licensed cosmetologist and owner of Hair Classique in Monkton, Vermont. "Aveda makes excellent color conditioners from the roots of plants." Irish adds that a color conditioner may be a good idea even if you like looking frosty. "If you glory in your gray, you can use a blue color conditioner. It enhances gray hair."

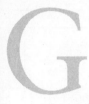

GUM PAIN

Ways to keep yourself in the pink

Your gums can suffer from lots of hard knocks. Ill-fitting dentures can rub against them and cause soreness and bleeding. Cigarettes, as well as medications from cold medicines to oral contraceptives, can puff up your gums. And so can the coursing hormones of a woman's menstrual period.

But the biggest cause of sore and bleeding gums is the dental disease gingivitis, an inflammation that comes from the buildup of a sticky mixture of food particles and bacteria called plaque. "It works the way a splinter in your finger does," says Gregory L. Baker, D.D.S., an orthodontist in private practice in Woodstock, Vermont, and West Lebanon and New London, New Hampshire. "Your finger will swell up and redden as a reaction to the foreign body of a splinter. Plaque is a foreign body in your mouth. When it accumulates on your teeth, it eventually touches the gums and irritates them." Some 44 percent of American mouths are gummed up with gingivitis.

Although gingivitis by itself rarely leads to tooth loss, Dr. Baker says, some cases turn into periodontitis—a disease that can cause teeth to loosen and eventually fall out. If your gums bleed, that's a sign you should work on improving your dental techniques.

Here's how.

Floss, Floss, Floss

"You don't have to floss all your teeth—just the ones you want to keep," Dr. Baker says. In other words, if you want to avoid losing your teeth to gum disease, floss them all daily.

Ignore the Gore

"Some people say they can't clean their gums because the gums bleed," Dr. Baker notes. "If your gums bleed, it's because the stimulation of the flossing causes blood to accumulate in the irritated tissue and then leak out. If you begin cleaning your teeth properly, with brushing twice a day and daily flossing, the bleeding will be markedly reduced within a week."

Get a Handle on Flossing

A device called a flosser—a plastic handle with a stretch of floss at the end of it—makes it easier to get to those hard-to-reach places. Flossers are available at most drugstores.

Stop Dragging

"Periodontal disease is three times higher in smokers than in nonsmokers," notes Gregory Colpitts, D.M.D., a dentist in private practice in Franklin, New Hampshire. "Even smokers with great dental habits can't keep their teeth clean enough to prevent gum disease." That's because nicotine, the addictive drug in cigarette smoke, restricts blood vessels in the gums and causes breakdown of the delicate tissue. There's one more reason to stop.

Fluoridate

Toothpaste that contains stannous fluoride, a well-known cavity fighter, can also help prevent gum disease, according to a study by dentists at Indiana University's Oral Health Research Institute. "Check the label to see that your toothpaste is approved by the American Dental Association," Dr. Baker says. "That ensures that you're getting the proper kind of fluoride."

Switch the Tube

Many common toothpastes contain ingredients that set some people's gums aflame. Well, maybe that's putting it a bit strongly, but if your gums are sensitive to allergy-causing ingredients in toothpastes, try switching brands. The most common culprits are preservatives and flavorings such as cinnamon and peppermint, according to researchers.

Flavor Your Gums

Dr. Colpitts recommends soothing your sore gums with an old-time remedy for teething babies: ground cloves. "You can buy ground gloves in the supermarket or grind your own," he says. "Put a pinch of ground cloves on a hard, smooth surface, such as the back of a glass baking pan. Mix in a little water, then add more ground cloves bit by bit until you have a thick paste. Apply it to your gums, and they should feel better immediately."

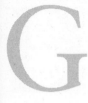

Pinch the Pain

"Make a tiny compress by rolling up a pinch of echinacea powder in damp gauze," suggests Rosemary Gladstar, an herbalist in East Barre, Vermont, and author of *Herbal Healing for Women*. You can buy echinacea—the root of purple coneflower—at herbal and health food stores. "Apply it directly to the painful spot, and it will help fight an infection," Gladstar says. Skip this treatment if you're allergic to ragweed, however; the plants are close relatives.

Let Your Mouth Nap

"Be sure you are well-rested," Dr. Colpitts says. "If you aren't getting enough sleep, the quality and amount of saliva you produce can change, and the saliva can lose some of its lubricants. In that kind of dry mouth, bacteria go crazy. You can get rampant decay around the gum line."

Buy Some Spit

"Drinking more water won't alleviate the problem of a dry mouth," Dr. Colpitts says. "Oral saliva substitutes are available over the counter. Ask your dentist or pharmacist to recommend one that will work best for you."

Check the Pills

"Some drugs, such as antidepressants, antihistamines, and blood pressure medication, may change the chemistry in your mouth, allowing bacteria to proliferate," Dr. Colpitts warns. "If you're having gum problems despite good brushing and flossing habits, check with your doctor about adjusting your medication."

H

HAIR LOSS

Is your tub drain getting hairy?
Here are some highbrow solutions

If your garden flowers lasted as long as the hairs on your head, you'd be thrilled. A healthy scalp hair grows about one-third millimeter a day for 3 to 10 years before it finally stops growing and falls out—only to be replaced, in most cases, by a new hair that grows out of the same follicle. "We normally lose 75 to 100 hairs per day," says Charles Hammer, M.D., a dermatologist with the North Country Outreach Program of the Lahey Hitchcock Clinic in St. Johnsbury, Vermont. "If you have a healthy head of hair, your scalp replaces hairs at the same rate you lose them."

If you lose more than 100 hairs a day, you have a problem: The new hairs just can't keep up. There are several possible causes, according to Dr. Hammer. Medication such as chemotherapy for cancer can cause you to lose your hair temporarily. A hormonal imbalance, a protein deficiency, or stress can make hair fall out. Remove the cause, and your hair normally grows back.

Another cause of hair loss: Women often find that their hair thins after they go through childbirth. "This hair loss is also temporary," Dr. Hammer says.

A severe scalp burn or injury, or a disease such as lupus, can sometimes destroy hair follicles, causing permanent hair loss. But in most cases, if you find your hair thinning over the years, genetics is to blame. "If your father was bald, you have

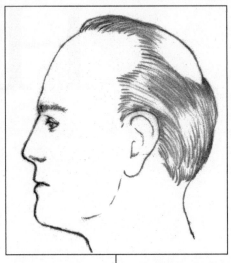

A classic case of male pattern baldness: loss of hair on the back of the head. Usually, you can blame your dad's genes.

a good chance of being bald as well," Dr. Hammer explains. About 40 percent of women age 60 or over also find their hair noticeably thinning—and you can blame genes in many of these cases.

If you'd prefer to keep the fur, try these remedies.

Guard Those Hairs

Don't scrub your head too hard with a towel after you get out of the shower, Dr. Hammer advises. You could yank out hairs with that kind of enthusiasm. "And a comb is gentler on your hair than a brush," he says. If you feel the need to use a brush, try to work out those tangles with your fingers first, rather than tugging at them with the brush, he adds.

Hang On

"Over-the-counter Rogaine—and its much less expensive generic version, minoxidil—help you keep the hair you have," says Owen Reynolds, M.D., a dermatologist in private practice in North Andover, Massachusetts. "Men with male pattern baldness—a receding hairline and thinning on top of the head—can't regain their lost hair with minoxidil. But by using these products, they can prevent further loss." Dr. Reynolds notes that minoxidil also can slow the march of female pattern baldness, in which a woman loses some hair at the temples.

Save Your Hair, Not Your Wallet

"Don't try to save money on shampoos," says Mary-Catherine Gennaro, D.O., a family osteopath in Warren, New Hampshire. "Buy your shampoo from a salon. Salon products do a better job than most drugstore shampoos, which tend to dry your hair out and make it look thinner."

TIME TO SEE THE DOCTOR

Is Your Hair Falling Out in Patches?

IF YOU'RE starting to see bare patches over your scalp within a few weeks after noticing the first bald spot, get a doctor to check you out, says Charles Hammer, M.D., a dermatologist with the North Country Outreach Program of the Lahey Hitchcock Clinic in St. Johnsbury, Vermont. "Any of several treatable causes could be the culprit. But delay of therapy can reduce your chances of success."

HAIR LOSS

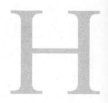

Ask for Layers

"Rather than combing over your thin spots, ask your barber for a layer cut," says Lorie Warren, a barber at Jack's Barber Shop in Ellsworth, Maine. "This kind of cut makes thin hair look fuller."

Dr. Gennaro says that a layer cut works as well for women as for men. "If my hair were thinning, I'd definitely get a short cut with lots of layers," she says. "Long hair weighs itself down and looks flatter."

Stock Up

"If you're worried about hair loss, make sure you're getting all the vitamins and minerals your body needs," Dr. Gennaro says. "A good multivitamin, available over the counter at drugstores and grocery stores, can provide you with added vitamin insurance."

HAIR PROBLEMS IN GENERAL
How to part with your uppermost sorrows

Is that mop on top a tangle of trouble? Elsewhere in this book, our country doctors recommend cures for tangled and graying hair and for hair loss. If your problems don't fit any of these categories, check out the remedies below.

Cut the Mineral Buildup

"If you live in an area with hard water, it will leave a buildup of minerals on your hair," says Valerie Major, a licensed cosmetologist and manager of Beth's Salon in Woodstock, Vermont. "The accumulation will make your hair look dragged down and lifeless." The cure: "Use clean cider vinegar in your last rinse after you shampoo. The vinegar will wash away the minerals." Major notes that you should rinse out the vinegar thoroughly in the shower to keep from smelling like a salad. And vinegar can lighten some people's hair. If you find your own hair turning an undesirable color, drop the vinegar.

Just a Quick Cut, Please

Up through the eighteenth century, barbers did a lot more than cut hair. They also regularly "bled" patients—drew small amounts of blood in the belief that the practice would restore the natural balance to a body that was out of whack. Barbers often performed complicated surgery as well. Doctors in those days were limited to advising their patients and left physical procedures up to barbers and others. Even as late as the Civil War (1861–1865), many barbers offered to pull teeth as well as cut hair.

These days, surgery is left to trained surgeons. But the next time you see a small child crying during a haircut, tell the kid, "Hey, it could be worse."

Kill the Chlorine

"Chlorine from pool water, or even from tap water, can build up in your hair," notes Cara Calomb-Down, co-owner of the Keene Beauty Academy in Keene, New Hampshire. Calomb-Down says that cheaply made or improperly used hair care products also can leave a residue on your hair. "A tablespoon of baking soda in a cup of water will help remove the buildup," she says. "Use the baking soda mixture as a rinse between your shampoo and conditioner."

By Gum, Here's an Idea

Has some little prankster put gum in your hair? Or has a curious child done it to herself? The answer is oil, according to Calomb-Down. Peanut butter, which contains peanut oil, is an old remedy. So is vegetable oil. "Massage the oil or peanut butter into the gum," Calomb-Down says. "The oil will break down the gum. Use a comb to remove the gum, starting at the hair ends with outward strokes. Then slowly work your way toward the scalp, removing all traces of gum." Calomb-Down notes that an alternative is to hold an ice cube against the gum, hardening it to the breaking point, and then removing the pieces.

Give Yourself Permanent Protection

"Your permanent can relax when you go out in the sun," Calomb-Down warns. "Wear a hat when you go outside. And if you try a tanning bed, wrap your hair in a towel for protection while you tan."

HAIR TANGLES
What to do
when it's a jungle up there

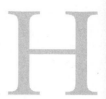

If birds are eyeing your head with the notion of taking up residence, you can blame any number of causes: dry air, a close brush with a hair dryer, and—ironically—many of the products you use to fix yourself up, such as shampoos, dyes, and permanents. Such foreign substances can coat the individual hairs, making them head in almost every direction but the one you want.

Here are ways to get your hair's act together.

Use Good Technique

If your hair is hard to brush, the last thing you want to do is make things worse with improper brushing, says Cara Calomb-Down, co-owner of the Keene Beauty Academy in Keene, New Hampshire. "To remove tangles, always start at the end and work inward," she says. "Focus on small sections, working each tangle out from the hair's end. Once the end is free, move toward the scalp, again in small sections." The most important thing is to stay calm, Calomb-Down says. Brushing can be painful. To make it hurt less, hold your hair between the tangle and your scalp to prevent pulling.

Calomb-Down suggests that you teach your children to brush their hair properly, just as you show them good toothbrushing technique. "Children have a tendency to comb only the top layer of hair to conceal tangles," she says. "You need to teach them patience."

Untangle First

"Before you wash your hair—or, especially, if you're about to wash your child's hair—brush out the tangles first," says Valerie Major, a licensed cosmetologist and manager of Beth's Salon in Woodstock, Vermont. "You'll get the hair cleaner and more manageable that way."

Don't Do It Wet

"Your hair is very stretchy and flexible when it is wet," says Debbie Irish, a licensed cosmetologist and owner of Hair Classique in Monkton, Vermont. "Brushing your hair when

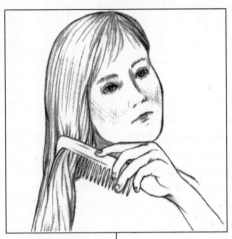

The right teeth are important when it comes to untangling hair. Start with a wide-tooth comb, then switch to a finer-tooth version.

it is wet is a no-no. That'll only split the ends more."

Open Wide

When you comb your hair, start with a wide-tooth comb to get out the worst tangles, Calomb-Down advises. Once you have the messes straightened out, switch to a finer-tooth comb.

Go Soft

Do not use stiff combs and hard-bristle brushes for hair tangles, says Barbara Alibozek, manager of the Clip Shop, with locations in Williamstown and Pittsfield, Massachusetts, and Bennington, Vermont. "Use a brush with flexible, bendable bristles and a rubber base."

HAMMERED THUMB

How to cope when your digit looks smashing

Even the most skilled among us occasionally find carpentry to be a hit-or-miss affair. A smashed thumb is a time-honored injury, a way that our forefathers have handed down foul language from time immemorial.

Often the injury will break the small blood vessels underneath the nail, causing a painful buildup of blood. "The pain comes from the hematoma, or bleeding, into a closed space, causing pressure to build up," says Brewster Martin, M.D., a retired family doctor in Chelsea, Vermont.

Once in a while, a lustily swung hammer can break a finger bone. "The tips of your thumbs and fingers are well padded, but it's still possible to break them," says John Dunn, M.D., an emergency room physician at the North-

---

western Medical Center in St. Albans, Vermont, and author of *Winterwise: A Backpacker's Guide*—a book that tells how to enjoy the season and deal with some of its medical challenges. In most thumb-bashing cases—even when small bones are broken—a doctor is unnecessary, Dr. Dunn says. Here's what you can do on your own.

Start with Ice

"If you hammer a finger or thumb, apply ice for no more than 10 minutes and keep the finger elevated," Dr. Dunn advises. "If it is broken, taping it to a splint or a neighboring finger will immobilize the bone and help it to heal."

Try the Paper Clip Trick . . .

"If there is blood under the nail and there is no indication of a fracture, heat the end of a straightened paper clip in a flame until the metal is red-hot," says Hugh P. Hermann, M.D., a family physician in Woodstock, Vermont. "Hold the clip with a piece of cloth so you don't burn your other hand.

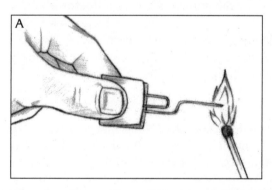

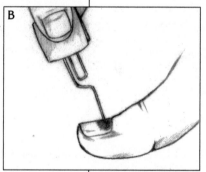

Then gently rest the red-hot tip of the paper clip on your blue, discolored nail. The metal will burn through the nail without pain or pressure, and a small fountain of blood will escape. This will result in much greater comfort for the patient."

. . . Then Soak Your Digit

"After you've relieved the pressure with a paper clip, soak your thumb or finger in warm salt water three times daily for a few days," Dr. Hermann says. "This will keep the wound draining until all is resolved."

The paper clip trick looks gory, but it's a painless way to remove blood from under a nail. Heat the metal until it's red (A), then burn through the nail (B) until blood comes out.

H

HAMMERTOE
Nailing a problem that starts when your feet take a pounding

Does your toe curl back in elfin fashion, looking more like a carpentry tool than a part of your anatomy? If so, you may have a hammertoe—a deformed digit that gets worse as your shoes rub against your feet.

"Hammertoes are usually caused by excessive pronation—a type of splaying or partial collapse of the feet," says Nicholas Vachon, D.P.M., a podiatrist in private practice in Ellsworth, Maine. "This is usually a genetically inherited characteristic."

Although home remedies can control pronation and keep your hammertoe from getting worse, "they will not reverse the damage," Dr. Vachon says. He recommends seeing a doctor about a cure. "Permanent reduction of digital deformities usually requires minor surgery."

On the other hand (or foot), you can ease the pounding of a hammertoe with these remedies.

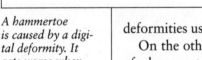

HAMMERTOE

A hammertoe is caused by a digital deformity. It gets worse when it's rubbed the wrong way.

Get Shod

"It is better to change shoes than to change your feet," Dr. Vachon says. "Buy wider shoes with a deep toe box. Specialty stores can make shoes for you."

Or Modify Your Shoe

"If your hammertoes are severe, you may need an extra-deep shoe," says Ralph McCoy, a certified shoe technician and owner of the Shoetorium shoe store in Lebanon, New Hampshire. "You can also have the inside of your shoe modified so that a plastic mold with a pad underneath can be fit into the shoe. You need the pad to give your toes something soft to come down on." Ask your doctor about the modification that works best for your toes.

"A pad on the top and the bottom would be beneficial," confirms Laurence Bouchard, D.O., an osteopathic family physician in Narragansett, Rhode Island. "A toe that sticks up also gets pushed down by the shoe, which can cause blisters or calluses below."

Walk Like a Man

"Women with hammertoes may be more comfortable in men's shoes, which run in wider sizes," says Eugene Hunt, a cobbler at Simon the Tanner in Island Pond, Vermont. "Men's shoes also tend to have a good, deep toe box."

Pad Your Paws

"To prevent irritation of the toe, buy soft pads such as Dr. Scholl's Foot Pads over the counter," Dr. Vachon suggests. Like moleskin, these adhesive pads provide a soft barrier between your shoe and your toe.

HANGNAILS
Put a stop to skin that's on a tear

Are you discovering loose ends in your life—the kind that hang from your fingers? Then you're suffering from those unattractive and sometimes bloody little annoyances called hangnails.

Hangnails aren't nails, of course. They're pieces of wayward skin that hang *from* your nails. Dry skin is the reason.

One way to execute a hangnail is simply to cut it off. Bad idea, says Daniel Caloras, M.D., a family doctor in private practice in Charlestown, New Hampshire. "Cutting a hangnail often makes it worse," he says. But there are plenty of better cures.

Salt Away

"I recommend a warm-water soak with Epsom salts for problem hangnails," Dr. Caloras says. Soak your fingers two or three times a day for 10 to 15 minutes at a time. "You can buy Epsom salts over the counter at the drugstore," he says. "I tell my patients to soak in salts, and I don't see many of them complaining of the problem again."

TIME TO SEE THE DOCTOR

Does Your Hangnail Look Hammered?

IF YOUR hangnail feels hot and is red and mean-looking, see a doctor," says Daniel Caloras, M.D., a family doctor in private practice in Charlestown, New Hampshire. "You may have an infection that needs an antibiotic to clear it up."

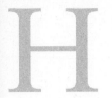

Take a "Q"

"Use a wet Q-Tip to push the skin away from the nail two or three times a day," Dr. Caloras advises. "That will free the nail from the skin and should resolve your problem in a couple of days."

Soften Up

"Put lotion on hangnails—your children's as well as your own," says Patricia Edwards, M.D., a pediatrician in private practice in Concord, New Hampshire. "You also need to be diligent about reminding your children not to get in the bad habit of picking their hangnails. Watch them like a hawk."

See Orange

"Use an orangewood stick to push your cuticles back after a bath or shower," says Valerie Major, a licensed cosmetologist and manager of Beth's Salon in Woodstock, Vermont. "An orange stick is just soft enough to avoid further damaging your skin, but it's firm enough to do the job." You can buy orangewood sticks at most pharmacies.

Toe the Line

"Hangnails can be a big problem on your big toe," says John C. Robinson, M.D., a pediatrician in private practice in Quincy, Massachusetts. "The most common cause of a toe hangnail is cutting the toenail back too far. The hangnail can become infected, requiring antibiotics until the nail can grow out over the margin of the nail bed. The key is prevention: Don't cut your toenails too short—especially the one on the big toe."

HANGOVER
What to do when the party's over and your head is still dancing

A hangover is like a stern parent chastising you for your sins the night before. You overdid it, and now, by golly, you're paying for it with a headache that pounds worse than the band you were bopping to.

What's the cause? Alcohol saps your body of water. The dehydration shrinks brain tissue and dilates blood vessels, which in turn tug at pain receptors. Ooh, what a headache. "Overindulgence in alcohol also can make you vomit, causing even worse dehydration," says Laurie Duncan, M.D., an internist who moved from Cooperstown, New York, to Washington, D.C. "Alcohol-induced dehydration and vomiting can be severe enough to require admission to a hospital," she adds.

In most cases, though, the ultimate cure is time. "Because of the way alcohol is metabolized, you can only wait for a hangover to go away," says David Whitaker, D.O., campus physician at the University of Rhode Island in Kingston. "That can take anywhere from several to many hours, depending on the amount of alcohol consumed."

Here's what you can do to make the wait tolerable.

Buffer That Aspirin

"My recommendation for hangovers is buffered aspirin and lots of fluids," says Paul Lena, M.D., a retired physician of internal medicine in Concord, New Hampshire. "Liquids restore the fluids, while aspirin reduces the pain." Take buffered aspirin to avoid an upset stomach.

Take a Strong Moral Dose

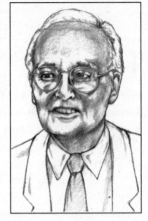

BEFORE I retired from my practice as a family doctor in Chelsea, Vermont, I used to take care of inmates in the Orange County (Vermont) Jail. For 20 years, I made daily rounds of the prisoners— an average of 15 of them at a time. A lot were in jail for drunkenness.

My treatment for their giant-size hangovers: I made them drink one glass of water every hour on the hour all day. And no aspirin. I wanted them to have all the agony and pain of a hangover so they might learn from it. If you mask the discomfort of a hangover, you aren't addressing the fundamental problem of alcoholism.

BREWSTER MARTIN, M.D., *a retired family doctor in Chelsea, Vermont (population 1,166), and cofounder of the Chelsea Family Health Center. He was named Vermont Doctor of the Year in 1991.*

Drink a Steady Trickle

"Take small amounts of fluids at frequent intervals, sipping slowly," says Lawrence H. Bernstein, M.D., a former family doctor who is the medical director at Jewish Geriatric Services in Longmeadow, Massachusetts. "Your body needs a lot of water, but you don't want to overstress it by gulping too much at once. That can make you vomit, worsening your dehydration. Let your body absorb the water at a moderate pace."

HAY FEVER

*Advice that eases
the wheezes and sneezes*

Ah, spring, when a body's fancy turns to . . . ah-CHOO. What is *that* all about?

What's happening is a serious case of mistaken identity. Your body is wonderful at fending off all kinds of invaders, from bacteria to viruses. The problem is, it can't always tell the bad guys—disease-causing attackers—from more benign substances. And so when some pollen or mold enters your body through your eyes, nose, or throat, your immune system kicks into overdrive. It produces powerful disease fighters called antibodies that head straight for the new substances, or allergens. The antibodies run smack into the allergens, and the resulting melee causes the release of chemicals, including histamine—the stuff that makes your sinuses swell, your eyes itch like crazy, and your nose feel as if it's about to ex . . . ex . . . ah-CHOO . . . explode.

"You can tell a hay fever sufferer from someone with a cold by the nose," says Robert F. Wilson, M.D., a pediatrician who is retired from his practice in Dover, New Hampshire. "The allergic nose itches and wiggles like a rabbit's. People with hay fever often wipe their noses straight up with the backs or palms of their hands. This stretches the tissue inside the nose, making them feel better." Dr. Wilson calls this form of scratching "the allergic salute."

It's the classic gesture for what doctors call allergic rhinitis, and what the rest of us call hay fever—an allergic reaction that hits more than 14 million Americans every year. Tree pollen is a common trigger in the early spring. Later in the summer, you get the pollen from grasses. Despite what your grandmother told you, most flowers won't make you sneeze. The pollen of most flowering species is too heavy to be carried by the wind into your nose. "People come in and tell me they have rose fever," says Wilfred Beaucher, M.D., an internist, allergist, and immunologist in Chelmsford, Massachusetts, and Nashua, New Hampshire. "But they're actually allergic to something else. Roses and other flowering plants have sticky pollen that needs bees to carry it from flower to flower. It is the plants with light, wind-borne pollen that cause most hay fever."

Plants may not be your problem, however. You may be allergic to molds instead—the fungi on spoiled bread or fruit, or the mildew on your old sneakers. Molds are all over the place, from your houseplants to the leaves on the ground to the natural ingredients in cheese and wine. Throw in pet dander, minuscule insect parts, and dust blowing from your house's heating system, and it's no wonder your immune system gets confused now and then.

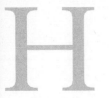

"The best indoor environment has no plants to collect dust and harbor mold in damp soil, no pets, and clean kitchens and bathrooms," Dr. Beaucher says. You could ditch your beloved plants and pets if you're a truly miserable allergy sufferer. In most cases, though, the remedies below are enough to help peace reign.

Get at the Pollen

"High-efficiency particulate filters, available from home and building supply stores, can help clean pollen from the air inside your house," says Sandra McCormack, A.R.N.P, a nurse-practitioner with Allergy Associates of New Hampshire in Portsmouth. "Install one in your bedroom."

Mug the Rug

"If you suffer from allergies, it is best not to have carpeting in your bedroom," McCormack says. "But if you do, sprinkle on either tannic acid or Acrosan—both available over the counter at drugstores and agricultural supply stores. These products denature the protein in dust mites and kill them." Dust mites, she explains, drop tiny feces that spark the immune systems in some allergy sufferers. Tannic acid can stain some rugs, McCormack warns, so you should experiment first on an obscure part of your carpet, such as the area under a chair.

Another way to blast the dust mites: "Put your scatter rugs outside for two days in the middle of winter," McCormack says. "The cold will kill the mites."

Dampen the Dust

"Don't vacuum the bare floor in the room of an allergy sufferer," McCormack warns. "A vacuum cleaner just pushes dust around. Instead, use a damp mop or dust cloth to pick up the dust."

Get Out Late

"Pollen counts are highest during the early-morning hours," Dr. Beaucher says. "If you have hay fever, jog in the afternoon or early evening. Or, better yet, save your run for a rainy day. Windy, dry days are the worst for hay fever sufferers."

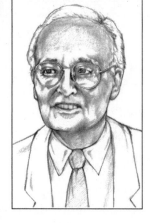

The Rug That Took Up a Collection

IN MY medical office, I had my old wall-to-wall carpeting replaced in the foyer and waiting room. It had been kept scrupulously clean, but after several years of heavy use was looking a bit threadbare in places.

When the workmen came to take it up, I asked them to sweep up what they found beneath the rug and matting and to weigh the results. From those two rooms, they collected 10 pounds of silt and dust—ideal habitat for allergy-causing dust mites.

If you have bad allergies, get rid of your wall-to-wall carpeting and stick to rugs you can sweep under. No matter how cleanly you live, dust mites will find safe harbor underneath a carpet if you can't get to the floor frequently.

BREWSTER MARTIN, M.D., *a retired family doctor in Chelsea, Vermont (population 1,166), and cofounder of the Chelsea Family Health Center. He was named Vermont Doctor of the Year in 1991.*

Dodge the Draft

"If you have hay fever, 'good fresh air' isn't good for you," Dr. Beaucher says. "You need to keep your windows closed tight and use an air conditioner with the vent closed."

Go Incognito

If you have hay fever and can't get someone else to mow your lawn, don't fire up the mower until you put on a pollen mask, Dr. Beaucher says. You can get pollen masks at your local drugstore.

Take a Drug

To combat the histamine by-product of your body's fight with allergens, you can take a variety of over-the-counter antihistamines. "The classic varieties are Benadryl and Chlor-Trimeton," Dr. Beaucher says. "They are inexpensive, but

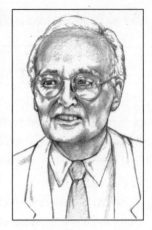

My Wife Screened My Calls

MY WIFE, Clara, was a marvelous doctor's wife. During the 40 years I ran our community's health center, she would answer the phone when patients called our home. It wasn't an easy job.

"Can I tell the doctor what the problem is?" she would ask. Some of these old farmers were pretty reticent about describing their problems to a woman. So Clara developed the technique of asking around the question. "Should I tell the doctor to bring the catheter or something to look in your ear?" she'd ask. "Is your problem above or below the belly button?" Clara died in 1990, the year before the University of Vermont gave me its Doctor of the Year award. I accepted it on behalf of both of us.

Clara knew the first technique of doctoring, and it's one you should use on your family as well: Know how to ask the right questions.

BREWSTER MARTIN, M.D., *a retired family doctor in Chelsea, Vermont (population 1,166), and cofounder of the Chelsea Family Health Center. He was named Vermont Doctor of the Year in 1991.*

they tend to make people drowsy." Alternatively, ask your physician for a nonsedating prescription antihistamine.

Chill Your Peepers

"If hay fever is making your eyes itchy, make a cool compress with a wet washcloth and cover your closed eyes with it," says Peter Mason, M.D., a family doctor in Lebanon, New Hampshire. "Another soothing remedy is a resealable plastic bag with crushed ice. Hold it against your eyes. The cold constricts the blood vessels, which helps reduce the swelling and itching." But be sure to place a thin towel between your skin and the bag and to leave the bag in place for no more than 15 minutes. The ice can actually freeze your skin if left on too long.

Salt Your Schnoz

"A nasal spray can help relieve the symptoms of hay fever by soothing your irritated mucous membranes," Dr. Mason says. "The spray also can ease congestion by clearing the discharge. Mix up eight ounces of warm water and half a teaspoon of salt. Stir until the salt dissolves and then put it in the refrigerator. You can use this mixture repeatedly in a nasal sprayer, which you can buy at your drugstore." If you can't find a sprayer, you can reuse the bottle from a store brand. Just be sure to clean it thoroughly.

Swallow Heat

To clear out the congestion of hay fever, grate some horseradish, mix it with a little honey, and eat it on a cracker, says Rosemary Gladstar, an herbalist in East Barre, Vermont, and author of *Herbal Healing for Women.*

HAYING OR LAWN-MOWING DISCOMFORT

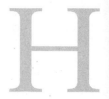

Stopping the itch that makes you say, "No mow!"

Nothing says summer and sunshine in the country more than haying—the age-old practice of cutting grass and putting it up in bales. It's beautiful to watch farmers mow their fields and wrestle the big bales onto their trucks or horse-drawn wagons. But if you've ever tried it yourself—or, more likely, if you've experienced the modern equivalent in mowing your lawn or raking dried grass—it may not seem so romantic. The hard, sweaty work can make you drier than—well, than the hay. Even worse is the prickly itch you can get from haying. Some people who are especially sensitive can develop a nasty rash.

"Generally, what causes haying discomfort is the bristliness of the cut hay," says Susie Tann, R.N., an elementary school nurse in Bradford, Vermont, and a breeder of Percheron draft horses. "Once you cut and dry the hay, the ends of the stems are scratchy. In addition, some people are allergic to timothy grass, which is a common form of hay.

The result is what doctors call contact dermatitis." Tann and her husband like to hay their 30 acres with horses, so they know what it is to itch. But they and their fellow country experts can tell you just what to do about it—even if *your* mowing problems stem from your own lawn.

Dress Up

"Some people are much more sensitive to hay than others," Tann notes. "My husband can hay bare-chested without any trouble. I think that is because he has a lot of hair on his chest and arms. I've known very few women to hay in a tank top." Tann wears a long-sleeved shirt when she hays. "The hay can really cut you and cause a rash that feels like nettles," she explains.

A WORD FROM DR. MARTIN

My Dad Thought I Was a Slacker

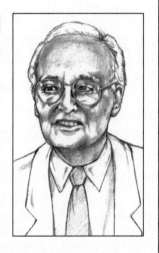

WHEN I was growing up on a Vermont farm, one of my summer chores was to even out the piles of hay in the hayloft. I had terrible hay fever and couldn't even breathe when I was up in that loft. I'd have to stop just to keep from fainting.

In those days, allergies were poorly understood. "This isn't a hotel," my father would say when he caught me stopping. "If you can't help with the haying, get yourself a job."

And that's exactly what I did. When I was 12, I found work peeling vegetables and washing dishes at a summer camp. I never spent another summer at home on the farm.

These days, I can take antihistamines for hay fever. But your best bet is to try to avoid what's making you miserable. I have a friend who has a big organic dairy operation, and I like to help out with the chores occasionally—except for anything having to do with hay. You still couldn't pay me to fork hay.

BREWSTER MARTIN, M.D., *a retired family doctor in Chelsea, Vermont (population 1,166), and cofounder of the Chelsea Family Health Center. He was named Vermont Doctor of the Year in 1991.*

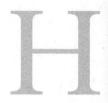

Or Try Soda

Kenneth Elder, an octogenarian and former dairy farmer in Lyme Center, New Hampshire, still does his mowing by hand. "If you're itchy when you're done haying, mix up baking soda and water and apply it wherever you itch," Elder says. "Leave it on for an hour or so, then wipe it off."

Go Jump in the Creek

"If I get all itchy after loading hay bales in the barn, I just go jump in the brook," says Timothy Bent, an emergency medical technician and farmer in Hanover, New Hampshire.

Mary-Catherine Gennaro, D.O., a family osteopath in Warren, New Hampshire, notes that both this watery remedy and the baking soda cure work only if the discomfort is "topical"—that is, only the surface of your skin is irritated. "If your itchiness is caused by an allergic reaction to breathing in grass pollen, you need to take an antihistamine," she says.

Stop the Allergy

To alleviate a skin rash that comes from a too-close encounter with hay, swallow 25 milligrams of the over-the-counter antihistamine Benadryl, says Paul Lena, M.D., a retired physician of internal medicine in Concord, New Hampshire.

HEADACHES
Ways to keep your lid from blowing

Chances are good that you've had a headache within the last month, especially if you're a woman. So there's no need to describe what it feels like and how it can ruin a perfectly good day. But not all headaches are alike, and for maximum effectiveness, the cures you choose should match the ache. Most headaches are tension headaches, which feel like a tight band around your head. The infamous migraine—a pulsing pain that usually hits one side of your head—is thought to stem from constricting and expanding blood vessels.

Lots of triggers cause other types of headaches, from a lack of water or blood sugar to a dying nerve in a tooth to eating something cold too fast. Sinus infections or a cold or

Even Puritans Got Headaches

BEFORE the medical world knew about caffeine, doctors were unwittingly prescribing the drug to cure headaches. "A Dish of Coffee;—yea and of Tea also . . . is a frequent Releef to Pains of the Head," wrote Cotton Mather, the famous Massachusetts Puritan.

"Caffeine does work for many kinds of headaches," confirms Richard Nordgren, M.D., a pediatric neurologist at the Dartmouth-Hitchcock Medical Center in Lebanon, New Hampshire. "You'll find caffeine in a great many over-the-counter headache remedies."

The early New Englanders didn't know everything about headaches, though. Mather also recommended anointing the temples with oil of nutmeg. "'Tis a famous Prescription," he said. And he approved of stopping a headache sufferer's nostrils with wool. Another early American remedy: hanging the head of a buzzard around your neck. "I wouldn't recommend it myself," Dr. Nordgren says.

the flu are other common causes, along with more serious illnesses such as Lyme disease, high blood pressure, a brain hemorrhage, or a stroke. A small group of sufferers, especially men ages 30 to 60, get nasty cluster headaches—pain that comes in waves that can last for months. "If you think you have cluster headaches, you should see your doctor," says Richard Nordgren, M.D., a pediatric neurologist at the Dartmouth-Hitchcock Medical Center in Lebanon, New Hampshire.

For most people, though, a headache is an annoying visitor that you'd rather not see coming. Here's how to show your pate pounder the door.

Take a Cure

"Acetaminophen, ibuprofen, and aspirin continue to be good over-the-counter remedies for most headaches," Dr. Nordgren says. "But don't give aspirin to children because of the risk of Reye's syndrome."

Chow Early

"Most of the headaches I see in kids before lunch are caused by their failing to eat breakfast," says Susie Tann, R.N., an

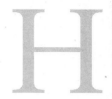

elementary school nurse in Bradford, Vermont. "I see far fewer headaches in the afternoon, because most kids eat at least something at lunchtime. Low blood sugar is a common cause of headaches. Make sure you keep yourself well-fueled throughout the day."

"Eating a good breakfast—plus a good lunch and dinner and maybe an apple for an afternoon snack—is a good idea," Dr. Nordgren confirms. "Low blood sugar can occasionally cause headaches."

Soak Your Head

"If a child comes in to see me with a headache, I prescribe water," Tann says. "The brain is among the first indicators of dehydration." Tann notes that an adult should drink at least two quarts of water during the day. "One third-grade teacher in our school tried an experiment," she says. "He put a squirt water bottle on each kid's desk so the students could drink throughout the day. The number of headaches went way down."

Get All 40 Winks

"I see many more children with headaches on Monday than on any other day, because they haven't gotten enough sleep over the weekend," Tann says. "You'll get fewer headaches if you get adequate rest."

Dr. Nordgren agrees. "Sleep is important in preventing headaches," he says.

Check the Eyes

"Once I've ruled out dehydration, low blood sugar, and lack of sleep, I ask headachy children about their eyes," Tann notes. "If they have glasses, have they been wearing them? If you're an adult with frequent headaches, you probably should get your eyes checked as well. Many headaches are caused by eyestrain."

TIME TO SEE THE DOCTOR

Don't Ignore a Hot Headache

IF YOUR headache is accompanied by a fever, you should consult your doctor, says Richard Nordgren, M.D., a pediatric neurologist at the Dartmouth-Hitchcock Medical Center in Lebanon, New Hampshire.

You also should get immediate medical attention if you have any of the following symptoms.
- Your headaches are getting worse.
- A headache wakes you in the night.
- You're also vomiting violently.
- You have a stiff neck.
- You're having trouble talking or with your coordination or vision.

And Paw Your Jaw

"Some headaches result from muscle tension caused by a mis-aligned jaw," says Robert Keene, D.M.D., a dentist in Hanover, New Hampshire. "To test your own jaw, lie flat on the floor. While holding the tip of your tongue up and back toward the roof of your mouth, let your lower jaw become rubbery and relaxed. Keep your tongue positioned back and up." Now gently close your back teeth together with a light tapping action. "Your back upper and lower teeth should all touch evenly at the same time on both sides of the mouth," Dr. Keene says. "If they don't, you should ask your dentist to evaluate your bite in what is called the centric relation position."

Take a Computer Break

"Staring at a computer screen can cause a tension headache," Dr. Nordgren says. "If you feel one coming on, move around a bit and try looking up and away from the computer every few minutes."

Go to Decaf Slowly

"Many headaches are caused by excessive amounts of caffeine or by caffeine withdrawal," Dr. Nordgren says. "Almost anyone who has been drinking four to six cups of coffee a day will get a headache if they suddenly stop drinking coffee. Try reducing your coffee intake gradually, over the span of a month. That way, you should be able to avoid caffeine withdrawal headaches."

HEAD LICE
Here's how you can quit the nits

A head louse is a small, flat insect that travels easily among children.

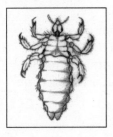

If your young one starts clawing his head as if he wants to get at its contents, it's time for a scalp examination. He could be harboring a healthy population of *Pediculus humanus capitis,* aka head lice.

"No way!" you protest. Your child is the epitome of hygiene. You enforce regular bath times, and his hair is kept as clean as any normal child's could be. You've always thought of head lice as the problem of poor or poorly supervised children.

Think again. "My practice provides coverage to 11 summer camps," says Mark Harris, M.D., a pediatrician in private practice in Bradford, Vermont. "Every single camp has an epidemic of head lice every year. These are girls from families who can afford to pay $4,500 for seven weeks of camp, and some of them show up with lice. Camp nurses now check the girls as they get off the bus."

Head lice travel easily. They get passed along when kids wrestle with each other or just share common space, such as a playroom. All it takes is a pioneering louse or two to establish a beachhead on your child's scalp.

Lice are small, flat insects that suck blood for nutrition. A chemical in their saliva prevents blood from clotting, making it easier for the louse to get its meal. This anticoagulant causes an allergic reaction in human skin, which is what your child's scratching is all about. The adult lice lay eggs, called nits, that stick like glue to shafts of hair close to the scalp. You can spot nits with the naked eye by plucking a few hairs from your kid's head and looking at them up close. (Wear gloves to keep the nits off you; head lice sometimes infest the body as well as the head.)

If you find nits, it's time for some serious debugging. Here's how to do it.

Nix 'Em

Nix, a cream rinse available over the counter at drugstores, "is the best thing there is for getting rid of lice," says Patricia Edwards, M.D., a pediatrician in private practice in Concord, New Hampshire. "All it should take is one application. If you still have a problem with your scalp a week later, talk to a doctor. Don't repeat the application."

Get Relief at Lash

Head lice can occupy your eyelashes as well as the hair on your head, according to Eugene J. Bernal, O.D., an op-

---

ANNALS OF MEDICINE

Whale Oil Didn't Work Either

THE kerosene from our grandparents' lamps was once a popular cure for head lice. "You'd put kerosene or coal oil on the kid's head, wrap the head up, and send the kid to school," says Everett Orbeton, M.D., a retired pediatrician who practiced in Portland, Maine. "The poison would kill the lice and nits dead as a doornail within 12 hours." That's the good news. The bad news is, kerosene can irritate the eyes and cause lung damage. That's why modern doctors would never recommend the treatment.

The Woman Who Saw the Point

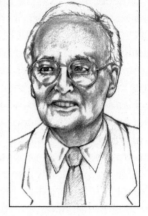

SCHOOLS go through epidemics of head lice. When that happened in my town, the school nurse would send a note home telling the parents to treat the infected child's head. The child couldn't return without a note from a parent saying that the lice had been treated.

One child kept coming in with lice over and over again, despite notes from her mother saying the girl had been treated. Finally, the school nurse refused to readmit the kid until she and her mother came to see me. I was the health officer for the area.

The mother admitted that she hadn't been treating her daughter. "I'm legally blind," she said. "I can't see well enough to do it."

"How did you get here?" I asked her.

"I drove," she said.

Without saying anything, I picked up the phone and started dialing.

"What are you doing?" she asked.

"I'm calling the state motor vehicles office," I replied. "If you can't see well enough to get the nits out of your daughter's hair, you're in no condition to drive."

"All right, all right, I'll do the delousing!" the mother said. And she did. Her daughter had no more lice problems after that.

Treating head lice properly is bothersome but very important. Don't procrastinate or make excuses.

BREWSTER MARTIN, M.D., *a retired family doctor in Chelsea, Vermont (population 1,166), and cofounder of the Chelsea Family Health Center. He was named Vermont Doctor of the Year in 1991.*

tometrist in White River Junction, Vermont. "Most louse remedies will irritate the corneas," Dr. Bernal says. "You can treat eyelashes by simply putting petroleum jelly on them at bedtime. It works by smothering the lice. Smear on petroleum jelly once a day for five to seven days." Really stubborn critters may have to be spotted—and removed—under a special ophthalmologist's microscope. "Your family doctor might not have one, in which case you can go to your eye doctor," Dr. Bernal says.

Outwit the Nits

Even if the nits are dead, they may be hard to remove. "They glue themselves in place," Dr. Edwards explains. "So try this trick. The morning after you've treated your hair with Nix, rinse it with vinegar. Then wrap your head in a towel for 20 minutes. That will allow the vinegar to loosen the glue. You can comb the nits right out."

Don't Let the Bugs Bite

If your child has had head lice, follow up the youngster's treatment with some serious washing of bedsheets and clothing, Dr. Harris advises. "Any cloth that's been in contact with your child should be put through the washing machine," he says. Also do a thorough vacuuming job on the bedroom and playroom.

"You don't have to overreact, though," Dr. Harris says. "An infestation of lice will go away if it has nothing to feed on. A louse that's gone without blood for 72 hours is incapable of infesting anyone." So a lingering louse or two on the floor will be harmless after a few days, even if your vacuum cleaner missed it.

HEARING LOSS
Sound strategies for dealing with an all-too-quiet world

You may be in top shape, with a full head of hair, all your own teeth, and a youthful waistline, but one of Father Time's calling cards is nearly impossible to avoid: a problem hearing sounds, especially those in the high-frequency range. The twittering of birds, the shrill of a piccolo, even the voices of children cause you to cock your head and strain to hear.

"High-frequency hearing loss is associated with age," says Robert Fagelson, M.D., an otolaryngologist in private practice in Brattleboro, Vermont. By age 60, Dr. Fagelson says, most people suffer some degree of hearing loss, and the decline proceeds steadily after age 70. "You can't cure this kind of hearing loss, but you can treat it and learn to live with it," he says.

You also can keep Old Man Time from arriving early by protecting your ears from sound assaults. "The degree of damage your ears sustain from loud noises depends on both the volume of the sound and how long it lasts," Dr. Fagelson notes.

Not all hearing loss is progressive or inevitable. A ruptured eardrum can cause sudden deafness. Calcium growth in the inner ear, called otosclerosis, can block hearing. Certain antibiotics can cause some people to lose their hearing. Ear infections can turn down your hearing volume. A change of air pressure in the inner ears, caused by an airplane flight, diseases such as inflamed tonsils or enlarged adenoids, or even the grunting effort of sports such as weight lifting, can cause temporary hearing loss, according to Paul Lena, M.D., a retired physician of internal medicine in Concord, New Hampshire. "A change in the air pressure in the ear canal pushes the eardrum against the bones of your inner ear, causing a hearing problem," Dr. Lena says. And, of course,

---

TIME TO SEE THE DOCTOR

Has the Sound Been Turned Down Suddenly?

ANY unexplained, sudden hearing loss should send you to the doctor," says Paul Lena, M.D., a retired physician of internal medicine in Concord, New Hampshire. "A specialist can examine your eardrum and the three bones in the ear for possible disease that can be corrected by microsurgery."

If you're suddenly having trouble hearing low-frequency sounds, such as a dog's low growl, the problem could be something blocking your ear passages, Dr. Lena says. If your low-frequency problem comes on gradually, the loss may be hereditary. A problem in hearing both low- and high-frequency sounds "will arouse the doctor's suspicion of a problem with the eardrum or the mechanism behind the drum," Dr. Lena adds. "That's fixable."

So is a thickened eardrum, caused by repeated ear infections during childhood, which make the drum move sluggishly, diminishing hearing. "In that case, the eardrum can be replaced to improve hearing," Dr. Lena notes.

My Son Played His Cards Right

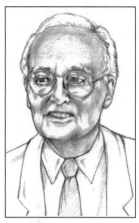

MY SON David was born severely hearing impaired. He was an unusually smart kid as well. Even as a little boy, he loved to play cards, and by the age of 11, he was good enough to be called upon by the older women in the town to make up a fourth for bridge.

David more than held his own against his more experienced opponents. He quickly acquired a reputation for reading the minds of players—seeming to know exactly what cards were in their hands. But it wasn't their minds he was reading; it was their lips. He noticed that some players mumbled, seemingly incoherently, when they looked at their cards. Being an excellent lip-reader, he could understand everything they said. He was an exceptional card counter as well, a useful skill in bridge. No one could ever say David was handicapped at cards.

Play to your strengths and don't dwell on your weaknesses. David has lived this advice.

BREWSTER MARTIN, M.D., *a retired family doctor in Chelsea, Vermont (population 1,166), and cofounder of the Chelsea Family Health Center. He was named Vermont Doctor of the Year in 1991.*

anything stuck in the ear—from wax buildup to a piece from a child's toy—can stop hearing as effectively as a store-bought earplug.

Here's what you can do when the world gets uncomfortably quieter.

Ditch the Wax

"The most common cause of sudden hearing loss is a buildup of earwax," Dr. Lena says. "You should avoid the use of Q-Tips, which tend to push wax back down into the ear canal. Most ear canals are about three-quarters the diameter of an eraser on a Number 2 pencil, so it doesn't take too much of a buildup to block the entrance."

H

Dr. Lena says that before he retired, he saw many patients with earwax that had built up so much it had become impacted. He even equipped his office with special surgical instruments so that he and a nurse could remove the wax. "We saved the trouble and expense of sending the patient to a specialist," he says. "It's a simple procedure that can seem miraculous to a patient whose hearing is blocked by wax."

Seek Aids

Hearing loss that can't be fixed mechanically can often be corrected by a hearing aid, Dr. Fagelson notes. He recommends getting examined by a doctor first to eliminate any correctable problems and to get advice on the most suitable equipment for you.

Hear ye, hear ye: Aids come in many designs, including one that's anchored behind the ear (A) and another that fits entirely inside (B).

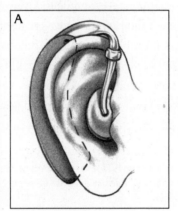
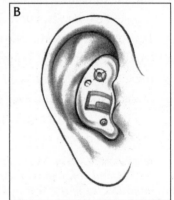

Use Your Eyes

"One of my sons is deaf," says Brewster Martin, M.D., a retired family doctor in Chelsea, Vermont. "My wife had German measles when she was six weeks pregnant, which destroyed the boy's hearing. He went away to school when he was three to learn sign language and to lip-read." Dr. Martin notes that it's never too late to improve your lip-reading skills. "Teach yourself to examine faces closely when people talk to you," he says. "We all lip-read to a certain degree, whether we admit it or not. As you age, you need to be more aware of that skill and to use it to your advantage."

Give Your Ear a Plug

Earplugs are an excellent way of reducing the impact of loud machinery such as a lawn mower or chain saw, Dr. Fagelson

HEARING LOSS

says. To prevent any further deterioration of your hearing, it would be smart to consider wearing them even at loud concerts, though it may be a tad hard to convince your teenager of that. A rock group can generate almost as much sound as a jet engine.

The best earplugs to buy are made of silicone. "Work each earplug with your fingers until it's pliable, then make a little bump on one side of the plug—the side that goes into the ear canal," Dr. Fagelson says. Leave the other side large. "That keeps the plug from going too deep into the ear canal and causing damage." A popular brand is Mack's Earplugs, available in six- and four-pair sets at drugstores across the nation.

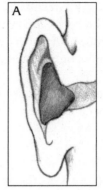
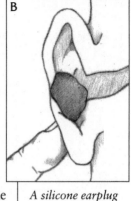

A silicone earplug can be molded into the proper shape to fit the entrance of the ear canal (A). When the noise ends, you just push from the back of the ear and out pops the plug (B).

HEARTBURN

When you can't stand the heat that starts in the kitchen

It's bad enough that you regret pigging out on that pepperoni pizza. Half an hour to an hour later, your body metes out severe punishment: a nasty burning behind your sternum, or chest bone.

So what's the pain doing up there if your stomach is the organ that took the abuse? The problem started in your abdomen, all right. Gastric acid, which can be about as strong as battery acid, builds up after a big or spicy meal and creeps upward in a process called reflux. Usually the acid is stopped from heading beyond the stomach into the esophagus by the lower esophageal sphincter, a muscle. But if the acid builds up too much, or if the sphincter isn't in top shape, the burn can spread upward, giving you that nasty burning feeling.

You may not be the one to blame. If you're pregnant or over 40, your sphincter probably doesn't have the spring it had when you were young, which is why you suffer heartburn more than some other people. You also can get heartburn from chronic digestion problems. "Another common cause of chest pain is muscular or skeletal in origin," says

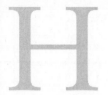

Mark Greenberg, M.D., a cardiologist at the Dartmouth-Hitchcock Medical Center in Lebanon, New Hampshire. "If your pain is sharp and lasts about a second, and if it hurts to press on your chest, you could have a muscle pull or an inflamed cartilage. The pain can be relieved with some acetaminophen or aspirin and a warm bath." (Don't give aspirin to children because of the risk of Reye's syndrome.)

More serious is angina, a sharp pain or a feeling of heaviness in the chest that comes from coronary artery disease. "If you can't pinpoint the cause of your chest pain, get yourself to a doctor immediately," Dr. Greenberg says. "Significant chest discomfort that lasts for more than 15 minutes may indicate a heart attack."

According to Linda B. Dacey, M.D., an internist at the Dartmouth-Hitchcock Medical Center in Lebanon, New Hampshire, if it hurts to lie down or bend over, you probably have plain old heartburn, which you can ease with these home remedies.

Retire on Empty

"Don't eat a big meal just before bedtime," Dr. Greenberg cautions. "Eat two or three hours before you sack out." When you eat, your stomach produces acid to digest the food. "If you lie down soon after eating, you're more likely to get reflux," he says.

Eat Small

It's a good idea to avoid giant meals altogether, according to Peter Mason, M.D., a family doctor in Lebanon, New Hampshire. "Overeating stimulates the stomach to put out even more acid than is necessary, causing a condition called rebound hyperacidity. Your stomach prepares for the next big meal by producing extra acid, and the acid is the most important factor in producing heartburn."

Skip the Aspirin

"Avoid aspirin if you suffer from heartburn," says Lawrence H. Bernstein, M.D., a former family doctor who is the medical director at Jewish Geriatric Services in Longmeadow, Massachusetts. "Aspirin can mess up the mucous lining in your esophagus, making acid reflux worse."

Is It a Burn or an Attack?

YOUR chest pain may not be heartburn at all—it could be a sign of coronary heart disease, the leading cause of death in the United States. How can you tell whether you're having a heart attack or suffering from plain old indigestion?

"A heart attack may involve a whole constellation of symptoms, not just chest pain," says Laurie Duncan, M.D., an internist who moved from Cooperstown, New York, to Washington, D.C. "Among the signs that your chest pain is a heart attack are pain across your upper stomach, nausea, sweating, heart palpitations, pain down the back or inside of the arm, pain in the left side of the jaw, pain across the back or the shoulders, or just a sharp pain in the elbows.

"Sometimes a heart attack may present as indigestion. If you're having persistent and unremitting indigestion, you should be evaluated in an emergency room by a physician."

Other signs of heart trouble:

- The pain increases with any physical activity and feels better when you rest.
- You're suffering from shortness of breath.
- You feel dizzy or light-headed.

"When in doubt, get to a doctor right away," Dr. Duncan advises, "especially if you or your family has a history of heart trouble."

Avoid the Ups and Downs

"Stay away from caffeine and alcohol," Dr. Bernstein says. "Both are bad for digestion, and bad digestion often means heartburn."

Sleep on a Slope

"Elevate the head of your bed four to six inches by putting blocks of wood or bricks under the bedposts at the head of the bed," Dr. Bernstein advises. "You want to sleep with your stomach on a slant. You can't do that by propping yourself up with pillows, because that position still brings your esophagus and ribs together, opening the lower esophageal sphincter and letting acid creep up."

Act on the Acid

"Take antacids at bedtime if you tend to suffer from heartburn at night," Dr. Bernstein says. "Pepcid AC and Tagamet

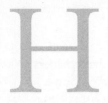

HB work well. They're available over the counter, and they can help heartburn dramatically."

Deal With Stress

"Much of our acid production is hereditary in nature, but stress does play a role," Dr. Mason notes. "Anxiety can cause your stomach to produce more acid. And if you are under stress, you may be more likely to indulge in bad habits that hurt digestion, such as smoking, drinking, and overeating." Reduce your stress, he suggests, and you may be able to cure your heartburn at the same time.

HEART PALPITATIONS

*Help when your heart travels
to the beat of a different drummer*

Does your ticker occasionally mark time in some strange ways—skipping a beat once in a while, thumping dramatically, or perhaps racing in high gear? Chances are, your condition isn't life threatening. "Irregular heartbeats are quite common, and many need no treatment," says Robert G. Page, M.D., a retired cardiologist who lives in Londonderry, Vermont.

But don't assume your heart is pumping perfectly until you get it checked. "Some palpitations are dangerous," Dr. Page warns. "If you can't set a metronome to your heartbeat, you need to see a doctor."

Dr. Page also recommends regular checkups if you're one of the 40 percent of Americans who suffer from paroxysmal atrial tachycardia, or PAT. This is when your heart occasionally kicks into high gear, beating 120, 140, even 220 times a minute for as long as half an hour. You don't need to fear for your heart—all that racing rarely does serious damage. But your high-paced ticker could be suffering from some other problem, he says.

Here are some ways to deal with the discomforts of PAT and other forms of heart palpitations. Before you try any of these remedies, of course, you should receive an okay from your doctor.

Shyness Was the Mother of Invention

IN 1816, a French doctor named René Théophile Hyacinthe La'nnec invented the stethoscope as a modest way to listen to the heart of a young woman. In those days, even doctors—respectable ones, anyway—didn't just press an ear to a patient's chest. So La'nnec rolled up some papers and listened through the tube. To his amazement, he heard the woman's heart more clearly than he ever had with the naked ear. He refined the instrument by making a wooden version with separate pieces for the chest and ear. The modern, two-eared version with flexible tubing was the invention of an American doctor, George P. Cammann, in 1852.

The shy doctor's experiment with rolled papers (A) inspired him to make a sturdier stethoscope. That wooden version (B) was the precursor of the modern instrument. And so modesty served medicine.

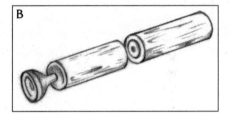

Hold Your Breath

If you have a bout of PAT, you may be able to get your heart rate down by taking a deep breath, holding it and bearing down for about 10 seconds, and then suddenly letting it go, Dr. Page says.

Live Right

"Heart palpitations can be caused by smoking, drinking, caffeine, or stress," says Mark Greenberg, M.D., a cardiologist at the Dartmouth-Hitchcock Medical Center in Lebanon, New Hampshire. "Avoid these heart strainers, and you may find that your palpitations are gone."

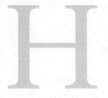

HEAT EXHAUSTION
Keeping hot weather from bringing you down

Summertime, and the living is easy—unless too much outdoor life makes you feel like something the cat dragged in. An overdose of sun and an underdose of liquids can combine to give you a powerful thirst along with a few more discomforts. "As you begin to overheat, you tend to sweat, feel a bit weak and dizzy, and maybe feel a little queasy in your stomach," says John Dunn, M.D., an emergency room physician at the Northwestern Medical Center in St. Albans, Vermont. Headache, stomachache, and muscle cramps are

---

TIME TO SEE THE DOCTOR
When the Sweating Stops

Heat exhaustion can usually be treated in the field," says John Dunn, M.D., an emergency room physician at the Northwestern Medical Center in St. Albans, Vermont. "But heatstroke is a medical emergency. You need help as soon as possible." Signs of heatstroke include dizziness, trouble walking, confusion, and blacking out after long exposure to heat or sun. Heatstroke victims also have dry skin and often seem sleepy.

The differences between heat exhaustion and heatstroke are body temperature and sweat. "You sweat with heat exhaustion. With heatstroke, you don't," Dr. Dunn says. He explains that with heatstroke, the body's cooling mechanisms have shut down and the temperature soars to 104°F or higher. A fever that high can

be life threatening, so aggressive treatment is necessary. That means providing rapid cooling, Dr. Dunn says. "Call an ambulance, then splash cool water on the person. If you're in the woods, immersion in a cold stream is best. If you're in civilization, get into an air-conditioned room right away."

Dr. Dunn once helped treat a heatstroke victim about as far from air-conditioning as you can get—at the Appalachian Mountain Club's Greenleaf Hut in the White Mountain National Forest of New Hampshire, several hours away from the nearest road. "We put him in the hut's water tank and then packed him in frozen food that the hut crew had packed in for dinner," he recalls. "It saved the man's life and thawed out our dinner at the same time."

---

common symptoms of heat exhaustion, and the feeling of nausea can even lead to a bout of vomiting.

If you're with someone who has heat exhaustion, watch him closely. "Some other illnesses exhibit the same symptoms," Dr. Dunn explains. One of those illnesses is heart trouble. "Shortness of breath or a squeezing pain in the heart is cause for getting someone to the hospital as quickly as possible."

For the run-of-the-mill sweaty fatigue that spells heat exhaustion, here are some cooling cures. "People usually respond quickly to treatments for heat exhaustion," Dr. Dunn notes. "You should start feeling better in 15 to 20 minutes."

Get to Shade

"The first thing to do for heat exhaustion is to get out of the sun," says Harry Rowe, M.D., a family doctor in Wells River, Vermont. "Get to a cool place and drink a lot of fluid. I don't see as much heat exhaustion as I used to. Most people don't work hard outside anymore. I do see some people who play too hard, though."

Make Some Weather

"The best way to cool down someone suffering from heat exhaustion is to spray her with water and then have her sit or lie in front of a fan," says Douglas Deaett, M.D., an emergency room physician at the Alice Peck Day Memorial Hospital in Lebanon, New Hampshire. "The fan helps evaporate the water for instant cooling."

Towel Up

"If you are overheating, put a wet towel on your head and loosely tie cool, wet cloths around your neck and wrists," says Sarah Johansen, M.D., medical di-

Cool aid can be yours in the form of wet cloths on your head, neck, and wrists.

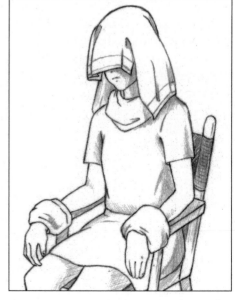

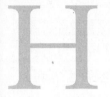

rector of emergency services at New London Hospital in New London, New Hampshire. "Even if you can't get out of the sun, a wet cloth can be surprisingly cooling."

Change Shape

"If you tend to suffer from heat exhaustion a lot, you might need to lose weight," Dr. Deaett says. "The round bodies of obese people are the most efficient for retaining heat."

HEAT RASH

Got the summer pricklies?
Here's how to chill out

One un-air-conditioned bus ride, and you feel prickly all over. And then you see spots—on you, no less!

Don't get even hotter under the collar. Your itchy spots are probably just a heat rash, also called prickly heat. According to Kathryn A. Zug, M.D., a dermatologist at the Dartmouth-Hitchcock Medical Center in Lebanon, New Hampshire, "A heat rash comes from sweating too much. Moisture gets trapped in the sweat glands, causing a rash that doctors call miliaria. You can see little blisters, often with tiny red dots, and your skin feels irritated."

Seek these remedies for your overheated hide.

Get the Temp Down

"Take a cool bath as soon as you can," Dr. Zug advises. "Lowering your skin's temperature will help get rid of the blistering and prickliness."

AN OUNCE OF PREVENTION

Do Some Shedding

I SEE a lot of heat rash in children in the spring," says Patricia Edwards, M.D., a pediatrician in private practice in Concord, New Hampshire. "Parents are still bundling up their babies, while the sun really heats up the car. Dress your child for the temperature of the place he's in."

Get Help from the Kitchen Cupboard

"Lightly dust skin that has a heat rash with cornstarch," says Patricia Edwards, M.D., a pediatrician in private practice in Concord, New Hampshire. "That will help soak up some of the excess sweat, relieving the problem that caused the rash in the first place."

Stop the Itch

"If the heat rash is very itchy," Dr. Zug says, "try taking over-the-counter Benadryl for some relief." Benadryl is an antihistamine that counters your skin's allergic reaction to summer substances around you.

Get in the Pink

"For an itchy heat rash, you can dab on some calamine lotion," says John C. Robinson, M.D., a pediatrician in private practice in Quincy, Massachusetts. Calamine soothes itchy skin, he explains.

Start a Smear Campaign

"A very bland moisturizer can help relieve the dry, scaly, itchy kind of rash," Dr. Zug says. She warns her patients away from more expensive moisturizers, especially those that are heavily perfumed. "Scents used in over-the-counter preparations can cause allergic reactions in some people." It's also a good idea to stay away from products that contain essential oils. "The concentrations of these oils are often high and may cause allergic reactions in some people," Dr. Zug notes.

HEMORRHOIDS

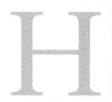

Bringing your rear troubles to an end

Cotton Mather, the great Massachusetts Puritan and amateur physician, wrote so movingly about hemorrhoids that you can't help thinking he must have suffered from them himself. "The Patient ought certainly to humble himself before God and Man, and walk softly under the Humiliations of such a Malady. The Seat of it, in the Parts of Dishonour, which can't be mentioned among people of any Breeding without a sort of Blush, seems to oblige the Sufferer unto Self-Abasement," he said, noting that a whole nation of "Wicked People" in the Bible were "smote in the Hinder Parts."

You know what "walking softly" is all about if you've experienced the pain and itching of hemorrhoids. Awful as they are, though, their causes—and cures—aren't terribly com-

H

plicated. (Mather recommended swallowing the sweaty leather of a ground-up shoe, but better cures have been developed since then.) Hemorrhoids are nothing more than swollen veins in the "hinder parts." "They're simply varicose veins," says Thomas Roy, M.D., a former New England cardiologist who now practices in Minocqua, Wisconsin. "You don't get varicose veins just in the legs."

Hemorrhoids often show up just outside the anus, where you can see them. At other times, they grow inside the rectum, where only a doctor can scope them out. Either way, the most common way to get them is by straining—either to pass a stool or to give birth to a child. The straining forces blood into the veins, which causes them to swell and become varicose. Overzealous wiping also can damage the veins, which explains why doctors think diarrhea as well as constipation might be a factor in causing hemorrhoids.

TIME TO SEE THE DOCTOR

Are You Seeing Red?

HAVE your doctor take a look if you're seeing blood in your stools or on your toilet paper. Also get a checkup if you experience a change in your bowel habits.

And what can you do about them? Our country doctors offer some comforting hints.

Get at the Sore

"What I find works best is an over-the-counter suppository called Anusol," says Laurence Bouchard, D.O., an osteopathic family physician in private practice in Narragansett, Rhode Island. "You can get it at most drugstores. Just follow the directions on the label."

Meet Hazel

"I tell people to put a dab of witch hazel on their toilet paper and apply it directly to their hemorrhoids," Dr. Bouchard says. "It's very soothing." Witch hazel can be found at most pharmacies and health food stores.

Clean Up

"Cleanse the hemorrhoids as best you can," Dr. Bouchard advises. "Use wipes such as Tucks, which contain alcohol to help dry the sores. The alcohol may cause a little burning, but anything is better than the itching."

Bulk Up

"You can help your hemorrhoids heal, and prevent new ones from coming in, by getting more fiber in your diet," Dr. Bouchard says. Cruciferous vegetables such as brussels sprouts, broccoli, and cabbage are high in fiber. So are salad mixings such as carrots and beans, along with bran muffins, any whole grain bread, squash, potatoes, and apples.

Or Buy Your Fiber

"Take two teaspoons of over-the-counter Metamucil, a natural form of fiber, before bedtime," Dr. Bouchard says. "Add a teaspoon or two more after a couple of weeks if your stomach doesn't object."

HICCUPS
Boo! Still doing the hics?
Then try these cures

Early New Englanders called it "the Hicket" or "hiccoughs" and prescribed sneezing as a surefire cure. You've doubtless had friends recommend remedies of their own, some of them worse than the hiccups themselves.

That may be because most cures tend to work—at least once. "Hiccups are a spasm of the diaphragm, the muscle that controls your breathing," says David Sigelman, M.D., a pediatrician with Holyoke Pediatric Associates in Holyoke, Massachusetts. "They usually go away on their own within half an hour, so anything you did just before your hiccups stopped looks like the ideal cure."

Doctors aren't sure why people get hiccups in the first place—they don't perform any practical function. Spicy or gassy foods can bring on a bout. A sudden gulp of air can bring them on. So can an emotional upset. Whatever the cause, here's how you can nix the hics.

Give 'Em a Push

"Push down with your innards as if you were having a bowel movement," says Lawrence H. Bernstein, M.D., medical director at Jewish Geriatric Services in Longmeadow, Massa-

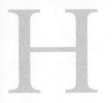

H

chusetts. "This technique, which doctors call the Valsalva maneuver, squeezes the diaphragm and can stop the spasms."

Try This Gag

"Stick your finger partway down your throat to make yourself gag," Dr. Bernstein says. "By retching a bit, you can change the signals your brain sends to the diaphragm, stopping the hiccups."

Sweeten Up

"Swallow one teaspoon of dry sugar," says Brewster Martin, M.D., a retired family doctor in Chelsea, Vermont. "This is a tried-and-true remedy. I don't know why it works, but it does."

Cover Up

"Put your hands over your face and breathe in and out fast," says Robert F. Wilson, M.D., a retired pediatrician who practiced for 37 years in Dover, New Hampshire. "It's the old paper bag trick, only you don't need the bag. The rapid breathing and the buildup of carbon dioxide change the pattern of your diaphragm rhythm."

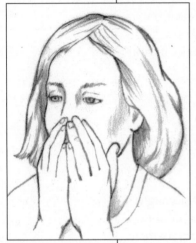

To get rid of hiccups, catch your breath—literally.

HIGH BLOOD PRESSURE

Turn down the volume on your overstressed system

Doctors call high blood pressure the silent killer because it may not cause you any trouble—right up to the moment when heart or kidney trouble strikes. Shortness of breath and severe headaches can be a sign that your pressure is in the danger zone, but "the only sure way to tell your blood pressure is to get it checked," says Robert G. Page, M.D., a retired cardiologist in Londonderry, Vermont. It's a good idea to check your pressure at least once a year. See your doctor for the checkup, try one of the blood pressure machines available at many pharmacies, or watch the newspaper for the

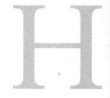

next public health fair, where pressure checks are usually done for free. If you're a normal, healthy person, your pressure should register less than 140 over 90.

Thanks in part to doctors' increasing understanding of high blood pressure and ways to treat it, deaths from heart attack and stroke have been declining for the past several decades. It's important to consult your doctor if you suffer from high blood pressure. She may put you on prescription medication. You also may be able to help things along with these down-home approaches to turning down the pressure.

A WORD FROM DR. MARTIN

Swing Low, Sweet Blood Pressure

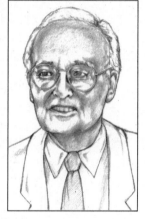

WHEN I was a young doctor of 40, I went for my usual pressure check. The diagnosis: high blood pressure. That's a tough diagnosis at that age. The chances of a 40-year-old male with high blood pressure getting heart disease are higher than for a man with normal pressure, unless he takes care of himself. If he has three other risk factors—such as a bad diet, lack of exercise, and a family history of heart trouble—his chances of having a heart attack within eight years are as high as 70 percent.

So I took care of myself. I got thoroughly tested and made sure it was okay to exercise without danger. Exercise is great for high blood pressure because it dilates the blood vessels, opening things up. It also releases your body's endorphins—natural painkillers that help lower stress.

Ever since that diagnosis, I have worked out an hour every day. I jogged for years. I still ride my bike 15 to 20 miles a day in the summer. In the winter, I cross-country ski. In between, I walk five miles a day. I am now over 70 years old and still addicted to exercise. That's a pretty good addiction to have.

BREWSTER MARTIN, M.D., *a retired family doctor in Chelsea, Vermont (population 1,166), and cofounder of the Chelsea Family Health Center. He was named Vermont Doctor of the Year in 1991.*

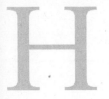

Let Go the Shaker

"If you have high blood pressure, you need to watch your salt intake," says F. Daniel Golyan, M.D., a former New Englander who is now an electrophysiologist in private practice on Long Island. "Read the labels on prepared foods. There is a great deal of salt in canned sodas, canned beans, and especially canned soups." Your doctor may tell you to restrict your salt to four grams of sodium a day—or to less than half that if you have a serious pressure problem.

Free Yourself of Fat

"Losing weight will help reduce your blood pressure," says Mark Greenberg, M.D., a cardiologist at the Dartmouth-Hitchcock Medical Center in Lebanon, New Hampshire. "Lose weight gradually, though, with your doctor's guidance."

Forget Your Pet Peeves—Get a Pet

"Stress and anger can raise your blood pressure," says Sarah Johansen, M.D., medical director of emergency services at New London Hospital in New London, New Hampshire. "Anything that relieves stress is good for your blood pressure. Keeping a pet may be good for you. Make sure you get out and see friends. And keep laughing."

Walk Your Heart

"You need to exercise to lower your blood pressure," Dr. Golyan says. "Take a brisk walk for 30 to 45 minutes at least three times a week. Walk steadily without a break. The point is to exercise your heart over a sustained period."

HIGH CHOLESTEROL
There's good and there's bad.
Here's how to maximize the good

It seems as if everyone is talking about cholesterol these days, and for good reason. Cholesterol, a fatty, gunky substance in your blood, is a leading cause of heart disease, and heart disease is the leading cause of death in this country. If you want to lower your chances of having heart trouble, or if you

How High Is Your Risk?

A DOCTOR's checkup will determine whether you have a cholesterol problem. If your LDL cholesterol is higher than 200, your doctor will suggest ways to bring it down—which may include prescription medicines.

The doctor also might suggest drugs if your high cholesterol is accompanied by one or more other risk factors for heart disease, including the following:

- A family history of heart problems
- High blood pressure
- A smoking habit
- Diabetes

If you already have been diagnosed with heart disease, and you have two or more risk factors, your doctor may want to get your LDL cholesterol below 160—a process that may take months of changes in your diet and lifestyle as well as medication.

---

want to ease existing heart problems, you need to get your cholesterol down.

That is, you need to get your *bad* cholesterol down. There's also a good kind, called high-density lipoprotein, or HDL, cholesterol. Low-density lipoprotein, or LDL, cholesterol, is the bad stuff that can gunk up your heart, veins, and arteries. "The LDL particles stick to the lining of your blood vessels and narrow the passageways, restricting blood flow much as rust in your pipes slows the flow of water in your bathroom," says Hugh P. Hermann, M.D., a family doctor in private practice in Woodstock, Vermont. "Sometimes a piece of this deposited plaque can break off and block a smaller vessel. This can cause a heart attack or stroke."

For reasons still largely a mystery to medical science, HDL helps to counteract the effects of LDL. "You want your HDL, or good, cholesterol to be over 40, and your LDL, or bad, cholesterol to be below 130," Dr. Hermann says. By contrast, an HDL under 40 combined with an LDL over 200 can put you at risk for heart disease.

The only way to tell whether you have too much bad cholesterol is to have your doctor send a blood sample to a medical laboratory, which tests the concentration of both HDL and LDL cholesterol (in milligrams per decaliter) in your blood. "A high-fat diet is a big factor in giving people a high

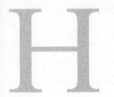

LDL count," Dr. Hermann says. "So are your genes. If your parents had a high count, chances are you do, too." He adds that overweight people tend to have higher counts than thin people.

Strangely enough, though, some *extremely* thin people have high cholesterol. "Too little fat can give you high cholesterol levels, just as too much fat can," says Marcia Herrin, Ed.D., M.P.H., R.D., coordinator of the Nutrition Education Program at Dartmouth College in Hanover, New Hampshire. "One way to tell whether a person has anorexia nervosa—starving herself to get skinny—is to test for a high cholesterol level. If your teenager has high cholesterol and has lost weight, you should be talking to a doctor."

For most of us, however, lowering cholesterol is mostly a matter of following the advice of our country doctors.

Don't Drop All Fat

"You want to lower your fat intake to lower your cholesterol," Dr. Herrin says. "But don't go to extremes, or you might lower your good cholesterol along with your bad." Most Americans take in nearly 40 percent of their calories in the form of fat. "You'd do a lot better eating about 20 to 30 percent fat," she says. "But don't go below 20 percent unless your doctor prescribes it."

If the math gets too complicated for you, Dr. Herrin says you should ask your doctor to tell you how many grams of fat you should be eating per day. "For most people, 40 to 60 grams of fat a day is healthy. Most of the food you buy in the supermarket is labeled for fat content. Determining how much you're taking in each day is a simple matter of addition if you eat mostly labeled food."

Sacrifice Your Breath

"To lower your bad cholesterol, eat lots of garlic or take an over-the-counter garlic supplement, available at health food stores and many grocery stores," Dr. Herrin says. "I cook with garlic all the time." In laboratory studies, garlic has been shown to reduce cholesterol levels in the blood.

Go to Sea

"Fish oil has been shown to lower LDL cholesterol while increasing beneficial HDL cholesterol in the blood," Dr. Herrin says. "Eating fish at least two or three times a week can help bring your levels to where you want them. That doesn't mean you have to eat fish dinners all the time. A tuna fish sandwich at lunch—watch the mayo—does the same thing."

Take a Walk-On Part

"A great way to increase your good HDL cholesterol is to exercise," says Mary-Catherine Gennaro, D.O., a family osteopath in Warren, New Hampshire. "If you don't want to spend money on fancy health clubs, go for a daily walk of at least 20 minutes." Researchers say that a fast walk works better than a meandering stroll.

Increase Your Roughage

"Adding more fiber to your diet can lower your cholesterol count," Dr. Gennaro says. "A really tasty way to do this without adding fat is to bake bran muffins, replacing the oil in the recipe with the same amount of applesauce. You also can eat a high-fiber cereal. I snack on Kellogg's Raisin Squares—shredded wheat with raisins in the middle. I eat them instead of potato chips."

Do This Regularly

"For high cholesterol, try taking Metamucil, an over-the-counter fiber remedy for constipation," Dr. Gennaro advises. "Take one teaspoonful two or three times a day to flush your system of cholesterol."

HIP PAIN

Too sore to hula?
Get hip to these remedies

You'd think that pain in such a big joint would be easy to pinpoint, but the hip is a tricky place for hurts, says Raymond Rocco Monto, M.D., an orthopedic surgeon at Martha's Vineyard Orthopedic Surgery and Sports Medicine in Oak Bluffs, Massachusetts. "A problem in the hip can cause pain somewhere else, such as your groin or your knee. And pain that starts elsewhere in your body also can be felt in your hip. Doctors call that referred pain."

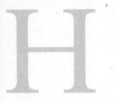H Improperly fitting shoes, a poor mattress, a knee injury, obesity, running, and weight-training exercises can all throw your hip out of whack, Dr. Monto says. "People with legs of uneven length also get pain in their hips," he says. "Physical therapy and shoe inserts often solve the problem, but sometimes corrective surgery is necessary."

Another common cause of pain is arthritis. Or your hip pain may be caused by bursitis, an inflammation of the fluid-filled sacs called bursae that help lubricate the hip joint. "You can tell bursitis from other kinds of hip problems by pinpointing the pain," Dr. Monto says. "If your hip feels tender on the outermost, curvy part, then bursitis is a good guess. If the pain is close to or on your groin, it's probably something other than bursitis."

If hip pain is curtailing your dancing, here's what you can do.

Take Ice and "I"

"The first thing to try for managing hip pain is ice and an over-the-counter anti-inflammatory medicine such as ibuprofen," says Dr. Monto. You can make an ice pack by putting cubes in a plastic bag, wrapping the bag in a towel, and propping the pack next to you while you sit in a chair.

Why Athletes Need Big Closets

"You can get hip pain from your sneakers," Dr. Monto says. "Sneakers are designed for such specific purposes now that you have to make sure you have the right pair for the right activity. For instance, you shouldn't play tennis in jogging shoes—the heel is too narrow, causing you to run awkwardly, which can inflame your hip. Get running shoes for running, walking shoes for walking, tennis shoes for tennis, or basketball shoes for basketball."

Pace Yourself

"If you've taken up running or increased your distance recently, cut back when you start to feel pain in your hip," Dr.

Monto advises. "Rest for a few days, then return to your activity at a slower pace. Gradually increase your speed and distance if your hip pain is gone."

Get Off the Machine

"The hip machines you see in gyms these days can give you trouble," Dr. Monto says. "Watch out for the hip adduction machine in particular. It may not hurt while you're using it, but you can feel the strain the next day. Take it easy on those machines. And if the pain lasts for more than a day, stop using them."

Choose Your Stick Carefully

"If you need to use a cane, make sure it's the right size," says Gary Venman-Clay, M.D., a family doctor in Bellows Falls, Vermont. "The wrong cane can worsen your hip problems." To make sure your cane is the proper height, prop it straight up against a wall. Stand next to the cane with your arm hanging down. The top of the cane should come just to the

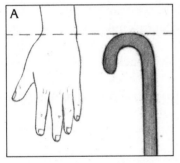 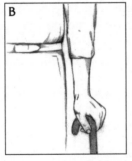 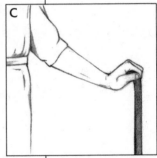

fold in your wrist. "Also be sure to carry the cane on the opposite side from the sore leg or hip joint," Dr. Venman-Clay says. "If your left hip hurts, use the cane with your right hand."

Lie Firmly

"A firm mattress is important to prevent hip problems," says Randal Schaetzke, D.C., a chiropractor at the Wholistic Health Center in Quechee, Vermont. "You also want a mattress that's even all the way across." Dr. Schaetzke says you should be sure that your mattress store has a liberal return policy; it's often impossible to tell whether the mattress is right for you until you've slept all night on it. "Return it immediately if it doesn't work for you," he says.

The top of a correctly sized cane comes to the fold in your wrist (A). If you can hold your arm at your side and still grip the top of the cane (B), it's the right height. If you have to bend your arm to hold it (C), the cane is too tall.

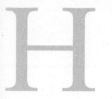

Heads Up

"When you are walking, look up and ahead instead of at your feet," Dr. Schaetzke recommends. "That will improve your posture and your stride, which will make things easier on your hips."

Stride On

"Particularly with older people, the best thing for hip pain is to keep moving," says Tiffany Renaud, D.C., a chiropractor in South Burlington, Vermont. "Take a daily walk unless the pain is incapacitating."

Take a Load Off

"Non-weight-bearing exercise is very helpful for hip pain," says Gerard Bozuwa, M.D., a retired family doctor in Wakefield, New Hampshire. "Try taking a water aerobics class, in which you do exercises in a swimming pool."

Pull a Couple of Knees

"For hip pain, try stretching," Dr. Renaud advises. "When you get up in the morning, step into a hot shower and bend forward gently with your hands on your hips, letting the hot water loosen your hips and lower back." Then, when you get out of the shower, lie flat on your back and pull one knee to your chest. Gently lower that leg and pull up the other one. Now pull both legs up together. This helps ease the hurt.

HIVES
Cures for when an allergy gets under your skin

You may think hay fever is bad until you join the one in five Americans who get the skin version of an allergic attack. Doctors call it urticaria; laypeople call it hives. Sufferers often don't say anything at all—they're too busy trying not to scratch their itchy, red-spotted skin.

What causes this maddening rash? In most cases, the culprit is something—last night's dinner, a dusty room, your neighbor's overly friendly dog—that stimulates an allergic reaction. "Most of the time, you can't pinpoint the cause,"

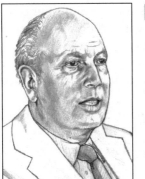

Pharmacists Didn't Have to Read My Handwriting

BECAUSE I practiced in an area with no drugstore, I simply followed what my predecessors had done: They dispensed their own medicine. That was the norm. That changed only after I'd been practicing for 10 years, when a drugstore was established in my town.

A country doctor in those earlier days brought his own pills with him on house calls. He didn't write prescriptions, because there was no place to get them filled.

Back then, I used to have my own little medical laboratory in my home. I also ran my own drugstore out of my house, selling the drugs my patients most commonly needed. (I wrote prescriptions for the drugs I didn't have on hand.) I was too busy to set a price on each different medicine, so I set a standard price of $4 for every prescription. That price never changed. I figure I made money on some drugs and lost money on others. It all evened out in the end.

You might say I sold "generic" drugs. These days, laws and regulations make it much more difficult to obtain drugs outside a pharmacy. But it's still a good idea to ask your pharmacist if a generic version of a drug is cheaper than the heavily advertised kind.

GERARD BOZUWA, M.D., *retired after 36 years as the sole family doctor for the town of Wakefield, New Hampshire.*

says Lawrence H. Bernstein, M.D., a former family doctor who is the medical director at Jewish Geriatric Services in Longmeadow, Massachusetts. "That's the maddening thing about hives. All kinds of things can trigger it."

Whatever the cause, your immune system senses a hostile invader and kicks into overdrive. The first line of defense, of course, is the skin. Tiny blood vessels begin to leak a protein-rich, itch-causing fluid. It's the buildup of fluid under the skin that makes the red dots characteristic of hives. Individual

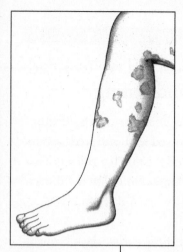

Fluid under the skin causes the itchy, red dots of hives.

welts rarely last more than a day or two at a time, although the rash can move around your skin for weeks. Some people with chronic urticaria even suffer from skin rashes for months.

Your skin, being the sensitive organ that it is, sometimes doesn't need an allergy-causing substance to bring up a rash. A job interview, a first date, or an argument with your teenage daughter—any form of emotional stress—can set you to itching. A hot summer day, a chilly morning on the ski slopes, fever, a few cocktails, premenstrual syndrome, or problems with your thyroid can make a mild attack of hives seem almost unbearable.

Fortunately, you don't have to start from scratch in searching for a remedy. Our Yankee doctors offer some time-tested solutions.

Treat the Allergy

"The antihistamine Benadryl is our first line of defense," says Stephen Blair, M.D., a pediatrician in private practice in Claremont, New Hampshire. "You can buy it over the counter in any drugstore. In most cases, it'll make your hives go away in two to four days. If you're still suffering, see your doctor about a prescription for Atarax, an antianxiety drug that's also a powerful antihistamine."

Stay Cool While You Soak

"Take a cool or lukewarm bath to relieve the itching of hives," says Kathryn A. Zug, M.D., a dermatologist at the Dartmouth-Hitchcock Medical Center in Lebanon, New Hampshire. "Avoid taking your usual hot shower. The skin of some people gets itchier from the beating of hot water against it."

Or Go for the Big Chill

"Ice massage is a marvelous thing for hives," says Brewster Martin, M.D., a retired family doctor in Chelsea, Vermont. Wrap several ice cubes in a clean cloth and stroke it slowly and gently against the rash. "The cold will send a mild pain message to your brain," Dr. Martin says. "Itching is carried on the same nerves as pain, so the ice will disrupt the itching message."

Get a Cold Foot

Here's a great way to cool down your itches, according to Dr. Martin: Fill a clean tube sock with uncooked rice, sew the sock shut, and put it in the freezer for two hours. Then hold the cold pack against your rash. The chilly rice is reusable, and it won't melt—making it less messy than ice.

Play Detective

Although it's often difficult to find the cause of hives, some experimentation is worth the effort if you're suffering from frequent rashes. Keep a food diary and consult it to see what you've eaten the day before a skin reaction. Common causes are eggs, wheat, shellfish, soy, peanuts, and milk.

Pitch the Rubber

Ironically, the latex gloves that you use to protect your hands when you do the dishes can cause allergic skin reactions, say researchers. Hives and other skin problems are increasing among hospital workers, who must use latex gloves often. If you find yourself getting rashes after wearing latex, buy gloves lined with cotton or use vinyl gloves as an alternative. Both are available at most pharmacies.

TIME TO SEE THE DOCTOR

When Itching Isn't Your Only Problem

You should get medical attention if, along with hives, you're suffering from any of these symptoms.
- A constantly running nose
- A tendency to bruise easily
- Aching or swollen joints
- Dark-colored urine
- Difficulty urinating
- Fatigue
- Fluid leaking from your vagina
- Night sweats
- Pale stools
- Sinus pain
- Swollen glands
- Tooth pain
- Weight loss
- Yellow skin

HOARSENESS

How to cope when you're dogged by a husky voice

It's a wonder the voice box works at all, what with the abuse it takes. Your voice box is actually just two small ligaments called the vocal cords, stretched behind the Adam's apple. They move apart when you breathe and vibrate when you

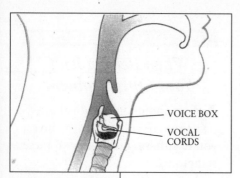

Yell or sing a little too loudly, and the vocal cords can be affected. The result: You're hoarse, of course.

talk or sing. Rev up the vibrations into overdrive, as when you yell for the home team or belt out the high notes in *Oklahoma!,* and the cords can become irritated or swollen. When they fail to vibrate properly, the result can be a raspy or breathy voice.

A viral infection such as a cold or the flu also can give you that husky voice. Cigarette smoke, irritating gases, hay fever, and sometimes even hormonal changes during the menstrual cycle can alter your sound. Older people in particular tend to lose their voices to nighttime acid reflux, when stomach acid creeps up into the esophagus during sleep. They wake up the next morning with hoarseness and, occasionally, a lumpy feeling in their throats. Usually the voice improves during the day as the voice box recovers from the acid.

Sometimes hoarseness fails to go away quickly. People who tend to keep their voices in high gear, such as singers, teachers, and ministers, can develop tiny, calluslike nodules on their vocal cords that keep the cords from vibrating properly. "Vocal nodules are the most common cause of hoarseness in children," says Dudley Weider, M.D., an otolaryngologist at the Dartmouth-Hitchcock Medical Center in Lebanon, New Hampshire. "One evening's yelling at a basketball game when you already have laryngitis can start vocal nodules. Once started, nodules are difficult to stop. The only effective treatment is voice rest. That means 10 days without talking."

If you owe your husky voice only to a cold or a good yell, here's some help for restoring those dulcet tones.

Shut Up

"If hoarseness is a result of a cold or the flu, it should resolve itself in a week," says Richard Lee, M.D., an otolaryngologist in private practice in Laconia, New Hampshire. "During that time,

---

TIME TO SEE THE DOCTOR

Watch for Danger Signs

CALL your doctor if your hoarseness lasts for more than two weeks. Call even sooner (or have someone call for you) if you're also:
• Coughing up blood
• Having difficulty swallowing
• Feeling a lump in your neck

If you're chronically hoarse when you get up in the morning, ask your doctor to examine you for acid reflux, the backing up of acid from your stomach into your esophagus and throat. Effective remedies are available by prescription.

HOARSENESS

you should rest the voice. Talk as little as possible." If you're
still croaky after a week has passed, see your doctor.

Stay Juiced

"You need to be hydrated," Dr. Weider notes. "Drink water
and fruit juice. Avoid coffee or anything else with caffeine."
Caffeine is a diuretic that makes you urinate, causing the loss
of more fluid and drying up the voice box.

Spray on Some Kids' Stuff

"If you are hoarse and absolutely must talk—if you're giving
a big speech or a sales presentation—try using this kids'
remedy," Dr. Weider says. "Buy some over-the-counter Benadryl liquid and mix it with an equal amount of water. Buy
an atomizer from your drugstore. That's a spray bottle with
a rubber end on the squirter mechanism. Squirt the Benadryl-
water mixture on the back of your throat. That will coat the
vocal cords and give them a slight topical anesthetic for a
short period." Dr. Weider warns, though, that any talking
will delay your voice box's full recovery.

HOT FLASHES
Douse the flames of menopause

Most women go through the change of life in their late forties or early fifties, although some enter menopause as early
as age 40. During this time, your ovaries produce less of the
female hormone estrogen. Eventually, the drop in estrogen
will cause your monthly periods to stop altogether. In the
meantime, your body may seem to play tricks on you. Your
periods might become irregular and produce unusually light
or heavy flows. You could have mood swings, especially before your period. Some women suffer from sleep problems,
vaginal dryness, and changes in their skin. And many women
get hot flashes.

They start with an uncomfortably warm, flushed feeling
that begins in the chest and spreads to the neck and face. The
sensation, which can last anywhere from a few seconds to
several minutes, can occur as often as 20 times in a 24-hour
period—continuing into the wee hours of the morning with

How Firewood Cooled
My Aunt Kate

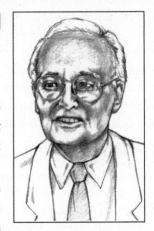

WOMEN have been putting up with hot flashes for centuries. A generation or two ago, at least in rural Vermont, women just wouldn't talk about it.

I had an aunt who, although she was a nurse, wasn't about to mention her personal discomforts. Aunt Kate's face would get bright red every once in a while, and she'd immediately excuse herself. "I need to get a stick of wood from the wood box," she'd say, and it would be a while before she'd come back in from the cold.

Aunt Kate dealt with her menopause in the best way she knew. Now there are many more things a doctor can do if the discomfort gets to be too much.

BREWSTER MARTIN, M.D., *a retired family doctor in Chelsea, Vermont (population 1,166), and cofounder of the Chelsea Family Health Center. He was named Vermont Doctor of the Year in 1991.*

those night sweats that mess up your sleep. Some women euphemistically call hot flashes power surges. Many women would just as soon do without them.

This time of change in your body—with hot flashes thrown in for good measure—usually lasts for about two years, but you might get recurring hot flashes for six years or even longer. Between one-tenth and one-third of menopausal women find their hot flashes severe enough to disrupt their lives.

Doctors aren't entirely sure what causes hot flashes. The drop in estrogen seems to bring about changes in metabolism, disrupting the vasomotor system that controls the blood vessels. Your vessels suddenly open up, causing a temporary rush of warm blood, which in turn warms up your skin by several degrees. That's the "hot" in the hot flash.

"It is hard for women going through hot flashes to realize that they are a normal part of life and will eventually pass," says Brewster Martin, M.D., a retired family doctor in Chelsea, Vermont. "But they really do go away eventually." In the meantime, here's how to stay relatively cool and comfortable.

Weather Your Veins

"Caffeine and alcohol are vasodilators, which can trigger a hot flash," says Paul Lena, M.D., a retired physician of internal medicine in Concord, New Hampshire. "Nicotine, on the other hand, is a vasoconstrictor. It causes the tightening of blood vessels, which can make a hot flash worse." If you're suffering from frequent hot flashes, steer clear of all three substances.

Eat Asian

"Many plants produce estrogen-like substances called phytoestrogens," says Hope Ricciotti, M.D., an obstetrician-gynecologist at the Beth Israel Deaconess Medical Center in Boston. "These are very helpful for preventing hot flashes." Foods especially rich in phytoestrogens include soy products such as tofu or tempeh, lentils, sushi, and dried seaweed. Asian women, who eat a diet rich in soy, have fewer hot flashes than American women, Dr. Ricciotti says.

Get Replacements

"I am a very strong advocate of hormone replacement," Dr. Lena says. "The hormone estrogen is the most effective treatment for hot flashes." Your doctor can measure your hormone levels and recommend proper therapy—while helping you weigh the risks of possible side effects of medication.

HYPERACTIVITY
Help for when your child's lack of focus drives you to distraction

Time was when a kid who consistently leaped before he looked was considered a product of his upbringing. These days, when a child is bouncing off the walls, doctors are at least as likely to blame his genes. The name they give the problem is attention deficit hyperactivity disorder, or ADHD.

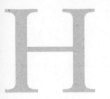H"A child with ADHD tends to sleep a lot less than his classmates, and he keeps disrupting others at home or at school," says Richard Nordgren, M.D., a pediatric neurologist at the Dartmouth-Hitchcock Medical Center in Lebanon, New Hampshire. "A boy is five times more likely than a girl to have the disorder."

Dr. Nordgren notes that the number of diagnoses increased dramatically from the 1960s through the 1980s before leveling off in the 1990s. That doesn't necessarily mean that more kids are bouncing off the walls. "The increased number of children being diagnosed is most certainly a reflection of increased awareness of the condition rather than an increase in the number of children with the disorder," he says. "Researchers now estimate that ADHD affects 1 out of every 20 kids."

Just because your child is more Huck Finn than Goody Two-Shoes doesn't mean he has a certifiable disorder, however. "Hyperactivity is in the eye of the beholder," Dr. Nordgren notes. "Some kids may just be more active than others. And a kid may be hyperactive without having ADHD." Lots of factors—from a faulty thyroid to partial deafness to emotional problems—can start a kid jumping.

Doctors aren't sure what causes the specific ADHD disorder. "It may have something to do with a chemical imbalance in the brain's frontal cortex, which helps determine a person's attention span," Dr. Nordgren says. ADHD tends to run in families. Although there is some evidence that other factors may be involved, such as competition between brothers and sisters, a hyperactive parent is much more likely than someone else to have a hyperactive kid.

If you think your child's chemicals are out of balance, "you should seek professional help," Dr. Nordgren says. "Your family may need counseling, and your child may benefit from prescription medication such as Ritalin—its generic name is methylphenidate." Ritalin helps tone down the heebie-jeebies and lengthens the child's attention span.

Here are some other ways to help a distracted child focus.

Enforce Stability

"Before you assume that your child has ADHD, make sure that the problem isn't coming from a chaotic household,"

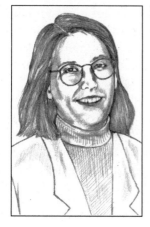

Few Two-Year-Olds Are Placid

WHEN I worked in an emergency room, frazzled mothers would bring in their two-year-olds asking me to cure them.

"He's terribly hyperactive," a mother would say about her son as he bounced off the walls. "Can you give him something?"

It's very difficult to tell whether a two-year-old really suffers from an attention deficit disorder. Of all the two-year-olds I've run across in my practice, I've met only one who truly needed treatment: a little girl who had not yet learned to speak. She couldn't concentrate long enough to pick up language.

All toddlers are hyperactive compared to their parents. It's as if our kids suck the energy out of us. They get into everything, they have to touch everything, and they can be real handfuls. But before you ask your doctor for prescription drugs, try this "cure" for an overly rambunctious two-year-old: discipline that's loving and consistent.

If your child has done something especially naughty or refuses to listen to you, punish him with a timeout by making him sit quietly in a chair for two to five minutes. (Two minutes can seem an eternity to a two-year-old.)

"But he won't sit still!" mothers say when I suggest a timeout. In that case, hold the child firmly in the chair just long enough for the child to sit still. Do this once or twice a day as needed, and within a few days, the child will get the message that inappropriate behavior won't be tolerated.

MARY-CATHERINE GENNARO, D.O., *a family osteopath who makes house calls in Warren, New Hampshire.*

says Kathleen Kovner-Kline, M.D., a child psychiatrist at the Dartmouth-Hitchcock Medical Center in Lebanon, New Hampshire. "It's a lot of work to be a good parent. If your child appears to be hyperactive but still has the capacity to sit quietly and complete a task, he probably doesn't need Ritalin—he needs structure."

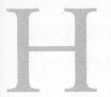

Dr. Kovner-Kline says that every child would benefit from a set bedtime, a daily routine, clear expectations for chores and behavior, "and consistent rewards and consequences. Don't threaten a punishment unless you intend to follow through. Kids do best when they know their boundaries."

Go Step by Step

"You can't expect a child with ADHD to improve overnight," Dr. Kovner-Kline says. "Make small changes over time, and pick your priorities." For example, the first step may be a regular time of waking up and getting dressed in the morning. "When the child can accomplish that, add making the bed to the list of morning duties."

Sell Short

"If your child has trouble sitting still for a story," Dr. Kovner-Kline says, "read him very short stories. Over time, build up to longer and longer reading periods."

Get Close

"The classic tool that teachers use for hyperactive children is to seat them in the first row of the class," Dr. Kovner-Kline notes. "This is a tried-and-true technique. It not only allows the teacher to keep an eye on the student, but it also makes it easier for the child to concentrate." She suggests that if your child has ADHD, you request front-row seating at the beginning of the school year.

Toss the Junk

"It never hurts to try limiting sugar and refined carbohydrates—the sort of ingredients found in many packaged snack foods," Dr. Kovner-Kline says. "It is misleading to attribute ADHD to sugar or additives, but a subset of hyperactive children are sensitive to these ingredients." She suggests getting the whole family to reduce the junk food habit. "In our society, restricting just one family member can seem to be a severe form of punishment. Get everyone to bear the burden together."

Have Yourself Checked

If you have a child with ADHD, you might consider getting yourself tested for the disorder. "It used to be thought that people outgrew hyperactivity, but that has proven to be untrue," says John C. Robinson, M.D., a pediatrician in private practice in Quincy, Massachusetts. "In fact, a child may do well from elementary school through high school and not have problems until college. And some people have hyperactivity problems throughout their lives."

Dr. Robinson recalls a mother who brought in a little boy who was doing poorly in school. "We tested the boy and then put him on Ritalin. His grades immediately improved. Then the mother got to wondering about her husband, who seemed to have problems focusing his attention. She brought him in for testing as well. The dad is now on Ritalin, too, and according to his wife, he's doing much better."

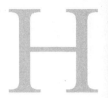

HYPERVENTILATION
Cures to help you breathe easy

When you're feeling anxious about a big exam, a business presentation, or even the prospect of appearing on the beach in a new bathing suit, sometimes you might feel yourself breathing rapidly with short, shallow breaths. You might even get light-headed. Your mouth and fingertips may feel tingly, and your lips may turn blue.

"These are the classic signs of hyperventilation," says Mark Greenberg, M.D., a cardiologist at the Dartmouth-Hitchcock Medical Center in Lebanon, New Hampshire. Dr. Greenberg explains that humans are programmed to breathe rapidly when they feel anxious or panicky. The response might be inherited from the days when we had to flee or fight predators and needed a quick dose of oxygen.

These days, Dr. Greenberg says, "we may not even know when we hyperventilate." But the symptoms are readily apparent. "Rapid, shallow breathing causes a change in the pH, or acidity level, of the blood, causing it to become more alkaline," he explains. "This in turn reduces the amount of ionized calcium, causing decreased blood flow to the lips and fingers." In other words, your hyperventilating temporarily messes up your circulation.

In some cases, hyperventilation is just one symptom of a larger problem. At least three percent of the population suffers from regular anxiety attacks, a condition doctors call

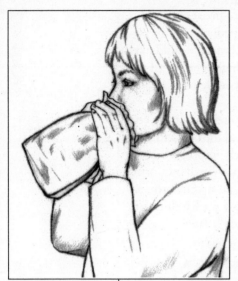

Breathe into a paper bag to bring your blood chemistry back to normal.

panic disorder. Other symptoms include chest pains, shakiness, chills, palpitations, nausea, and faintness. The good news is, your doctor can treat the condition with medication and psychotherapy.

More rarely, shortness of breath could indicate heart and lung disease. "If you have any trouble breathing, see your doctor," Dr. Greenberg says.

For the occasional bout with rapid breathing, try these remedies.

It Also Holds Your Lunch

The traditional cure for hyperventilation is a brown paper bag. "It works," Dr. Greenberg notes. "Breathe into a lunch bag, and it will raise your carbon dioxide level, restoring the blood chemistry to normal."

Chill Out

"I tell people who are hyperventilating to sit down and relax," says F. Daniel Golyan, M.D., a former New Englander who is now an electrophysiologist in private practice on Long Island. "Most people who hyperventilate are very nervous, and you need to counteract that."

I

IMPOTENCE
Reassuring remedies for a private problem

An erection is a complicated process involving an elaborate piece of machinery: the penis. It begins during sexual arousal or during the most intense periods of sleep at night. Stimulated by a complex set of signals from the brain, central nervous system, and endocrine glands, muscles lining the shaft of the penis relax, allowing blood to flow in. A band of muscle at the base of the penis shaft constricts, keeping blood from flowing back out. The penis becomes engorged with blood and ready for sex. Detumescence, or the softening of the penis, happens when the process goes into reverse. The constricting band relaxes, the muscles in the penis shaft contract, and more blood flows out of the penis than in.

It's a wonder that something so complicated works as often as it does. And it's no surprise that most men suffer from occasional impotence—the inability to become erect enough for sexual intercourse. Men who are tired, under stress, or distracted during the act may find themselves unable to achieve an erection. But doctors say there is no cause for concern unless the problem occurs often.

In that case, what's wrong? Physical causes are to blame for an estimated 50 percent of all cases of chronic impotence. Brain or spinal injury, drug side effects, heart or vascular disease, and diabetes are among the most common causes. At

I least half of all men over age 50 with diabetes mellitus suffer from impotence.

The remaining 50 percent of impotence cases are caused by psychological factors. "An erection is a fragile thing," says Stephen Rous, M.D., chief of urology at the Veterans Administration Medical Center in White River Junction, Vermont. "In the absence of an encouraging woman, a man who wants intercourse but thinks his partner doesn't may be unable to maintain an erection." Feelings of guilt, inadequacy, boredom, or just plain lack of desire also can stop an erection. "If impotence comes on gradually—with failure to achieve an erection happening more and more frequently—an organic problem is the most likely cause. If impotence comes on suddenly and you haven't recently had a traumatic injury, the cause is likely a problem in the mind."

Dr. Rous discounts the old husbands' tale of "use it or lose it." If a man does not have sex frequently, his chances of experiencing impotence are no greater than for a man who enjoys intercourse regularly, he says. "During the rapid eye movement period of sleep, when sleep is most intense, most men will experience erections—often several times during a single night," he explains. "In other words, even without intercourse, men tend to have several erections a day. Even without sex, you're using it, so a lack of intercourse is unlikely to be the cause of losing it."

Here are some remedies to try if you're not getting enough of the using it part.

Ask about Your Medications

"If you are suffering from impotence, the first thing you should do is talk with your primary care physician about any medications you are taking," Dr. Rous says. "It is very common to see a patient over the age of 50 or 60 taking 10 or 15 different prescription drugs. People at particular risk of impotence are those patients who have diabetes or are being treated for heart disease or high blood pressure." Two categories of drugs—antidepressants and medication for high blood pressure such as beta-blockers—can be especially troubling to your sex life, Dr. Rous notes. Ask your doctor to change your medications if they seem to be contributing to your impotence, he says.

Get on the Pill

On the other hand, a different kind of medication may be just what the doctor orders to treat an impotence problem. You probably have heard of Viagra, a prescription pill made by the Pfizer pharmaceutical company that can help men achieve erections.

"We doctors call it the 'Pfizer Riser,'" Dr. Rous says. "Viagra increases the blood flow to the penis by enhancing the effect of nitric oxide, a naturally produced chemical in the body that enhances the erectile process." Once you get an erection from Viagra, Dr. Rous says you can count on its lasting 20 to 30 minutes, though your erection may well last up to an hour.

Despite the ecstatic reception that greeted its introduction to the marketplace, Viagra is no miracle drug, Dr. Rous cautions. For one thing, it won't magically produce an erection on its own. "You can't just take a pill and then read the newspaper," he says. "You need to take the pill an hour before intercourse, and begin sexual stimulation 20 to 30 minutes after taking the pill." And you should avoid the drug if you are taking any medication based on a nitrate compound such as nitroglycerin, Dr. Rous adds. Another drawback: expense. Even as prescription medicines go, this one is definitely not cheap.

"A lot of my patients think the cost is worth it, though," Dr. Rous says. See your doctor if you think Viagra might help you.

Skip the Bad Stuff

"Stay away from alcohol and avoid caffeine and smoking," says Brewster Martin, M.D., a retired family doctor in Chelsea, Vermont. "All three things can cause problems with circulation, and adequate circulation is a vital part of the erectile process."

Get Healthy

Regular exercise and a low-fat diet can keep your sex life humming along with the rest of your body, doctors say. Ask your physician about a diet and exercise program that's right for you.

Try a Pellet

Another alternative is a product developed by the California-based company Vivus. This device—a capsule filled with alprostadil—can be inserted into the urethra (the tube that ends in the hole at the tip of the penis). "Think of the injector as an eyedropper with a pellet in it," Dr. Rous says. "You insert the eyedropper about three centimeters into your urethra and then push the plunger. Then you massage your penis to cause absorption of the hormone." The liquid-filled pellet, called MUSE (which stands for Medicated Urethral System for Erection), is available only by prescription. See your doctor if you think this treatment might be appropriate for you.

INCONTINENCE
Preventing the embarrassment of an unpredictable leak

If you find yourself unable to stop an accidental discharge of urine, you probably have one of four kinds of urinary incontinence. "Both men and women can suffer from *overflow incontinence,*" says Stephen Rous, M.D., chief of urology at the Veterans Administration Medical Center in White River Junction, Vermont, and author of *The Prostate Book*. In overflow incontinence, the bladder is unable to empty completely when you go to the bathroom. The result is a constant dribbling of urine.

Urge incontinence is when you suddenly feel you have to urinate but don't have time to make it to the bathroom. "The accident could consist of anything from a few drops to a real flow," Dr. Rous says. "Just a bit of leaking may be a sign of a urinary tract infection."

"In *stress incontinence,* there is no urge to void, but urine nonetheless is passed when you cough, laugh, exercise, or sneeze," says Dr. Rous. "Women who have gone through childbirth or men who have had their prostates removed often have stress incontinence."

A fourth kind of incontinence is a *neurogenic bladder*. "This is a spasmlike release of urine," he says. "People with multiple sclerosis or spinal injuries often have this kind of incontinence, caused by a problem with the central nervous system."

Dr. Rous says that people who suffer from a combination of urge and stress incontinence should see a doctor. In fact, he notes that it's a good idea to have any incontinence problem checked out by a health professional.

Once your doctor has looked you over, here's what you can do at home.

Women: Do Your Kegels

"Childbirth is the most common cause of incontinence in women," says Hope Ricciotti, M.D., an obstetrician-gynecologist in Boston and coauthor of *The Pregnancy Cookbook*. "To regain the muscle tone you lost having children, you need to do Kegel exercises." Kegels work the sphincter muscles, which surround the anus and the urethra (the passageway that carries urine out of the body). When the sphincter muscles contract, they stop the flow of urine. A strong muscle is better equipped to provide a tight clamp against incontinence.

"To find your own muscle, make yourself shut off the flow while you're urinating," Dr. Ricciotti says. "That is the muscle you need. Practice using it while urinating. Once you get the hang of contracting the muscle, you can exercise it anywhere—while driving, reading, or cooking supper." She notes that you should contract the sphincter slowly, hold for 10 seconds, and then repeat the exercise 50 times in a row. "You want to do your Kegels every day for the rest of your life."

Watch the Antihistamines

"Antihistamines can cause borderline obstruction of your urinary tract," Dr. Rous says. "The drugs can narrow the channels the urine must flow through, making it difficult or impossible to void. The bladder becomes overfull, which can lead to acute retention. If you're having problems voiding, you might want to skip the antihistamines."

Wear a Pad

"A woman can wear a feminine hygiene pad, the kind you use when menstruating, to catch any wayward dribbling of urine," says Paul Lena, M.D., a retired physician of internal medicine in Concord, New Hampshire.

Get It All Out

"See a doctor for training in self-catheterization," Dr. Rous says. "The procedure is for those who cannot empty the bladder normally, leaving behind a lot of urine. It's also for people, mostly diabetics, who are unable to void. You can be taught to catheterize yourself five or six times a day by inserting a catheter—a very small tube—into your urethra and draining the bladder, then removing the catheter. This keeps you dry. And having an empty bladder, you are less prone to urinary tract infections."

Cure Your Constipation

"There is very little tissue between the rectum and the urethra," Dr. Rous notes. "If a person is chronically constipated, large feces can press on the urethra and cause voiding difficulty." To avoid constipation, he recommends that you eat foods especially high in fiber: any cruciferous vegetable, such as brussels sprouts, broccoli, and cabbage; salad fixings such as carrots and beans; bran muffins; any whole grain bread; and apples. Dr. Rous says that if increasing your dietary fiber doesn't solve the constipation problem, you should see a physician.

INDIGESTION
How to fix
your internal food processor

Do you have a gut feeling that your stomach didn't like what you ate? Chances are, you have some form of indigestion—a catchall term for any discomfort in the upper abdomen. You might find yourself burping a lot, or it could be your rumbling stomach making the noise. Pain, burning, and a bloated or sour feeling are other symptoms. So are heartburn and nausea.

If your indigestion is chronic, you should see a doctor—especially if your ache comes with exercise. "Your stomach trouble could really be heart trouble," says Lawrence H.

Bernstein, M.D., a former family doctor who is the medical director at Jewish Geriatric Services in Longmeadow, Massachusetts. "You should get it checked out."

For more occasional bellyaching, here are some cures that might cheer you up down there.

Skip the Stimulation

"Coffee, nicotine, tea, and chocolate all contain a chemical that relaxes the lower esophageal sphincter, contributing to indigestion," says Laurie Duncan, M.D., an internist who moved from Cooperstown, New York, to Washington, D.C. "If you have heartburn, you'll probably want to stay away from these stimulants."

Back Off on the Baking Soda

If your infant has indigestion, it's best to avoid the traditional cure of giving baking soda to help him burp. Too much baking soda can cause sodium bicarbonate intoxication in infants and small children, a condition that can be life threatening.

Don't Be a Pig

As almost anyone who stuffs herself on Thanksgiving knows, overeating is a great way to send your stomach into a tailspin. "What happens is, your stomach produces extra acid to help digest that big meal," says Peter Mason, M.D., a family doctor in Lebanon, New Hampshire. "Then it assumes you're going to have another big meal, so it produces even more acid. That causes what doctors call rebound hyperacidity, a form of acid indigestion." If your stomach gets bummed out from pigging out, try eating smaller amounts.

Get Digestive Help

"Try taking an over-the-counter digestive plant enzyme, such as maltase, lactase, protease, lipase, or sucrase," says

---

ANNALS OF MEDICINE

And It Makes a Heck of a Julep

OLD-TIME doctors believed that each organ of the body had qualities of hot or cold, as well as dry or moist. The stomach was said to be naturally cold and moist. Mint, doctors thought, was warm and dry, which made it a good plant to balance out an uncomfortably clammy digestion.

Peppermint is still widely recommended by herbalists, according to Corinne Martin, a certified clinical herbalist in Bridgton, Maine. Peppermint is an antispasmodic that helps to relieve an irritated stomach. "So try some peppermint tea, available at health food stores and some supermarkets, to soothe your indigestion," she says.

Lawrence Bronstein, D.C., a chiropractor and certified nutrition specialist in Great Barrington, Massachusetts. "You can also try papain, bromelain, or pepsin, all available at many drugstores or any health food store."

Suit Yourself to a Tea

"Catnip and chamomile make excellent teas for indigestion," says Corinne Martin, a certified clinical herbalist in Bridgton, Maine. "Both are available at health food stores."

Catnip (A) and chamomile (B) are traditional stomach soothers.

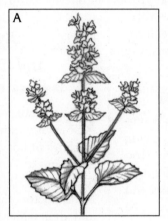
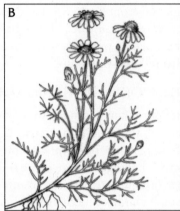

Go Bland

"Watch what you are eating if you tend to get indigestion after a meal," says Laurence Bouchard, D.O., an osteopathic family physician in private practice in Narragansett, Rhode Island. "Eat bland foods, such as cereal, bread, potatoes, and cooked vegetables. Avoid peppery sauces, orange juice, chili, and tomatoes."

Take Yogurt with Medicine

If your doctor has prescribed antibiotics, you might consider eating yogurt every day. Some commonly prescribed antibiotics, such as amoxicillin, can cause stomach problems. Yogurt with active lactobacillus cultures has been shown to reduce some of these side effects. Check the yogurt label for *Lactobacillus acidophilus.* "It helps a lot to eat yogurt with live acidophilus," says Mary-Catherine Gennaro, D.O., a family osteopath in Warren, New Hampshire. "Also, don't take antibiotics on an empty stomach if you're troubled by indigestion."

INGROWN HAIRS
Getting your hair to do its part

It's the greatest excuse there is for growing a beard: Some men have coarse, curly hairs on their faces that tend to take a U-turn and head right back into the skin. "It's a mechanical problem," says Owen Reynolds, M.D., a dermatologist in private practice in North Andover, Massachusetts. "When you push the razor against the skin to get a close shave, cutting the hair off below the surface, the skin may grow over the follicle before the hair grows out." Then you'll get a bump, which is an ingrown hair. "Doctors call the effect pseudofolliculitis barbae. It can be pretty painful," Dr. Reynolds adds. African-American men are more likely to have the problem because their hair tends to curl tightly.

Knowing the name doesn't make it hurt any less. Here are some solutions.

Electrify

"Some men who get ingrown hairs find that they get them less often after they switch to an electric razor," says Charles Hammer, M.D., a dermatologist with the North Country Outreach Program of the Lahey Hitchcock Clinic in St. Johnsbury, Vermont. "An electric razor doesn't cut the hair as close to the skin as a blade does. That makes the hair less likely to curl into the skin after it has been cut."

Harvest with the Grain

"Shave with the grain, running the razor in the direction your hair goes," Dr. Hammer says. "Run the blade over each part of your face just once. Don't repeat the stroke. Repeating may worsen the problem."

And Don't Sing

"Shave in the shower, when your hair is plump with moisture," Dr. Reynolds advises. "That makes your hair less likely to curl back." You can practice with a safety razor, or buy the kind of battery-operated electric razor made to work in the shower. If, like most men, you'd prefer to see what you're doing, check at your local hardware store for a special mirror that doesn't fog up in the shower.

Do a Lube Job

"Use a shaving cream that provides a lot of lubrication to keep the razor from forcing hairs to curl back," Dr. Reynolds says. "Edge and Aveeno, both commonly available at drugstores, have a lot of lubricant."

Do a Slow Burn

"You might try a chemical depilatory, such as Nair," Dr. Hammer says. "Be careful with it, though. It can irritate sensitive skin. Try just a bit of it on a small patch of your face before trying it over your whole beard. If you do choose to use it, do so as infrequently as possible and follow up with hydrocortisone cream to relieve the inflammation." Both Nair and hydrocortisone cream are readily available at drugstores without a prescription.

Use a sterilized needle to pull up on a stuck hair.

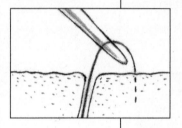

Free Your Hair

"You can carefully release an ingrown hair by using a clean needle that's been sterilized with rubbing alcohol," Dr. Hammer notes. "Insert the tip of the needle into the loop made by the hair, then gently pull upward."

Look Distinguished

"It may be simpler just to grow a beard," Dr. Hammer says.

INGROWN TOENAILS
Toe-saving advice from Yankee clippers

Usually, your toenails provide great armor against many of the abuses your feet suffer, such as stubbed toes or a night of dancing. But like any useful allies, toenails need to be treated with some respect, or they'll turn against you. Poor nail-trimming technique or ill-fitting shoes can cause a toenail to grow back toward your skin, sticking a sharp edge into your flesh. This nail invasion, like any other puncture, can cause an infection.

Even if things don't go quite that far, the pain of an ingrown nail is enough to make you seek some solutions. Here are some of the best.

Soak Your Sorrows

Add 1 tablespoon salt to 1 pint tepid water, soak a gauze pad in this solution, and apply it to your toe for 10 to 15 minutes, says Donald Helms, D.P.M., a podiatrist at the Dartmouth-Hitchcock Medical Center in Lebanon, New Hampshire. Do this several times a day until your toe feels better.

And Soak Your Bandage

"Try my wet-bandage cure for ingrown toenails," says Gerard Bozuwa, M.D., a retired family doctor in Wakefield, New Hampshire. "Place an adhesive bandage, such as a Band-Aid, over the ingrown nail. Wet the gauze with water and keep sprinkling water on it every few hours to keep it soaking. Replace the bandage daily. Over the course of a few days or a couple of weeks, the wet bandage will soften the nail and keep it from growing into the skin until the nail is long enough to be properly cut."

Get into Trim

"Using a nail file or emery board, try filing the curved middle part of your ingrown toenail to make it thinner," Dr. Bozuwa advises. "By thinning the nail, you can cause the edges to lift and stop growing into your toe."

Give the Nail a Lift

"Push a bit of cotton underneath the ingrown side of the nail to lift it from the skin," says Gary Venman-Clay, M.D., a family doctor in Bellows Falls, Vermont. "You might be able to redirect the nail so that it will stop growing into your flesh."

TIME TO SEE THE DOCTOR
Don't Operate on Yourself

If the sore area around your ingrown toenail gets swollen, bleeds, turns red, or starts to ooze pus, "don't be a bathroom surgeon," advises Nicholas Vachon, D.P.M., a podiatrist in private practice in Ellsworth, Maine. "Instead of trying to treat it yourself, see a doctor. I see a lot of patients who use improperly sterilized tools or remove too much toenail or tissue. That causes even worse problems. An infected ingrown toenail needs professional help."

To get things growing in a new direction, try slipping cotton under the edge of the nail.

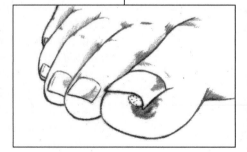

Cutting Remarks from a Medic

"Most ingrown toenails can be avoided if you care for your toes properly," says Gary Venman-Clay, M.D., a family doctor in Bellows Falls, Vermont. Here are some techniques to remember, according to Dr. Venman-Clay.

- When you use toenail clippers, squeeze, don't pull. The clippers should cut a straight edge, without any shards. If you're getting too many little pieces, buy a new, sharp pair of clippers.
- Make sure your toenail always has a white edge on the end. Don't cut too far.
- Cut straight across the nail. To get rid of sharp edges, buff them with a nail file. Remember: Don't cut those edges.

Pamper Your Dogs

"If you have ingrown toenails, get your feet measured by a podiatrist or a good shoe salesperson to make sure you have comfortable shoes," Dr. Bozuwa says.

INSECT BITES
Cures for what bugs you

You think *you* suffer from insect bites? Talk to Nick Yardley. Once when he was the director of the International Mountain Climbing School in North Conway, New Hampshire, Yardley went rock climbing on his state's Mount Willard. "It was a warm and breezy day, and we climbed in shorts," he recalls. "About 80 feet up, the wind suddenly died, and the blackflies came out. I just wanted to cut the rope and jump off the cliff. I got more than 500 bites." Yardley's climbing partner was so miserable that he lost two days of work.

Such horror stories abound in the Northwoods, where blackflies are joined by mosquitoes, no-see-ums, and deerflies. Down South they brag about the indefatigable chiggers. When these bugs bite you, the poison causes an allergic reaction, says Elizabeth Lowry, M.D., who is retired after 38 years as a pediatrician in Guilford, Connecticut. "Children can also get swollen glands behind the ears or on the back of the neck from blackfly and other insect bites. The bites will usually clear up in a few days, but the glands take longer to go down—sometimes a week or more." Toddlers tend to be more sensitive to bug bites, so you need to protect them more than other children.

All of us get chomped sooner or later. Here's what to do.

Wash Plainly

Avoid scented shampoos, says Michael Pelchat, an emergency medicine instructor and summer manager of Mount Washington State Park in New Hampshire. "Insects are attracted to sweet smells," he warns.

Have No Bananas

Bananas are especially appealing to mosquitoes and blackflies, Pelchat says. "I don't eat bananas in the summer."

Outwalk Bugs

A walking pace is usually enough to keep most insects away. "If you're hiking, you probably don't need a repellent," Pelchat says. "Just don't stop for very long."

Slop Softly

Avon's Skin-So-Soft, available at many drugstores and supermarkets, can help keep insects at bay, Pelchat notes. Avon doesn't promote its skin softener as an insect repellent, but bugs do drown in the goop.

Try a Homemade Concoction

Pamela Sorton, V.M.D., a veterinarian in Brattleboro, Vermont, protects horses and dogs from insects with a homemade ointment. "I use it on myself, too," she says. "It's great for preventing horsefly and blackfly bites." Buy a 1-pound jar of petroleum jelly. Melt it in the microwave oven, then stir in 1 ounce citronella, which you can buy in a hardware store. "Rub it on your skin to keep the bugs away," Dr. Sorton advises.

"B" Stops the Buzzing

"Take 25 to 50 milligrams of vitamin B_1 every day," says Harry Rowe, M.D., a family doctor in Wells River, Vermont. "Vitamin B gets into your system and makes your skin taste bad to a bug."

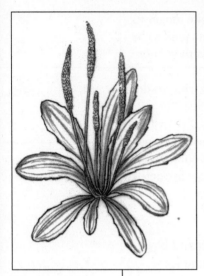

Here's something to chew on: Plantain is an old-time treatment that still works to soothe bug bites.

Add Cream

Over-the-counter hydrocortisone cream in a 1 percent solution can help relieve the itching of bug bites, according to Dr. Rowe, who was Vermont's Family Doctor of the Year in 1988 and 1996.

Try This Plant

"Pick a leaf of plantain, chew on it, and place the pulpy mass on the bite," says Susan Root, an herbalist in Sharon, Vermont. "It will draw out the poison." Plantain is a common weed that grows throughout much of the United States. It even springs up through the cracks in New York City sidewalks.

Bugged? Chill!

"If you've been bitten, grab an ice cube and put it in a plastic bag," says Lawrence H. Bernstein, M.D., a former family doctor who is the medical director at Jewish Geriatric Services in Longmeadow, Massachusetts. "Apply the ice to the bite. At first it will feel cold. Then it will hurt, then ache, and finally it'll get numb. Don't overdo it and freeze the skin. The itching should stop for a very long time. I find that ice is particularly helpful for bites on the toes."

Take Benadryl

"Liquid Benadryl, an easy-to-swallow antihistamine available over the counter, works on all kinds of allergic reactions, including insect bites," says Hugh P. Hermann, M.D., a family doctor in Woodstock, Vermont.

INSOMNIA
Count on these remedies instead of sheep

If you lie awake wondering how to get to sleep, your insomnia is no open-and-shut-(eye) case. "There are many, many causes," says Michael Sateia, M.D., director of the

Sleep Disorders Clinic at the Dartmouth-Hitchcock Medical Center in Lebanon, New Hampshire. "Stress may make you unable to fall asleep. Depression is another major cause. And physical problems, such as restless legs or the pain of arthritis, can keep you awake."

Hormonal cycles, especially in women, can affect sleep patterns. So can breathing problems or the mere process of aging. But a primary cause of insomnia, according to Dr. Sateia, "is habit. If you don't get to sleep at a normal time every night, or if you find yourself worrying about going to sleep, your bed can become a place of anxiety rather than a place of rest."

You have less to worry about, sleep-wise, than it may seem. Most insomniacs are only half an hour behind normal sleepers in the amount of shut-eye they get per night. And though all that tossing and turning seems to take hours, in most instances it lasts a mere 15 minutes. "In the sleep lab, we can tell that a lot of insomniacs are sleeping significantly more than they think," Dr. Sateia says.

If that isn't enough to ease your mind, close your eyes and picture these sleep-inducing remedies.

Get Up

"If you can't fall asleep within 20 minutes of going to bed, get up and do something else," Dr. Sateia says. "Read or watch television, or go for a short walk until you feel sleepy again. A lot of people fool themselves into thinking that they are about to fall asleep, and they lie awake waiting for sleep to happen. That just strengthens the pattern of insomnia."

And Get Up Again

"If you don't think you slept well the night before, don't stay in bed trying to regain lost sleep," Dr. Sateia says. "Get up at your regular time. Otherwise, you are training your body to go to sleep late and get up late."

Don't Face the Clock

"Remove the clocks from your bedroom," Dr. Sateia advises. "If you need an alarm, put one outside your door. Clock-watching feeds the pattern of insomnia—that anxiety that time is going by without your getting sleep."

Work Out Early

"Regular exercise is good for getting rid of insomnia," Dr. Sateia notes. "But don't exercise within two or three hours of going to bed. That can keep you awake."

Be a Bore

"Keep a reasonable buffer zone before bedtime," Dr. Sateia says. "Don't do your bills or study for an exam right before going to bed. Give yourself some wind-down time by doing something relaxing, such as reading or listening to soft music—or even doing something that bores you. Quiet time before bed can help you take your mind off your fear of losing sleep."

Nix the Siesta

"If you have trouble with insomnia, don't take naps during the day," Dr. Sateia says. "Napping can take the edge off your ability to sleep."

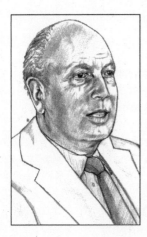

A WORD FROM DR. B.

I Really Didn't Mind the Midnight Calls

For most of my time as a family doctor, people would call me if they were sick and unable to leave home, and I'd go to them.

Then, in the late 1980s, the town got an ambulance. All of a sudden, people would call the ambulance instead of me. The ambulance would take them to the hospital in a nearby town, and the emergency room would call me in if I was needed. It hurt my feelings a little bit when I wasn't called every time.

On the other hand, I suppose I shouldn't have minded that I wasn't always needed. I just wouldn't get as many calls in the middle of the night, because the emergency room doctors could take care of things. I *wasn't* always needed.

GERARD BOZUWA, M.D., *retired after 36 years as the sole family doctor for the town of Wakefield, New Hampshire.*

Skip the Irish Coffee

"Alcohol does more harm than good in an insomniac," Dr. Sateia says. "It disrupts sleep patterns. And caffeine is definitely not useful. It's a stimulant, which is the last thing you need at bedtime."

Gobble This

"There are natural sedatives in some of the foods we eat," says Kathleen Kovner-Kline, M.D., a child psychiatrist at the Dartmouth-Hitchcock Medical Center in Lebanon, New Hampshire. "If you are having trouble sleeping, try having a turkey sandwich and a glass of milk an hour before going to bed. Turkey and milk both contain tryptophan, a chemical that causes drowsiness. That's probably why everyone feels like taking a nap after Thanksgiving dinner."

Stash the Smokes

Insomnia is yet another reason to give up smoking, according to John Bland, M.D., a rheumatologist in Cambridge, Vermont, and author of *Live Long, Die Fast: Playing the Aging Game to Win.* "Smokers have greater difficulty falling asleep because cigarettes raise blood pressure, increase the heart rate, and stimulate brain activity, all of which compromise normal sleep mechanisms," he says.

J

JAW CLICKING

*Stopping noise that may signal
bigger problems*

Do you sound like a robot when you chew, making mechanical noises as if your jaw needs a good dose of motor
oil? What you're hearing is the sound of dislocation or mis-
alignment in the hinge that connects your lower jaw to your
skull.

This hinge, which doctors call the temporomandibular
joint, or TMJ, is the most used joint in your body. You use
it to talk, eat, chew, even swallow. You can locate your TMJ
by putting a finger just in front of your ear and opening and
closing your jaw. Feel the hinge?

"The joint is seated like a ball and socket," says Gregory
L. Baker, D.D.S., an orthodontist in private practice in Woodstock, Vermont, and West Lebanon and New London, New
Hampshire. "Sometimes large fillings, skeletal differences, or
bad habits such as teeth grinding or gum chewing will cause
the jaw to seat improperly. Then when the person bites, the
jaw moves forward and pulls out of the socket. The muscles
compensate for the difference." Eventually, your jaw muscles stretch the ligaments or tough fibers that connect muscle
to bone. "Your ligaments don't spring back after they've been
overly stretched, and they tend to bunch up," Dr. Baker says.
"This creates a clicking sound—the same sound you get from
ligaments in a bad knee."

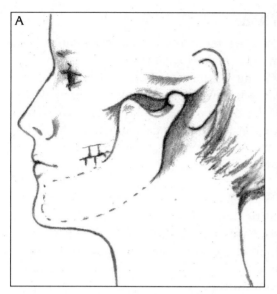
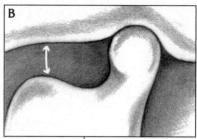
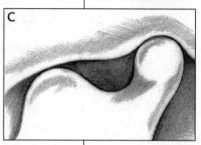

In your jaw, everything hinges on the temporomandibular joint (A), which allows you to open (B) and close (C) your mouth.

Serious deterioration of the TMJ can lead to worse problems than the annoying clicking. You can get an achy or locked jaw, headaches, ringing in the ears, chewing problems, and neck pain. "You may have just a muscle spasm, or you may have serious deterioration of the jaw," Dr. Baker says. "The only way to tell is to see your dentist."

Before things get that bad, here's how you can ease up on your overworked jaw.

Lay Off the Cud

"Avoid chewing gum," Dr. Baker says. "If you have jaw problems, chewing gum is like running on a bad knee—really bad news for the joint."

Back Off

"Sleep on your back rather than on your side if you have jaw problems," Dr. Baker advises. "If you lie on your side, you lie on your jaw and push it out of alignment."

Lick the Click

Dr. Baker recommends the painkiller ibuprofen to help stop your jaw from clicking. "It is not only a painkiller," he says. "It is also an anti-inflammatory and will reduce the swelling in your jaw muscles that can cause clicking."

Don't Open Wide

"If you have strained the muscle around the joint and you have inflammation there as well, the muscle is somewhat weak," says Gregory Colpitts, D.M.D., a dentist in private practice in Franklin, New Hampshire. "While it is weak, you could damage the joint. For two weeks, avoid opening your mouth too wide. And don't eat hard or chewy things like bagels." Also stay away from the candy called jawbreakers. "They're like rocks."

Stand Guard

"Wear an athletic mouth guard when you go to bed," Dr. Baker suggests. "Wearing a mouth guard will separate the top and bottom teeth and prevent nighttime grinding, allowing the muscles to relax." You can buy a mouth guard at a sporting goods store.

Pass on the Java

"Avoid caffeine," Dr. Baker says. "It stimulates your muscles, making them more likely to cause jaw clicking. You want them to relax."

Balance Chewing

If you tend to favor one side when you chew, practice working on both sides of the mouth to allow one side to rest.

Switch to the Guitar

A study by Finnish scientists showed that violin players tend to be more susceptible to jaw problems than the rest of us. If the clicking is providing unwanted percussion sounds, consider taking up another instrument.

JOINT PAIN
Stiff and sore?
Relief is just around the bend

From tennis elbow to housemaid's knee, there are lots of names and places for joint pain—and lots of causes as well. A fever or infection can make your joints hurt all over. Food allergies, diet deficiencies, and liver problems all can cause joint pain. Athletes who fail to drink enough liquids before they get sweaty can develop painful calcium crystals in their joints. Lyme disease, an infection spread primarily by the tiny deer tick, can cause terrible joint aching, swelling, and inflammation. The skin disease called psoriasis also can affect your joints, causing a deep ache.

But most joint pain comes from arthritis, injury, or just plain wear and tear. Just as your car's parts wear out after years of use, so can your joints after you've been around the block a few times. Overuse also can inflame the individual parts that make up your joints—muscles, tendons, ligaments, and bursae—the tiny, fluid-filled sacs that provide lubrication. An overly rough game of touch football or a missed step on a staircase can lead to joint pain. And gout, which is a common form of arthritis, can cause a sharp pain in a joint you may never have thought was so sensitive: your big toe.

"Sometimes you can get pain in your joints days after you've increased your activity level," says Raymond Rocco Monto, M.D., an orthopedic surgeon at Martha's Vineyard Orthopedic Surgery and Sports Medicine in Oak Bluffs, Massachusetts, and the physician for the Under 17 World Cup Soccer Team. "That two-mile jogging habit you've started may not hurt the next day, but a couple of days later you may find yourself a bit achy." Strangely enough, though, consistently active people such as runners tend to feel less, not more, joint pain later in life.

Which may be small consolation when your joints are jumpin' with feeling. Here are some ways to settle them down.

Take a Break

"The first thing to do for joint pain is to decrease the amount you use that joint for a while," says Dr. Monto. "If you have

---

---

tennis elbow, for example, avoid racket sports for a couple of weeks. Also try not to do too much hand shaking, hammering, or working with a screwdriver. If your knees or hips hurt from a daily jog or a two-mile walk to your office, take shorter walks, or take the elevator instead of climbing the stairs. If the pain goes away, you can gradually increase your amount of activity again."

Blast the Pain

"Ibuprofen is one of the most effective anti-inflammatories available," Dr. Monto says. "It will cut the pain and reduce the inflammation in your joints. But the kind you buy over the counter in remedies such as Advil and Nuprin is just one-quarter the strength of prescription ibuprofen—200 milligrams in the over-the-counter version versus 800 for the prescription kind. To treat your joint pain effectively, take 800 milligrams—four 200-milligram pills—of ibuprofen three times a day." He notes that it's wise to get your doctor's okay for this first. And never take ibuprofen on an empty stomach. Drink a glass of milk or orange juice when you take the pills, or down your ibuprofen after a meal.

Bottle It Up

"Put heat directly on your painful joints," says Daniel Caloras, M.D., a family doctor in private practice in Charlestown, New Hampshire. "I like heat for all kinds of joint pain—particularly moist heat, such as that from a hot-water bottle."

Drink Ahead

"At least an hour and a half before you exercise, drink plenty of water," Dr. Monto advises. "Calcium crystallization, the buildup of crystals in your joints, can be extremely painful, and dehydration is a major cause. An athlete should start drinking water six or seven hours before a big game."

Give It a Rub

"There are lots of balms and salves on the market to relieve joint pain, but I think there is more benefit in the rubbing than there is in the salve," Dr. Monto says. "Ask a partner to gently massage an aching joint."

K

KIDNEY STONES

*Dealing with those
painfully passing pellets*

A kidney stone usually isn't a problem until it starts to move, passing from one of your kidneys toward your bladder. To get from one organ to the other, the stone must travel through a tiny tube called the ureter. "The ureter is roughly three to four millimeters in diameter," says Stephen Rous, M.D., chief of urology at the Veterans Administration Medical Center in White River Junction, Vermont. "A stone five millimeters in diameter or less—and that accounts for 80 percent of all kidney stones—will usually squeeze through on its own." Eventually, the stone will exit with the urine.

The squeezing part is no laughing matter. The pain can be acute, though relief is quick once the stone passes. Men are four times more likely than women to suffer from this painful passage, according to Dr. Rous. If you've already had a stone, your chances of getting another are 50 percent greater.

So how on earth do those stones get their start in your body? Stones are actually crystals of uric acid, calcium, phosphates, or other minerals that form in your urine. That happens when the

To get from a kidney to the bladder, a stone has to pass through a tiny ureter.

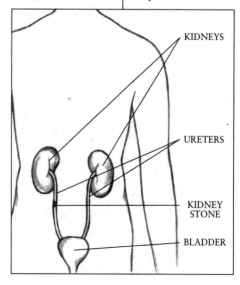

KIDNEYS

URETERS

KIDNEY
STONE

BLADDER

I Prefer the Stones, Thank You

IN COLONIAL times, barbers didn't just cut hair. The most common form of surgery was lithotomy, in which barber-surgeons called stone-cutters sliced patients open and removed kidney and bladder stones. The most popular stonecutters were the speediest in those painful days before anesthesia. One early-eighteenth-century surgeon, William Cheselden, won widespread fame for performing a lithotomy in less than half a minute.

Benjamin Franklin, understandably, preferred living with his kidney stones rather than undergoing surgery. He tried all sorts of cures, none of which worked—though he thought that blackberry jelly helped a bit. He ate it before going to bed every night.

Thank heaven we have more effective treatments today. "Franklin would have done better if he'd skipped the jelly and drunk a lot of water," says Stephen Rous, M.D., chief of urology at the Veterans Administration Medical Center in White River Junction, Vermont.

concentrations of these minerals get too high or the acidity level of your urine changes, making crystallization easier. Your doctor can examine your stones and urine to see which crystals you have. This will allow him to recommend appropriate treatment.

But you don't have to wait around for another stone to pass. Here's how to reduce your chances of feeling giant-size pain from tiny crystals.

See Clear

"If you can drink enough fluid so that your urine is always colorless, your body is much less likely to form stones," Dr. Rous says.

Acidify

"Some less common forms of kidney stones respond to changing acidity levels," Dr. Rous says. "Try taking citric acid in tablet form to change your body's pH."

Bag the Tea

"Tea is high in oxalic acid, a substance that can help the formation of crystals," Dr. Rous says. "That's why tea is best avoided by stone formers."

Don't Bone Up Too Much

"Be prudent about your calcium intake," says Laurie Duncan, M.D., an internist who moved from Cooperstown, New York, to Washington, D.C. Beware of too many supplements, such as calcium-filled Tums antacid. "Taking Tums as a supplement is fine," she says. "But some tablets contain 500 milligrams, which, added to a diet that's already high in calcium, can cause a calcium overload."

The recommended daily allowance of calcium for adults over age 25 is 800 milligrams of calcium per day, though women who are pregnant, nursing, or postmenopausal need more. "Don't overdo it with the cheese and yogurt if you're already taking calcium supplements," Dr. Duncan says. "Adding too much calcium and too little fluid to your diet could cause kidney stones."

KNEE PAIN

If your knee is needy, try these cures to cap your troubles

A trick knee makes you limp in stride with some 50 million other Americans. Pain usually comes to your knee in one or more of three ways: sudden injury, inflammation, or just plain wear and tear.

Many skiers know all too well about knee injuries. The most common sprain on the slopes is an injured anterior cruciate ligament—the tough fiber just in back of the kneecap. A sudden accidental twist when you hit a bump can make you hear a pop. That's your knee.

Inflammation often comes in the form of bursitis—an irritation in the bursae, or fluid-filled sacs that serve as natural ball bearings in your joints. Bursitis can arise from, among other things, hard use of your knees, such as crawling around on them for extended periods. Which is why bursitis in this all-important joint is traditionally called housemaid's knee.

A knee can signal that it's wearing out in a variety of ways. Overzealous joggers—especially those who up their running mileage too dramatically in a short period of time—can get chondromalacia patella, a fancy name for a wearing down of the cartilage at the back of the kneecap. If you jog and feel

Kknee pain, chondromalacia is the most likely reason. The pain in the back of your kneecap feels worst when you stand, climb stairs, or bend to pick up a quarter from the sidewalk. Another result of wear and tear over the years is arthritis.

Sometimes knee pain can arise from the way you walk. "Look at the alignment of your lower ankle," advises Daniel Wing, M.D., who practices physical medicine and rehabilitation throughout Vermont. "If it twists, causing your foot to turn in when you walk, that can cause problems in your knee by twisting it constantly. Too much downhill walking or stooping and kneeling can make knee pain worse. Injuries often arise when the muscles in your thighs are weak. The muscles that provide support to your knee bear an especially heavy burden, and if they're not up to the task, your ligaments and cartilage can bear too much strain."

Here's how you can lighten the burden and ease the pain.

Freeze!

"If your knee feels warm as well as sore, ice it," Dr. Wing advises. "Fill a plastic bag with ice and wrap a towel around it, then apply the towel to your sore knee. Leave it on for 10 minutes. Do this four times a day."

Say Aye to "I"

"Ibuprofen is good for reducing inflammation and swelling in your knee," says Laurence Bouchard, D.O., an osteopathic family physician in Narragansett, Rhode Island. But Dr. Bouchard says you need more ibuprofen for a hurt knee than you do for a headache. "A doctor's prescription of ibuprofen is generally at least four times stronger than the over-the-counter varieties," he says. "So if you're taking the over-the-counter kind, you need to take more. Take no less than two of the over-the-counter version at a time, and don't take it on an empty stomach." The common dosage in over-the-counter ibuprofen is 200 milligrams per tablet. A prescription ibuprofen pill can contain 800 milligrams.

TIME TO SEE THE DOCTOR

If Your Knee Is Swollen, Take It In

SEE a doctor immediately if you have any significant swelling of your knee," says Daniel Wing, M.D., who practices physical medicine and rehabilitation throughout Vermont. "You may have injured the ligaments of your knee or torn cartilage, either of which needs medical attention."

Brace Yourself

"Over-the-counter knee braces can be beneficial for people with knee pain, for three reasons," says Raymond Rocco Monto, M.D., an orthopedic surgeon at Martha's Vineyard Orthopedic Surgery and Sports Medicine in Oak Bluffs, Massachusetts. "First, the brace helps provide feedback to the brain on where the knee is—a sense of where it is in space, so your nervous system can react instantly to correct a twist. Second, a brace compresses a swollen knee and helps distribute the weight that the joint bears. And third, the brace helps keep the muscles around the knee warm, which prevents a strain that can cause further injury. Recent research suggests that a warm muscle can stretch farther and absorb more energy before injury than a cold muscle."

Arch Triumphantly

"If the soles of your shoes wear unevenly, that could mean you're pronating when you walk," says Gary Venman-Clay, M.D., a family doctor in Bellows Falls, Vermont. If you pronate, Dr. Venman-Clay explains, your feet turn in toward each other, putting extra strain on your knees. "Buy over-the-counter arch supports at your drugstore or shoe store," he says. "That may help you get rid of your knee pain." If it doesn't, he suggests that you see your doctor.

Try This Bandage for a Change

"If a child bangs her knee and it swells up, try to keep her from bending it," says Everett Orbeton, M.D., a retired pediatrician who practiced in Portland, Maine. "Put a big, bulky bandage on it—such as a disposable diaper—and hold it in place with a clean strip of cloth wrapped a few times around the knee. The bulk of the bandage is important. You want to hobble the kid for a few days so she'll stay off the knee."

AN OUNCE OF PREVENTION

A Thigh Is Not Just a Thigh

To avoid knee problems, make sure your thigh muscles are in good shape," says Raymond Rocco Monto, M.D., an orthopedic surgeon at Martha's Vineyard Orthopedic Surgery and Sports Medicine in Oak Bluffs, Massachusetts.

One of the best thigh exercises, according to Dr. Monto, is the squat. "Keeping your back straight and heels flat on the floor, squat down until your thighs are parallel to the ground. Repeat 15 to 20 times." If you find this exercise easy, Dr. Monto suggests holding some light weights, such as full soup cans, to your shoulders. Eventually, you may work your way up to five-pound dumbbells, he says.

Slow the Growing Pains

"If you have an active kid age 11 or 12 with sore knees, he could have Osgood-Schlatter disease," says John C. Robinson, M.D., a pediatrician in private practice in Quincy, Massachusetts. "You see it mostly in boys, and it's commonly called growing pains. A growth spurt along with some heavy use can cause some fraying in the tendons that attach the lower leg bone to the kneecap." The knee usually heals itself within a few months. "In the meantime, ice the knee three or four times a day, give ibuprofen for the pain, and have the child lay off the sports for a few weeks to give the knee some rest."

Get Behind Your Knee

"For a sore knee, massage the muscle that's right in back of your knee to help stabilize the knee and reduce the pain," says Randal Schaetzke, D.C., a chiropractor at the Wholistic Health Center in Quechee, Vermont. "Do it gently. There are nerves back there."

Pad Your Kneeling

"Wear knee pads when you garden," Dr. Schaetzke says. "Knees aren't designed for kneeling for long periods."

Drop Some Ballast

"If you have knee pain and you're overweight, you absolutely need to lose weight," says Michael Ackland, M.D., an orthopedic surgeon and sports medicine specialist in private practice in Hyannis, Massachusetts. "Weight is the number one factor behind knee problems—the stress you put on your knee can total as much as eight times your body weight. The more weight you lose, the easier it is on your knees." Dr. Ackland notes that he employs a nurse in his practice "whose only job is to help people with knee problems lose weight. It's that important."

L

LOW SEXUAL DESIRE

*How to keep "Not tonight,
Honey" from becoming
a permanent affair*

First of all, not everyone thinks it's such a bad thing to lose
that sexy feeling now and then. The ancient Greek philosopher Plato lost his altogether, and he claimed not to mind at
all, "Most joyfully did I escape it, as though I had run away
from a sort of frenzied and savage monster," he said, refer-
ring to his absent libido.

Even among those who still have it, sexual desire isn't dis-
tributed equally. "People have different levels of desire and
habits that may change over time," says Laurie Duncan,
M.D., an internist who moved from Cooperstown, New
York, to Washington, D.C.

Okay, but what is normal? "It's better to ask whether you
and your partner are happy," Dr. Duncan notes. "If you are
both satisfied with the frequency of sex and time of day, there
shouldn't be a problem."

But a problem can crop up occasionally. "Physical problems—such as the man's difficulty in maintaining an erection
or a lack of sufficient lubrication in the woman—can affect
people's mental attitudes toward sex," Dr. Duncan says. She
notes that emotional stress or an illness can temporarily put
a damper on desire.

For low libido that stays in the dumps, a common cause
is the blues. "You can suffer from long-term low libido if you

L are depressed," Dr. Duncan says. She adds that long-lasting low desire also can stem from decreased sexual hormones in your system—a problem that should be evaluated by an endocrinologist. "People with high blood pressure or diabetes also may find their libidos impaired," she says, adding that some medications can change libido as well.

If you're taking prescription medications, ask your doctor if they might be affecting your sexual desire. "Beta-blockers, prescribed to treat heart conditions, can affect your libido," says Hope Ricciotti, M.D., an obstetrician-gynecologist at the Beth Israel Deaconess Medical Center in Boston.

Sometimes, though, you just need to retune your sexual spark plugs. Here are some ways to do that.

Check Your Schedule

"A lot of the 'low sexual desire problems' I hear about from patients have to do with someone being worn-out from leading too busy lives," says Mary-Catherine Gennaro, D.O., a family osteopath in Warren, New Hampshire. "If a woman goes to bed at 9:30 and is sound asleep when her husband comes to bed at 11:00 and wants to make love, that isn't low sexual desire, that's bad timing. Schedule at least an hour or two a week when you're both wide-awake, alone, and undistracted."

Women: Stay Slick

"If you're going through menopause, or if you're past it, insert an applicator full of an over-the-counter lubricant before intercourse," Dr. Duncan says. "A lack of lubrication can make you feel as though you're too old for sex." A common and effective lubricant is K-Y Jelly, available over the counter at drugstores.

Rub the Right Way

"Massage is great for increasing sexual desire," Dr. Gennaro says. "You don't need to do anything fancy—just spend time with back rubs, even if one of you doesn't feel like having sex. At the very least, you come out of it with a great back rub."

Read Up

"Most of your body's sexual arousal is stimulated from the brain," Dr. Ricciotti says. "Try reading erotic literature an hour or two before you and your partner plan to have intercourse."

Liquor Isn't Quicker

"Avoid alcohol if you have low sexual desire," Dr. Ricciotti advises. "Heavy drinking can enhance the sex drive, but it

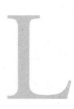

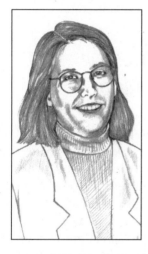

A WORD FROM DR. MANDY

The Wife Who Liked Her Husband as He Was

A COUPLE came in to see me. Actually, it was the man who was my patient, but he never showed up without his wife.

He was on some medication for high blood pressure, and one of the potential side effects of that particular medicine was impotence. I asked him whether he had had such a problem.

"No," said the wife.

The man cleared his throat and looked a bit embarrassed. So I pursued the point, telling the man that if impotence was a problem, I could change his medication. "Would you like me to do that?" I asked him.

"No," the wife said again. "It's fine the way it is. I *like* it this way."

The man stayed silent, so I had to leave things the way they were. But it was clear to me that whereas the man might have felt there was a problem, the wife lacked sexual desire. If you don't desire to have the desire, no doctor is going to butt in and "fix" things.

MARY-CATHERINE GENNARO, D.O., *a family osteopath who makes house calls in Warren, New Hampshire.*

---

decreases a woman's ability to have an orgasm and can block a man's erection. That doesn't help your desire at all."

Don't Blame Your Body

"There are plenty of heavy people who don't look like the models in women's magazines and have happy sex lives," Dr. Duncan notes. "But being too thin can inhibit sexual desire." She explains that a woman who loses too much fat will stop menstruating, and her body will not make enough sex hormones. The answer? Try to get your weight around where your doctor's chart says it should be. According to the Columbia University College of Physicians and Surgeons, you should weigh 100 pounds for the first 5 feet of height and 3 pounds for every inch over 5 feet. If you're under 5 feet, subtract 3 pounds for each inch under that height.

LYME DISEASE
*Dealing with a big problem
from a tiny tick*

You'd think that an ailment caused by a harmless-looking tick and named after a picturesque little town in Connecticut would be pretty benign. Alas, Lyme disease is one serious rash. If untreated, it can lead to arthritis-like symptoms and even paralysis.

The rash has spread throughout the United States and has become the most common disease spread by bugs in this country. Nationwide, more than 100,000 people have been diagnosed with the ailment since 1982. Connecticut (where it was first discovered) and Cape Cod, Massachusetts, are the most high-risk areas.

The culprit behind this nasty illness is usually the deer tick, a minuscule creature that looks like a tiny mole when it's on your skin. "Ticks are the most dangerous bugs in the United States," says

---

AN OUNCE OF PREVENTION

Be Picky

You can avoid all the problems associated with Lyme disease if you can get the tick off you. "You have very little chance of infection if you remove the tick within 24 hours," says Kathleen Kovner-Kline, M.D., a child psychiatrist at the Dartmouth-Hitchcock Medical Center in Lebanon, New Hampshire. "Check your children every night at bath time for ticks—especially during the spring and fall, when ticks are most active."

Laurence Bouchard, D.O., an osteopathic family physician in Narragansett, Rhode Island. More than a third of the deer ticks on the East Coast carry the disease, which enters your blood after the tick attaches itself to you.

The first sign that you have Lyme disease comes within five days to a week after your encounter with the tick. You may get a bull's-eye skin rash the size of a half-dollar and looking like a target, with a bright red border, red inner rings, and a tiny red mark in the center. You also may feel achy all over, as if you have the flu. And that's just the early stage. If left untreated, the disease can spread through the blood to the heart and the nervous system. Another sign of Lyme disease is Bell's palsy, in which one side of the face droops.

Okay, now for the good news: An infected deer tick usually has to ride around on your skin for at least 24 hours—long enough to settle in and actually bite you—before it can transmit the disease.

Even if you or your kid don't get to the ticks in time, Lyme disease is treatable with antibiotics, especially if you catch it early. "My family and I lived for several years in East Haddam, Connecticut, the next town over from Lyme—the town for which the disease is named," says Kathleen Kovner-Kline, M.D., a child psychiatrist at the Dartmouth-Hitchcock Medical Center in Lebanon, New Hampshire. "One of my sons got Lyme disease. I'd spotted a tick on him and watched him closely. The moment I saw the characteristic round rash, I started him on antibiotics. He never showed any other symptom because he got treated quickly enough."

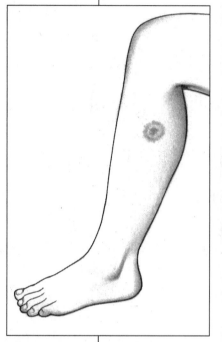

The first sign of Lyme disease: a rash that looks like a target.

Dr. Kovner-Kline's husband wasn't so lucky. He never saw what bit him. "We thought the terrible aches in his joints were caused by a tetanus booster shot," she says. "After five days of achy pains, he woke one morning covered with giant bull's-eyes all over his body, each five inches in diameter. He had classic Lyme disease throughout his body." Antibiotics cured him within a few weeks.

L

If you get a rash that looks like Lyme disease, see a doctor immediately, Dr. Kovner-Kline says. To keep the ticks from getting to you in the first place, follow these tips.

Hide Yourself

"If you're in an area with a lot of deer ticks, you should wear long socks, long pants, and long sleeves when you are walking through grassy areas," says Patricia Edwards, M.D., a pediatrician in private practice in Concord, New Hampshire. "That's where ticks hang out, waiting to land on you."

Get Ticked Off

If you see a tick on you, Dr. Kovner-Kline says, pull it off immediately. If the tick's head is already embedded in your skin, use tweezers. "Carefully probe underneath the tick, grab the tip of the head where it meets your body, and gently pull it off," she explains. "Take care not to grab the tick's body. That could squeeze blood from the tick's body back into you, increasing the likelihood of infection." You can buy special tick removal kits in drugstores. Most contain a magnifying glass along with tweezers or a small notched instrument that you use to pry the tick off. A cheaper solution is to buy tweezers and magnifier separately.

Beware of the Bull's-Eye

"If you've been bitten by a deer tick, look for the rash," says Peter Brassard, M.D., a family doctor on Block Island, Rhode Island. "If the rash is smaller than a 50-cent piece, that's not a sign of Lyme disease. But keep watching it. If it doubles in size in 24 hours, that probably *is* the disease." Other symptoms to watch for are "a stiff neck and a fever of around 103°F. Those three symptoms together equal Lyme disease unless proven otherwise."

Test the Tick

"If you find a tick embedded in you, it can be analyzed at a lab to see if it is carrying Lyme disease," Dr. Bouchard says. "Insurance companies won't pay for the test, but they will pay for starting you on antibiotics."

M

MENOPAUSE
Making the change of life worth living through

After age 40, a woman's ovaries produce less estrogen, the hormone that triggers menstruation. The drop in estrogen continues until her periods stop altogether. By age 48, half of American women have gone an entire year without menstruating—the official medical definition of menopause. Nearly all women have completed the change of life by age 54.

You can experience other changes in addition to a halt in periods. "Menopause usually takes two years from onset to completion," notes Eric A. Sailer, M.D., an obstetrician-gynecologist at the Dartmouth-Hitchcock Medical Center in Lebanon, New Hampshire. During this time, a woman may have hot flashes—a flushed feeling that starts in the chest and rises upward to the neck and face. Her vagina might feel dry and itchy, and intercourse can sometimes be painful. Urinary tract infections are more common in women going through the change. Some women gain weight. And some experience psychological changes: disturbed sleep and mood swings, for example.

As many as one-third of all women have a trouble-free transition, however, experiencing no uncomfortable symptoms whatsoever. "There is nothing a woman can do to prevent menopause," Dr. Sailer says. But here is what you can do to make the change smoother.

Know Beans

"Add soy and legumes—beans—to your diet," recommends Hope Ricciotti, M.D., an obstetrician-gynecologist at the Beth Israel Deaconess Medical Center in Boston. Soy and other kinds of beans appear to compensate partially for lowered estrogen levels, helping alleviate hot flashes and other symptoms, Dr. Ricciotti says.

Work Out

"The effect of exercise on mood changes is under study by medical researchers," Dr. Ricciotti notes. "Some people think exercise can help stabilize the mood swings that sometimes accompany the onset of menopause."

Replace the Hormone

Ask your doctor about the pros and cons of estrogen replacement therapy—prescription drugs that help compensate for less active ovaries. Prescribed estrogen has its risks: It can make you more susceptible to breast or uterine cancer, for example. By contrast, women on estrogen therapy tend to fall victim less frequently to heart disease and bone problems, and the drugs can greatly alleviate the discomforts of menopause, including hot flashes, urinary tract infections, and vaginal dryness.

MENSTRUAL CRAMPS
What to do about that pressing monthly engagement

Doctors used to believe that most "female concerns"—from headaches to nervous problems to cramps—stemmed from the uterus.

Well, they got the cramps part right. When your innards feel like one big knot, the cause is likely to be the uterus contracting as it sloughs off its lining of cells. More than half of all women get that uncomfortable crampy feeling just before and during menstrual bleeding. In 5 to 10 percent of women, the pain is enough to interfere with their lives.

If your own pain is bad enough to incapacitate you, it's best to see a doctor. Your cramps might be caused by something serious, such as endometriosis, an imbalance of hormones, a fibroid tumor, or a pelvic infection. Be thankful for modern medicine in this case. Doctors in the days before the Civil War might have applied some thirsty leeches to relieve your cramps.

If you're suffering from cramps of the run-of-the-mill, monthly variety, here's what you can do on your own.

Do a Preemptive Strike

"Take ibuprofen before you think your cramps will begin," says Hope Ricciotti, M.D., an obstetrician-gynecologist in Boston. "Ibuprofen will help if you take it once your cramps have begun. But if you take it ahead of time, you can actually prevent cramps altogether." Dr. Ricciotti explains that ibuprofen restricts your body's production of prostaglandin, the hormone that causes uterine contractions.

Take Your Tums

"Take three Tums every day, even when you're not having your period," Dr. Ricciotti advises. Tums is an over-the-counter antacid. Each tablet contains about 500 milligrams of calcium. "Over the long term—four to six weeks—calcium decreases the number of uterine contractions, which can work to reduce menstrual cramping," she says. "If you don't want to take Tums, you can take calcium supplements."

Put On the Heat

"Lie with a hot-water bottle against you," says Paul Lena, M.D., a retired physician of internal medicine in Concord, New Hampshire. "It will help make the cramps tolerable."

Ask about the Pill

"Many gynecologists now prescribe birth control pills for three to six months to regulate a woman's menstrual cycle and reduce cramping," Dr. Lena says. "A temporary dosage can get your body on track." Ask your doctor if birth control pills are right for you.

Shout for Bark

Maureen Williams, N.D., a naturopath in private practice in Hanover, New Hampshire, recommends cramp bark, a

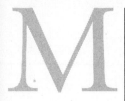

traditional remedy that, true to its name, is a muscle relaxant that helps soothe cramping. You can buy cramp bark, *Viburnum prunifolium,* at your local health food store.

MIGRAINES
You don't have to bow to the king of headaches

You'd think a headache that strikes only one side of your head would be only half as bad. But a migraine sufferer will tell you that this head banger beats all.

A migraine isn't just a headache. Besides the pain, most migraine sufferers also feel sick to their stomachs, sometimes even to the point of vomiting. During a migraine attack, you can have blurry vision, a stuffy nose, and ringing in the ears. Ahead of the migraine, many sufferers get weird visual signs called auras, lasting from a minute to half an hour. They see small bright or dark dots, flashes of light, or combinations of these.

"Not all auras are visual," says Lawrence H. Bernstein, M.D., a former family doctor who is the medical director at Jewish Geriatric Services in Longmeadow, Massachusetts. "Some auras come as a strange smell. Other people get a sense through their whole body that a migraine is coming."

Several German neurologists have speculated that Saint Paul had migraines. Some 3 out of 100 men and nearly three times as many women get them. The problem tends to run in families, and you're most likely to suffer your first migraine between the ages of 10 and 20. One of the consolations of old age is a reduction in the frequency of migraines. You're also less likely to get migraines when you're pregnant.

If you're in migraine prime time, however, you don't have to sit back and take it. For severe migraines, your doctor can give you a prescription medicine such as an ergotamine or Imitrex, which can stop a migraine cold. For less severe cases, these home remedies might do the trick.

Look on the Dark Side
"The best thing to do for a migraine—or any other headache, for that matter—is to take a painkiller such as ibuprofen and lie down with a cool, damp cloth on your forehead," says

Keep Your Fingers off the Triggers

MOST people with migraines quickly learn to identify their own personal triggers—substances or activities that cause their headaches —and learn to avoid them," says Sarah Johansen, M.D., medical director of emergency services at New London Hospital in New London, New Hampshire. "Migraines tend to be caused by vasodilation, the expansion of arteries in the head. So it's smart to avoid anything that causes vasodilation if you get migraines."

Common triggers, according to Dr. Johansen, include nitrates (often found in wine), too much coffee, chocolate, red wine, birth control pills, the flavor enhancer monosodium glutamate (MSG), ovulation during a woman's menstrual cycle, the onset of menstruation, dehydration, irregular sleep habits, too much sleep, menopause, psychological stress, and sudden withdrawal from coffee.

Laurie Duncan, M.D., an internist who moved from Cooperstown, New York, to Washington, D.C. "Turn off the lights. Most migraine sufferers are sensitive to light."

Up the Pressure

"During a migraine attack, try pressing your fingers against your temples," says Sarah Johansen, M.D., medical director of emergency services at New London Hospital in New London, New Hampshire. "The pressure decreases the flow of blood through the arteries and can bring some relief."

Eat Leaves

"The most common herbal treatment for migraines is to eat a leaf of feverfew every day," says Corinne Martin, a certified clinical herbalist in Bridgton, Maine. Feverfew has been a cure for thousands of years, but the ancients used it for menstruation problems, not headaches. Since the 1970s, herbalists have been singing the herb's praises for migraines. "You need to take it every day," Martin says. She notes that the leaves can cause mouth sores in some people, "in which case chew the leaves only every other day." You also can buy a tincture or freeze-dried capsules at health food stores.

Herbalists say chewing feverfew leaves can prevent migraines.

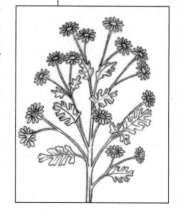

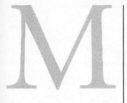

MORNING SICKNESS
Keeping the miracle of life
from making you queasy

If the early part of pregnancy is making you feel sick, don't add worry to your nausea. Your churning stomach is not a sign of illness but probably indicates a healthy dose of hormone. More than half of all pregnant women get morning sickness—an upset stomach that can hit at any time of the day but is especially likely to strike when you first wake up. The feeling is believed to be the body's reaction to the copious amounts of the female hormone estrogen that it produces during pregnancy, especially during the second and third months. Things generally settle down by the fourth month, when you can look at your husband's food without rushing to the bathroom.

In the meantime, there's a temptation to try anything that will ease your innards. But don't start popping pills until you've tried more homely cures, advises Thomas J. O'Connor III, M.D., an obstetrician-gynecologist in private practice in Rockport, Maine. "Treating morning sickness can be very tricky, because you're treating two people at once, the mother and the child," Dr. O'Connor says. "You should avoid medications if possible." Here are some techniques that are worth trying first.

Swallow Goldfish

"Keep something in your stomach at all times," Dr. O'Connor says. "Crackers and bread are easy to digest. I tell my patients to keep a little bag of plain Goldfish crackers beside the bed and to eat a handful before they get up."

Hold Your Nose

Dr. O'Connor says that it's wise to avoid the smell of food altogether. "Let someone else do the cooking. And improve the ventilation of the kitchen while you're in it by opening a window."

Hold the Joe

"Caffeine, nicotine, and alcohol are all stomach irritants," Dr. O'Connor says. "Avoid coffee, smoking, and drinking."

Don't Be Tepid

For some reason, lukewarm liquids seem to upset the stomach more than hot or cold liquids do. "Drink your drinks while they're hot or cold," says Eric A. Sailer, M.D., an obstetrician-gynecologist at the Dartmouth-Hitchcock Medical Center in Lebanon, New Hampshire.

Walk Away

"When my wife was pregnant with each of our four children, the old doctor who cared for her made her walk a mile every single day," says Brewster Martin, M.D., a retired family doctor in Chelsea, Vermont. "That's still a good idea. Exercise helps morning sickness, I think, because it causes your body to produce natural morphine, a chemical that kills pain and nausea."

Stand Slowly

"Move slowly as you get out of bed," Dr. O'Connor says. "Take yourself gradually from a lying to a sitting position, and then from sitting to standing. Your blood vessels relax when you are pregnant, making it harder to get blood to the brain.

Let Your Blender Calm Your Stomach

My FAVORITE remedy for nausea during pregnancy is a cantaloupe-banana shake that my husband and I developed," says Hope Ricciotti, a Boston obstetrician-gynecologist and coauthor of *The Pregnancy Cookbook*. "Some women are so nauseated that they have to be on a liquid diet for a while. Instead of sticking to juices and water, try our shake. It contains plenty of protein, carbohydrates, calcium, and vitamin C —in other words, just about everything your body needs when pregnant. And you can drink as many shakes as you want."

Here is the recipe for Dr. Ricciotti's cantaloupe-banana shake, adapted from her book.

1 large ripe banana, peeled, cut into chunks, wrapped tightly in plastic wrap, and frozen for 24 hours

1 cup cantaloupe chunks, covered tightly with plastic wrap and frozen for 24 hours

1¼ cups skim milk

½ cup nonfat dry milk

1 teaspoon vanilla

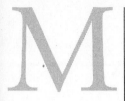

The result is a phenomenon called postural hypotension, when blood pools in certain places. By moving slowly, you can allow your blood to circulate to the brain, avoiding the dizziness and nausea you might otherwise feel when you get up."

MOTION SICKNESS
Ways to find
your sea (and car) legs

It's the bane of many a cruise passenger. When the sea gets up, the ship goes one way, your stomach goes another, and you end up doing the old heave-ho.

But you don't have to be at sea to get sick. "You can get a headache, dizziness, and nausea when traveling by car, plane, boat, train, even on amusement park rides," says Laurie Duncan, M.D., an internist who moved from Cooperstown, New York, to Washington, D.C. One Swiss researcher has coined the term *ski sickness* for the queasy feeling that some people get schussing down snowy slopes.

What's going on? Motion sickness is caused by what airline pilots call an instrumentation problem—only the malfunctioning instruments are in your body, not the plane. To tell you where you are and which end is up, your nervous system uses five sensitive detectors: your inner ears, eyes, sense of touch, muscles, and brain. Usually, these "instruments" work in sync. But in the dining room of a cruise ship, your inner ears and muscles may feel the ship tossing while your eyes see motionless walls. The same thing happens when you try to read a book in a moving car. Your brain gets mixed messages, and the confusion goes to your stomach.

Internal problems can make some people especially susceptible to motion sickness. Damage to the inner ear can make you feel almost constantly queasy. And, for reasons that doctors don't entirely understand, children who tend to get carsick often suffer from migraines as well.

There are ways to keep your stomach from traveling on its own. Here are some of the best.

Swallow Early

"Take an over-the-counter motion sickness medicine, such as Dramamine, before you travel," says Linda B. Dacey, M.D., an internist at the Dartmouth-Hitchcock Medical Center in Lebanon, New Hampshire. But don't take it if you're the driver, she adds. Dramamine can make you drowsy.

Avoid the Peanuts

The sort of snacks often served on airplanes could make your airsickness worse, according to researchers at the University of North Dakota College of Nursing. In a study of airline pilots, the researchers found that salty foods such as potato chips and preserved meats were most implicated in airsickness. Foods high in the mineral thiamine, such as beef, pork, eggs, and fish, also seemed to be triggers. So were high-protein foods such as milk and cheese. You might want to stick to fruit when you snack on the move.

Change Seats

"Put children in seats where they are least likely to get sick," advises John C. Robinson, M.D., a pediatrician in Quincy, Massachusetts. "My son was always fine in the front seat, but if we put him in the back, he'd be vomiting within 20 minutes."

Get Some Airtime

"Try driving with the windows down, even just a little bit, if you suffer from motion sickness," Dr. Robinson says. "The fresh air can help relieve the nausea. And if someone is feeling queasy in the car, keep the heat off. Heat may bother some people with motion sickness."

Fight an Allergy

"The antihistamine meclizine, sold as Bonine over the counter, helps overcome motion sickness," says Laurence Bouchard, D.O., an osteopathic family physician in private practice in Narragansett, Rhode Island.

Brace(let) Yourself

"I keep some special bracelets on my boat for people with motion sickness," Dr. Bouchard says. "You can buy them at a marine supply store. Each bracelet has a bead in the middle that presses against the inside of the wrist, applying acu-

---

TIME TO SEE THE DOCTOR
Is Your Nausea Accelerating?

GET medical attention if your episodes of motion sickness are getting worse or more frequent.

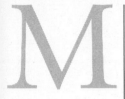

M

pressure that relieves nausea." Researchers at Humboldt State University in Arcata, California, found that applying pressure to the inside of the wrist seemed to prevent motion sickness in a group of patients.

Down Some Ginger

"Ginger tea is wonderful for motion sickness," says herbalist Jane Smolnik, owner of Crystal Garden Herbs in Springfield, Vermont. Ginger has been used by seasick sailors for thousands of years and is available in tea form at herbal or health food stores.

"It works," confirms Dr. Dacey.

MOUTH SORES

Cures for when you're feeling down in the mouth

In some ways, your mouth acts like a canary in a mine. At one time, miners used to take canaries with them into the mine shafts, on the presumption that if the air got bad, the little birds would keel over before the miners did. Your mouth does much the same thing—reacting to negative conditions and warning you before the rest of your body succumbs to oncoming ills.

That's one reason why mouth sores are so common. All sorts of problems can show up in the mouth first. Sores there can result from allergies to medication, bacterial infection, emotional stress, misuse of aspirin, addiction to chewing tobacco or snuff, poor-fitting dentures, an accidental chomp, nutritional deficiencies, or such serious diseases as tuberculosis, syphilis, and mouth cancer.

But the most common mouth miseries are not so serious: fever blisters (also called cold sores) and canker sores. People often use the terms interchangeably, and both of them can hurt a lot, but they're actually two very different ailments.

A canker sore is a painful little ulcer that appears on your tongue, the roof of your mouth, or inside a lip or cheek. Doctors aren't sure what causes it, but they think it may have to do with your body's immune system responding to stress, highly acidic foods such as oranges or tomatoes, or an accidentally bitten tongue or inside cheek. Women often get canker sores during the week before their menstrual periods. Whatever the cause, the ulcer usually disappears within 5 to 10 days.

A cold sore looks different from a canker sore. Whereas a canker sore is shaped like a shallow crater, a cold sore is a little fluid-filled bubble. The culprit in this kind of sore is the herpes simplex virus Type I—a highly contagious virus that's similar to genital herpes. Once you contract the virus in your mouth through kissing, sharing food, or touching your mouth with a hand that's touched the virus, you can have herpes simplex all your life. The first outbreak is the worst. You feel a tingling in your mouth, and sores break out, usually on your lips but sometimes on other parts of your mouth as well. You're most contagious from the time a blister ruptures until the sore is completely healed. The blisters pop on their own within hours, crust over, and are gone after 7 to 10 days. After that, the virus hangs out in your nervous system, causing cold sore breakouts at unpredictable times—which makes you contagious to other people.

Doctors know no way to prevent either canker or cold sores, but there are lots of remedies to ease the discomfort.

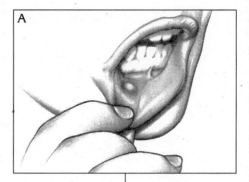

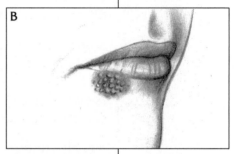

A canker sore (A) is a small, painful ulcer. A cold sore (B) is a fluid-filled blister.

Paint Your Sores

"To numb sores before eating and drinking, mix equal amounts of liquid Benadryl and Maalox," says Patricia Edwards, M.D., a pediatrician in Concord, New Hampshire. "Use a Q-Tip to paint the mixture on the sores." Both ingredients can soothe irritated tissue, she explains.

Bandage Your Mouth

"Try using over-the-counter Orabase for mouth sores," says Gregory Colpitts, D.M.D., a dentist in private practice in Franklin, New Hampshire. "It comes in a tube and will stick to a sore even when wet. Orabase acts like a bandage over the sore, protecting it from your roaming tongue."

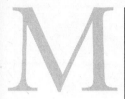

Can the Chaw

"Chewing tobacco can cause mouth sores, but that's not the worst part," Dr. Colpitts says. "Keep using it long enough, and you are going to get mouth cancer."

Beware of Movie Theaters

"With some gum inflammation and mouth sores, the culprit is popcorn hulls," says Peter Lodge, D.M.D., a dentist in Narragansett, Rhode Island. "The hulls get stuck below the gum line, hide out in the back of the mouth, and can irritate. After eating popcorn, try to rinse your mouth carefully."

Stop Playing Ketchup

"Some people's mouths react to acidic foods," Dr. Lodge says. "Drinking a lot of grapefruit juice or eating a lot of tomatoes may cause sores. If you're one of the sensitive types, you might cut back on these foods."

Switch Toothpastes

Some people develop mouth sores from their own toothpastes, according to a study by scientists in Finland. You might be allergic to any of some 30 compounds in toothpastes, from preservatives to cinnamon oil. If you get sores frequently, try switching your brand.

Eat Pineapple

A tried-and-true remedy for canker sores is pineapple. You can eat it fresh or apply the juice to the sore.

Don't Be Irritating

To keep from injuring the soft tissue and inviting mouth sores, doctors say it helps to avoid abrasive foods such as hard candy. Also, don't eat too much salt, and avoid talking while you chew to keep the food from slamming around in your mouth.

N

NAIL BITING

Chew on these remedies instead of yourself

Do you find it hard to keep from nibbling at your fingers? Doctors have a name for the nail-biting habit: onychophagia.

The problem often starts in childhood. "Some children become nail biters because their parents do it," says Robert F. Wilson, M.D., a pediatrician who is retired from his practice in Dover, New Hampshire. "It's especially annoying to see your own kid take up your bad habits."

Another cause is "pressure, anxiety, or nervousness," says Everett Orbeton, M.D., a pediatrician who is retired from his practice in Portland, Maine. "The easiest way to stop nail biting in yourself or your kid is relaxation."

There also are ways you can deal directly with the biting itself. Here's how to nip the habit in the bud.

Add a Layer

"Put sticky tape, such as duct tape, around each fingertip," says Elizabeth Lowry, M.D., who is retired after 38 years as a pediatrician in Guilford, Connecticut. "Let the biter work on the tape instead of his fingers. By the time he chews through the tape, he probably will have worked off the impulse to chew his nails."

A strategic application of duct tape can discourage nail biting.

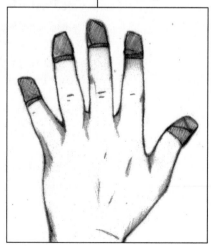

He Was Nothing if Not Flexible

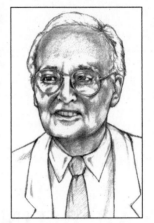

I ONCE treated a patient who benefited from a bad habit in a very strange way. He was an attorney on vacation in New England, and he came to see me with an injured ankle. While I examined him, I noticed that he chewed constantly on his fingernails.

I had his ankle x-rayed while I looked at another patient. The technician found me in the hallway. "You won't believe this," she said, "but that man from New York is sitting in a chair and biting his toenails!"

When his x-rays were developed, I went in to discuss them with the man. "I can't help noticing that your toenails look as if they've been chewed on," I said to him.

He looked a little sheepish and admitted, "Well, at night, if my fingernails are all gone, I go to work on my toenails."

I wouldn't recommend the habit, but his toenail biting must have been a great form of stretching. He was one of the most flexible people I've ever met.

BREWSTER MARTIN, M.D., *a retired family doctor in Chelsea, Vermont (population 1,166), and cofounder of the Chelsea Family Health Center. He was named Vermont Doctor of the Year in 1991.*

Get Positive

"Kids who bite their nails often do it unconsciously," Dr. Wilson says. "To get them to think about what they're doing, set up a reward system. Offer a small treat for every nail that grows long enough to cut."

Make Yourself Feel Pretty

"Try a regimen of regular manicures if you still have the nail-biting habit as an adult," suggests Cara Calomb-Down, co-owner of the Keene Beauty Academy in Keene, New Hampshire. "If you pay for your nails, you're less likely to bite them off."

NAUSEA
Ways to ease the quease

If what goes down feels as if it's coming back up, you can blame any one of a number of causes: a stomach bug, the tuna-with-mayo sandwich that spent a bit too much time outdoors, the novel you tried to read in the car, the flowing champagne at your cousin's wedding, your prescription medicine, or an attack of appendicitis.

"You can feel nauseous from something fatty like a pepperoni pizza or from an infection, ulcers, or pneumonia," says Laurie Duncan, M.D., an internist who moved from Cooperstown, New York, to Washington, D.C. "A migraine headache, a bad smell, and the first trimester of pregnancy are other common causes. Nausea also can be the first sign of a heart attack. If any kind of pain accompanies your queasiness or that queasy feeling just doesn't go away, see a doctor immediately."

For the occasional upset stomach, though, there are plenty of home cures.

Eat Breakfast

"As a school nurse, the number one cause of nausea I see is kids coming to school without having eaten any breakfast," says Susie Tann, R.N., an elementary school nurse in Bradford, Vermont. "A bowl of cereal and some juice are essential for getting the stomach off to a good start."

Have a Chaser

"Antibiotics and other prescription drugs can cause nausea," Dr. Duncan notes. "If the label says to take your medicine with food, do it. Drink a glass of milk with your pill or eat some crackers." Make sure it's okay to have food with your medicine, though. If you have any doubt, ask your doctor. And while you're at it, you also might ask if

---

TIME TO SEE THE DOCTOR
Follow Your Stomach

It's time to get checked out by your doctor when:

- You feel sick for more than two days.
- Your morning sickness from pregnancy keeps you from eating or drinking.
- You have a fever with your nausea.
- You haven't urinated all day.
- Your skin or the whites of your eyes have a yellow tinge.
- You have a sharp pain in your stomach.
- Your nausea comes and goes.

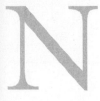

you can change prescriptions to one that's easier on your stomach, Dr. Duncan says.

Leave the Aspirin

"Aspirin and ibuprofen can upset your stomach and even cause ulcers," Dr. Duncan notes. "If you're taking a lot of over-the-counter painkillers and find yourself getting nauseated, switch to acetaminophen, which is gentler on your stomach."

Coke Is It

"Coke syrup—concentrated, uncarbonated Coca-Cola—is an old-time remedy for nausea, and it still works," says Sarah Johansen, M.D., medical director of emergency services at New London Hospital in New London, New Hampshire. "You can still buy Coke syrup in a little bottle at your pharmacy. Take a teaspoon every 20 minutes until your nausea subsides. But don't overdo it. Too much sugary syrup can have the side effect of causing a loose stool. Don't take more than six teaspoons a day."

If you don't have Coke syrup handy, Dr. Johansen suggests opening a can or bottle of cola and letting it go flat and lukewarm before drinking it. She notes, by the way, that a diet cola won't do the trick. You need the sugar to settle your stomach.

Fight the Acid

"If your nausea is caused by acid indigestion, take an over-the-counter antacid," Dr. Johansen advises. "Maalox is effective, for example." She adds that over-the-counter acid blockers also do the trick for some people. Sold as Pepcid AC, Zantac, and other brands, these drugs have the same ingredients as prescription drugs but in smaller doses.

Try Allergy Medicine

"Antihistamines such as Dramamine can help ease nausea, especially the kind caused by a food allergy," Dr. Johansen says. "Or try Bonine, an over-the-counter antihistamine that won't make you sleepy."

Have a Warm One

"Ginger tea with honey is great for nausea," says Jane Smolnik, owner of Crystal Garden Herbs in Springfield, Vermont. "It tastes like warm ginger ale." Ginger has been used as a digestive aid for thousands of years, and its stomach-soothing qualities have been confirmed in modern studies.

NECK PAIN

Is there a cramp in your rubbernecking style?

No wonder we use "pain in the neck" to describe an unbearable annoyance that just won't go away. Your neck has to support as much as 18 pounds of head while bending and twisting or being held perfectly still for hours in front of a computer screen or car windshield. Is it any wonder your neck hurts now and then?

What's more, a pain in the neck can start from lower down. Problems that originate in your back, such as a pull in a muscle or ligament, can radiate up to your neck. "If you have posture problems or some other trouble with your mid-back and shoulders, you'll probably feel it occasionally in the neck," says Gary Venman-Clay, M.D., a family doctor in Bellows Falls, Vermont. A poor alignment between the head and the back causes the neck to become an overworked fulcrum, Dr. Venman-Clay says. "As a result, a lot of neck pain has to do with muscles that go into spasm."

Another common form of neck pain crops up after your car gets rear-ended, or after an overenthusiastic tag in touch football. When your neck snaps back, the sudden stretch can tear some of your neck muscles, which bleed internally and cause painful swelling. The pain may build up gradually and not become severe until hours later, or even the next day. Emotional stress also can cause neck pain, from the constant unconscious tensing of neck muscles.

In most cases, though, neck pain or stiffness is no different from the kind you feel in your back, says Dr. Venman-

---

TIME TO SEE THE DOCTOR

Do You Feel It in Your Head?

IF YOU have a new, severe headache as well as neck pain, get medical attention quickly, says Gary Venman-Clay, M.D., a family doctor in Bellows Falls, Vermont. "You might have meningitis, a serious disease that can become a medical emergency," he says. Other signs of meningitis are neck pain along with drowsiness, confusion, or fever.

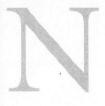Clay, and the cures can be much the same. Here are some specific remedies.

Some Like It Hot

"Neck pain that arises from muscular problems will be helped by any kind of heat," Dr. Venman-Clay notes. "Stand in a hot shower as long as you can, directing the stream right to your neck. The heat causes more blood to flow to the dam-

Are You Becoming a Working Stiff?
Try These Defensive Postures

A LOT of neck pain arises from holding a poor posture during a long-term activity, according to Laurence Bouchard, D.O., an osteopathic family physician in Narragansett, Rhode Island. That means there are plenty of things you can do to avoid the problem in the first place. Try these techniques.

• "When you do something in a seated position for a long period, such as reading a book or doing needlework, place a pillow in your lap and place the book or handwork on top of it," Dr. Bouchard says. "That will relieve your neck of the strain of bending."

• Position your computer screen so that your neck doesn't have to accommodate it. "The top of the screen should be level with your eyes," he says.

• If you have neck problems, skip the breaststroke when you swim. "The breaststroke hyperextends the neck and causes strain," Dr. Bouchard explains.

• Sit up when you watch television. "Never watch it lying down," he says. "When lying, you tend to put your neck in an awkward position and then hold it for long periods."

• Supplement your bifocals with glasses made only for reading. "The trouble with bifocals is that you have to tilt your head back when you look down," Dr. Bou-chard notes. "That's the worst position you can put your neck in."

• "Don't drive with your arm up on the window frame," he cautions. "That position jams the neck." Hold the steering wheel at the five o'clock and seven o'clock positions. Avoid gripping high up on the wheel. Most cars now have easy steering, allowing the lower grip.

• Watch your posture when you're on the phone. The phone should come to your ear; your ear shouldn't come to the phone. And never rest the receiver between

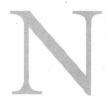

aged muscle, and the blood then carries away debris such as blood cells and damaged fiber from the injury, causing it to heal faster."

Get Your Back Up

"If you take good care of your mid-back and shoulders, your head will naturally sit right," Dr. Venman-Clay says. "Strengthen your back to help your neck." Here's a back-strengthening exercise that also works the shoulders: Lie on the floor—a soft rug or carpet helps. Place your hands at your sides, palms up. Now slowly lift your head, shoulders, and hands as far as you comfortably can—no more than a foot off the floor. Lower them gently, then repeat 10 times. Do this exercise 3 times a week to build supportive muscle in the back and shoulders.

Add Some Spice

"A gentle massage can work wonders on a sore neck," Dr. Venman-Clay says. "You don't have to use a fancy technique or expensive lotions. Just get a loved one to rub the sore area slowly for as long as she has the patience to do it."

If you want to use a massage cream, consider one such as Zostrix, made with capsaicin—the compound found in hot red peppers. Researchers with the U.S. Army in Texas got positive results when they had patients with chronic neck pain use capsaicin cream four times a day for a five-week period. But, Dr. Venman-Clay notes, "more important than the cream or lotion is the act of massaging it into your sore neck. That's the real reliever."

Let Fall

"A lot of neck pain arises from constant muscle tension," says Randal Schaetzke, D.C., a chiropractor at the Wholistic Health Center in Quechee, Vermont. "Practice relaxing your shoulders by letting them drop when they're bunched around your neck."

Pillow Fight the Pain

"Cervical pillows are great at relieving neck pain for some people," Dr. Schaetzke says. "You can buy them at medical supply stores. But they work only if you sleep on your back."

Hang In There

IF YOUR neck tends to be stiff in the morning, avoid the temptation to stretch it with the traditional 360-degree neck roll, says Tiffany Renaud, D.C., a chiropractor in South Burlington, Vermont. "Never allow your head to drop backward," she says. "You could damage muscle and nerve fiber." Instead, try Dr. Renaud's favorite neck stretch when you get out of bed. "It works even better if you do it in a hot shower," she notes.

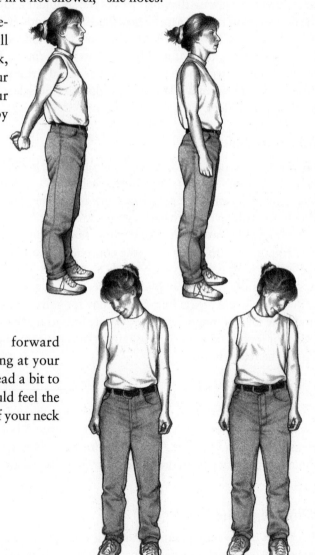

1. Grip your hands behind your back, pull your shoulders back, and then release your hands and let your arms hang limp by your sides.

2. Drop your head forward gently. While looking at your feet, stretch your head a bit to each side. You should feel the stretch in one side of your neck at a time.

Feed Your Neck

"To avoid muscle problems in your neck and other areas, make sure you're getting plenty of calcium and magnesium in your diet," Dr. Schaetzke says. "They act as a lubricant on the cellular level. You can get these minerals in dairy products, broccoli, dark green leafy vegetables such as spinach, and sardines."

NERVOUSNESS
Anxious for a cure? Try these

Waiting to hear if you got that job? Working up the courage to ask for your beloved's hand in marriage? Packing up for a cross-country move? You have a *right* to feel nervous. How you deal with your feelings of anxiety is another thing. Some people tend to breeze through life's cliff-hanging moments. Other poor souls suffer mightily from the same anxious times, losing sleep, constantly tensing their muscles, finding it difficult to concentrate, jumping at every sound. Or they might have an overall feeling of constant dread.

Usually, the feeling goes away with the source of fear. But in some cases, your nervousness can last for more than half a year, with no one identifiable cause. Doctors call this feeling "generalized anxiety disorder"—a condition that needs to be treated by a qualified therapist. Get medical help if you have suffered four or more panic attacks in the past month or if your feeling of nervousness lasts more than six months and doesn't have a single identifiable cause. "If you feel nervous because you're getting ready to head off to college or start a new job, that's normal," says Mary-Catherine Gennaro, D.O., a family osteopath in Warren, New Hampshire. "But if you panic every time the telephone rings, you need to talk to a doctor about it."

Long-lasting nervousness also can show itself in the form of occasional panic attacks, moments of terror when you may have trouble breathing, chest pain, a racing heart, choking, chills or hot flashes, or a feeling that you're losing control or going bonkers. "You can also experience sweating, dizziness, and a feeling that the room is closing in," says Kathleen Kovner-Kline, M.D., a child psychiatrist at the Dartmouth-

Practice AWAREness

IF YOU'RE experiencing a panic attack, remember the acronym AWARE, says Kathleen Kovner-Kline, M.D., a child psychiatrist at the Dartmouth-Hitchcock Medical Center in Lebanon, New Hampshire.

The first **A** stands for awareness: "Be aware of what's going on," Dr. Kovner-Kline says. "Label your feelings as a panic attack and remind yourself that you're not dying and that the attack will go away."

The **W** is for watchfulness. "Watch your symptoms," she explains. "All panic attacks have a pattern—the symptoms come on like a wave. I tell my patients to ride that wave and wait for it to pass. That kind of watchful detachment is reassuring in itself."

The next **A** stands for act. "Stay active through the attack. Don't stop what you're doing," Dr. Kovner-Kline says. "Try not to retreat from where you are."

R is for relax. "Learn relaxation techniques from your doctor," she advises. "These may include breathing exercises, distraction, and biofeedback."

E means enjoy life. "Don't let panic attacks rule you," she says.

Hitchcock Medical Center in Lebanon, New Hampshire. "A reminder of a past bad experience can cause a panic attack. So can intractable fears called phobias, or a biochemical imbalance in your system."

A passing panic attack is no cause for long-term alarm, Dr. Kovner-Kline says. For the occasional case of nerves, chill out with these remedies.

Plan Ahead

"Many nervous people find that having a lot of structure in their lives helps," Dr. Gennaro says. "Plan out your day or week so that you know what's ahead."

Expose Yourself

"Some phobias have to do with things you don't have to face very often," Dr. Kovner-Kline notes. "If you're terrified of tarantulas, for example, you probably don't need to treat that fear—just avoid the spiders." By contrast, a traveling salesperson who's afraid to fly might need to deal with the phobia.

An effective technique, according to Dr. Kovner-Kline, is what therapists call exposure. There are two kinds of exposure: gradual and flooding. "For the traveling salesperson, gradual exposure might mean seeing a movie about what goes on in an airplane cockpit, then visiting the airport, then going with a friend onto a plane but not riding on it, and finally taking a flight," she explains. If that's too difficult, flooding might be the best method to overcome the phobia. "Have the salesperson take eight flights in one day."

NIGHT BLINDNESS
Shedding light on your personal darkness

If you're having problems with night vision and you are over 40, it could just be that your baby blues aren't as young as they used to be. "Aging reduces the ability of the rods in your eyes—the structures that detect light—to distinguish shapes in the dark," says Eugene J. Bernal, O.D., an optometrist in private practice in White River Junction, Vermont. "Over time, your eye's retina becomes less sensitive. The lens also gets cloudier, and your eyes begin to have difficulty adapting to changes in light and darkness." By contrast, he says, some people are just born with less ability than others to see in the dark.

"If you're still in your teens or twenties, I suspect that you may be nearsighted at night," says Henry Kriegstein, M.D., an ophthalmologist in private practice in Hingham, Plymouth, and Sandwich, Massachusetts. "You might not be nearsighted in the daytime, but in the dark your eyes focus more closely, making you temporarily nearsighted."

Poor night vision also can stem from eye problems caused by diabetes, cataracts, or diseases of the retina. People in Third World countries (and sometimes in the United States) who suffer from a lack of vitamin A can develop night blindness.

Here's what you can do to brighten things up.

Take Your Vitamins
"Antioxidants—vitamins that help reduce the natural wear and tear on your body—seem to be important for the eye,"

The Cop Who Cured My Sight

EVERY year, one of my two daughters comes to visit me on the anniversary of my wife's death. On her most recent visit, we drove to the city of Montpelier, Vermont, to see a movie. We headed out into the night despite a bad rainstorm. Being Vermonters, we don't let weather hold us back. I drove.

"Can you see okay?" my daughter kept asking me, peering into the night.

"Sure, sure, pretty well," I said, and in fact I could see the middle of the road just fine. Problem was, I couldn't see the white line on the edge of the road at all. I didn't say anything, but I was convinced that I was getting night blindness—in my right eye, at least.

Just as we passed the city line in Montpelier, a policeman pulled us over. "Your right headlight is out," he said. I got a new bulb for the headlight, and I was cured!

Sometimes even a good doctor can benefit from a second opinion.

BREWSTER MARTIN, M.D., *a retired family doctor in Chelsea, Vermont (population 1,166), and cofounder of the Chelsea Family Health Center. He was named Vermont Doctor of the Year in 1991.*

says Stephen Moore, M.D., an ophthalmologist in Great Barrington, Massachusetts. "They might prevent cataracts and macular degeneration." Dr. Moore recommends a daily vitamin supplement called Ocuvite, which contains all the daily requirements for vitamins that help ensure good eyesight. Ocuvite is available over the counter at drugstores.

Focus on Your Glasses

"If you want to see in dim light, you need the best vision possible," Dr. Bernal says. "Get an eye exam once a year to make sure you have the right glasses."

Don't Be Reflective

Glasses with special nonreflective lenses that reduce glare "may increase the contrast between light and dark," Dr. Bernal says. "It isn't a miracle cure, but it may help some people who are having trouble with night vision."

Stub the Smokes

"Chronic use of tobacco can affect night vision," Dr. Bernal notes. Which is one of many reasons for seeing your way clear to kicking the habit.

And Skip the Nightcap

Excessive drinking of alcohol can harm your ability to see at night, Dr. Bernal says. Limit yourself to no more than two drinks a day.

Eat Brightly

Night blindness is one of the early symptoms of poor nutrition. "If you want your eyes to operate at maximum efficiency, eat a balanced diet with plenty of fruits and vegetables," Dr. Bernal advises.

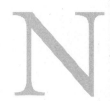

NIGHTMARES

Keeping sweet dreams
from going sour

"To sleep: perchance to dream," said Shakespeare's Hamlet. Sleep sounded pretty good to the melancholy Dane; it was the dreaming part that troubled him. Like many people who suffer from nightmares, Hamlet was under some stress.

"An occasional nightmare is normal," says Michael Sateia, M.D., director of the Sleep Disorders Clinic at the Dartmouth-Hitchcock Medical Center in Lebanon, New Hampshire. "Bad dreams reflect our day-to-day fears and anxiety. If they are more frequent, that may be a reflection of a psychiatric illness or distress. We see more frequent nightmares in individuals who have suffered some trauma—abuse, war, a natural disaster"—or, as in Hamlet's case, seeing your dad get bumped off by a rival for the Danish throne.

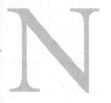

Most bearers of bad dreams happen to be younger than Hamlet. "Nightmares are most common in children," Dr. Sateia explains. "Kids are like sponges, soaking up information around them. But they often have trouble processing all the new stuff cognitively. And so frightening thoughts and new life experiences can bother kids more than adults."

Just how do dreams turn nightmarish? Dr. Sateia explains that most nightmares occur during periods of rapid eye movement (REM) sleep. You don't usually get bad dreams—or dreams of any kind—when you first fall asleep. You tend to sleep most deeply during the first hour to an hour and a half after you drop off. After that, your brain alternates between REM sleep and deeper sleep. The periods of REM sleep get longer as the night wanes. "That's why most nightmares occur toward morning," Dr. Sateia says.

Bad dreams or no bad dreams—that is the question. We offer some answers below.

Face the Mare

"I've always believed that nightmares are a child's way of working out unresolved conflicts from his waking hours," says Mark Harris, M.D., a pediatrician in private practice in Bradford, Vermont. Dr. Harris says that you should ask a nightmare-plagued child what is bothering him. The next step is to use what psychiatrists call imagery rehearsal—practicing turning a bad dream into a good one. "For example, if a child is having nightmares in which he is chased by a dog, give him a feeling of mastery over dogs," Dr. Harris says. "During the day, help him play with good dogs or give him stuffed toy dogs."

If the youngster can't specify just what the nightmare is all about, "look at the child's life for situations that may be troubling him—a divorce, a move, or an ill parent. Then try to help the child understand the situation in ways that don't threaten him."

TIME TO SEE THE DOCTOR

When Nightmares Get out of Hand

AN OCCASIONAL nightmare is normal, even in adults, but you should get medical attention if frequent nightmares make you afraid to fall asleep, says Michael Sateia, M.D., director of the Sleep Disorders Clinic at the Dartmouth-Hitchcock Medical Center in Lebanon, New Hampshire. "If the nightmares reflect a trauma, a psychiatrist can help you or your child face the trauma and work through it," he says. "We call that desensitizing therapy."

Remove the Scares

"Look at the content of your child's day if she's had a nightmare," says Kathleen Kovner-Kline, M.D., a child psychiatrist at the Dartmouth-Hitchcock Medical Center in Lebanon, New Hampshire. "If your child has just seen *Jurassic Park* and is having nightmares, she doesn't need drugs or fancy therapy—she needs to avoid scary movies. The brain has fewer inhibitions at night, so things a child can handle in the daytime may be too much for her when she's sleeping."

Get a Bedtime Ritual

"Make bedtime a safe time for your children," Dr. Kovner-Kline says. "Do the same things every night. Read comforting stories and say bedtime prayers together—preferably the same prayers. Children love ritual. I have a friend who whispers a prayer into her little boy's ear every night before he falls asleep. If she forgets, he tells her, 'Say the comforting words, Mama.'" Dr. Kovner-Kline says some well-practiced nighttime prayers to her own four children. The wife of an Episcopalian minister, she also has a master's degree in divinity from Yale University.

Wake Up!

"Some children have nightmares at the same time every night," says Patricia Edwards, M.D., a pediatrician in private practice in Concord, New Hampshire. "If your child has a regularly scheduled nightmare, try waking her a half hour before the nightmare time every night for a week. That should break the pattern."

Deal With the Terror

One form of nighttime trouble seems like a nightmare, but it tends to occur early in the night, it has to do with a single scary image, and it makes your child sit bolt upright,

---

ANNALS OF MEDICINE

It's Terrifying to Birds, Though

THE word *nightmare* comes from Mara, an old German demon that was said to suffocate people while they slept. The great Puritan clergyman Cotton Mather noted a popular remedy to keep nightmares off your chest: "a Swallows Head, worn about the Neck." He personally preferred the more pleasant remedy of drinking the syrup of peony in a glass of wine. Neither remedy is recommended by doctors today.

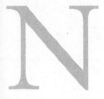

screaming. "That's a night terror," Dr. Edwards says. Like nightmares, night terrors tend to be caused by stress. A lack of sleep, fever, and some medications also can trigger terrors. "First," Dr. Edwards says, "check to make sure the screaming is caused by a terror and not a foot that got caught in the crib." That accomplished, "your best bet is to comfort the child and help him get back to sleep."

Don't Bottle Your Nightmares

"Watch your alcohol consumption at night if you're an adult who gets nightmares," says Mary-Catherine Gennaro, D.O., a family osteopath in Warren, New Hampshire. "Drinking can cause nightmares. Also, don't eat right before bed."

NOSEBLEED

Ways to stop the leak in your beak

Nosebleeds may look dramatic, but the gore usually isn't cause for alarm. "Most nosebleeds are due to minor trauma in the anterior nose—the part near the tip—which is rich in blood supply," says Dudley Weider, M.D., an otolaryngologist at the Dartmouth-Hitchcock Medical Center in Lebanon, New Hampshire. The hundreds of tiny blood vessels in that area are easily disturbed by a punch in the snout, a walk into a door, a cold or allergy, a vigorous honk into a handkerchief, a bout of nose picking, various medications, or just plain dry indoor air. As people age, their nasal membranes may dry out, contributing to spontaneous nosebleeds.

A small number of nosebleeds are in the back of the nose and allow blood to trickle down the throat. This could be a sign of a serious problem, says Richard Lee, M.D., an otolaryngologist in Laconia, New Hampshire. "First, try to pinch the soft part of the nose—the part right up front—for 10 to 20 minutes," Dr. Lee says. "If the bleeding won't stop, get to an emergency room. You need medical help if you can't stanch the bleeding."

For the more benign, front-of-the-nose versions, here's how you can stop the flow.

In a Pinch, This Will Work

"First, sit down in a chair and mellow out," says Peter Brassard, M.D., a family physician on Block Island, Rhode Island. "Rushing around will just make you bleed more." Sitting up also relieves the pressure on blood vessels, helping to slow the flow. Lean forward a bit to prevent the blood from going down the back of your throat. "Now gently pinch the softest part of your nostrils together," Dr. Brassard says. "Ninety percent of nosebleeds are in the anterior, or front, part of the nose, so the pinching will stop the bleeding there." He says to hold your nose for at least 10 minutes, preferably 20.

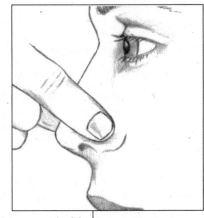

A gentle pinch usually stops the bleeding.

Stop the Bleeding Cold

"Use an ice-filled washcloth on the side of the bleeding nostril when you squeeze it," recommends David Sigelman, M.D., a pediatrician with Holyoke Pediatric Associates in

---

AN OUNCE OF PREVENTION

Pick a Fight with a Bad Habit

DOCTORS say that nose pickers are among the most common victims of nosebleeds. "That's because their noses never get a chance to heal," says Dudley Weider, M.D., an otolaryngologist at the Dartmouth-Hitchcock Medical Center in Lebanon, New Hampshire.

To prevent straying fingers in small children, Dr. Weider recommends putting gloves on them at night, when nose picking often reaches its peak. If the digging knows no hours, "put gloves on them in the daytime as well. I had a couple of kids who were so bad that I put boxing gloves on them until their noses healed."

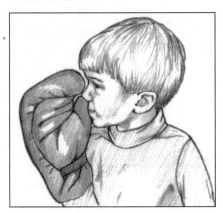

Talk about Your Stuffed-Up Nose

For centuries, doctors recommended relieving bloody noses by putting various materials up the nostrils. "Lint made into tents, dipped in Vinegar, stuffed up the Nose" is what Thomas Palmer, a seventeenth-century minister and country doctor, recommended in his guidebook, *The Admirable Secrets of Physick and Chyrurgery*. Vinegar is an astringent, which could reduce the bleeding. But these days, doctors recommend moisteners instead of astringents.

Holyoke, Massachusetts. "The cold will constrict the blood vessels inside your nose and help stop the bleeding."

Try Some Nostril Nostrums

"Put a dab of over-the-counter Bacitracin, an antibacterial ointment, on a small ball of cotton," Dr. Weider says. "Stick it in the nostril and leave it for 12 hours." Be sure to use Bacitracin, not another ointment.

Get Slick

Dr. Lee recommends moistening dried-out, bloody nostrils with K-Y Jelly, a product sold in drugstores to lubricate a woman's vagina for sexual intercourse. Apply it to the outside rim and just inside the nostrils.

Make Yourself a Humid Being

Because many nosebleeds are caused by the drying out of the delicate tissue inside your nostrils, doctors recommend keeping your home humid. Crack a window in your bedroom in the winter, place pans of water near radiators and stoves, or get a humidifier.

Take the Slow Cure

"Some nosebleeds are caused by anemia, a lack of iron in the blood," says Corinne Martin, a certified clinical herbalist in Bridgton, Maine. "If you have a tendency to be anemic, take a teaspoon of molasses several times a day." Molasses is high in iron, Martin explains.

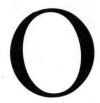

OVEREXERTION

*Healing steps to take
when you've pushed yourself too far*

If you find yourself gasping for breath after an unaccustomed
activity, you may have gone beyond what's appropriate for
your physical condition. "How much is
too much depends on the person," says
Daniel Caloras, M.D., a family doctor
in private practice in Charlestown, New
Hampshire. "If you run marathons, an
activity that makes you a bit tired might
kill someone else. I have a patient who
developed chest pains while making love
with his wife; that was overexertion
for him."

You can overdo it over long periods
as well. "One young fellow came in
looking awful," Dr. Caloras says. "He
had bags and dark circles under his eyes,
and he could hardly stand. Turns out he
was a real Yankee, working two physically demanding jobs. He would work
his 40-hour-a-week job and then moon-
light milking a herd of dairy cows. He
was home just six hours each day and
was probably sleeping only four hours
a night."

TIME TO SEE THE DOCTOR

Let Your Chest Be the Judge

IF YOU get pains in your chest
during an activity, see a doctor
immediately, says Sarah Johansen,
M.D., medical director of emergency services at New London
Hospital in New London, New
Hampshire. Also see your doctor if
you find breathing difficult when
you exert yourself or if you feel a
numbness radiating up your left
arm. "These signs are especially important if you are obese, smoke, or
have high cholesterol, high blood
pressure, or a family history of
heart disease," she says.

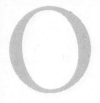

O

The only real cure for overexertion, of course, is rest. "Most people need to get at least seven to eight hours of sleep per night," Dr. Caloras says. "And if a single activity is too much for you, don't try to gut it out. Stop immediately."

To keep from getting to the shutdown point, follow these tips from hardworking country doctors.

Be Cool

"When exercising, always start out well-hydrated," says Sarah Johansen, M.D., medical director of emergency services at New London Hospital in New London, New Hampshire. "Drink about a quart of water at least an hour and a half before any sustained outdoor activity. Once you begin, be sure to take frequent breaks, and don't stay out in the sun too long. Overheating can easily make your overexertion worse."

Do a Proper Snow Job

"If you are not in good physical shape and you're older than 50, you might want to hire someone to shovel your snow for you," says Douglas Deaett, M.D., an emergency room physician at Alice Peck Day Memorial Hospital in Lebanon, New Hampshire. As an alternative, he says, use a small shovel—

When the only available snow mover is you, take some simple precautions: Use a small shovel, bend at the knees, and don't twist.

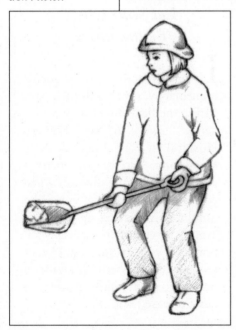

even one made for a child. Or if you must use a full-size shovel, at least avoid loading it all the way. "A load of snow in one of those big scoop shovels may weigh as much as 50 pounds," Dr. Deaett says. "Don't try to lift a shovel that heavy—fill it halfway."

When you do lift, use proper technique: Bend at the knees and hold your back straight. "Turn your feet to throw snow off to the side of your driveway or walk," Dr. Deaett says. "Do not pivot with your mid-body. That is very, very unsafe for your back." He adds that it's also a good idea to warm up beforehand, treating your shoveling job as if it were a sporting event. "Do some jumping jacks for 10 minutes, then stretch by touching your toes."

OVERWEIGHT

Lighten up! Shedding pounds doesn't have to be a grim affair

You've admitted to yourself that there's more of you to go around lately; the person in the mirror is you and then some. Well, join a very large crowd—the average weight of Americans has been on the rise over the past several decades. At any one moment, about a third of the American population is trying to lose weight. Some 35 million adults in this country are at least 20 percent fatter than the chart on the doctor's wall says they should be—which classifies them as officially obese.

And then there are the rest of us, who cringe a little when it's time to hit the beach in a bathing suit. If you've ever tried a diet plan to fit into that suit better, you probably ended up discouraged—along with millions of other dieting Americans who have lost weight only to regain it within the year. Oh, sure, you can often get dramatic results during the first two or three weeks of a diet, when your weight takes a gratifying dip. But those pounds you're shedding are mostly fluids. After that initial heady period, the only way to lose more weight is to lose actual fat. And that's the hard part. Dieting can slow down your metabolism—the rate at which your body naturally burns fuel. If you eat less and fail to move about more, a diet can actually train your body to need less food—and to convert the excess into the very fat you're trying to shed.

"Some people are worse off than others when it comes to being overweight," says Brewster Martin, M.D., a retired family doctor in Chelsea, Vermont. "You may have inher-

Say, Socrates, Won't You Stay for Dessert?

DANGEROUSLY wacky fad diets were taking people in for thousands of years before the development of the infomercial. The more gullible Romans in the third century A.D. were following milk-only diets, eating only water and figs, or avoiding liquids altogether.

If only they had listened to Socrates, the great Greek philosopher of the fifth century B.C. His diet prescription: Walk away from a meal when you're still slightly hungry. "That's not a bad idea," says Mary-Catherine Gennaro, D.O., a family osteopath in Warren, New Hampshire. "My generation was taught by our parents to be part of the Clean Plate Club, dooming us to a habit of eating too many calories. If you want to lose weight, push away from the table before you feel full."

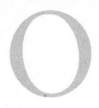ited a slow metabolic rate, making your body efficient at storing calories as fat. Or you may have been encouraged as a child to eat too much, acquiring a lifetime tendency toward being overweight."

Still, you know the importance of trying to lose that poundage. Even a mere 5 percent drop in weight can reduce or eliminate some of the illnesses caused by obesity, a Harvard Medical School study showed. As the great Benjamin Franklin asked, "Wouldst thou enjoy a long Life, a healthy Body, and a vigorous Mind?" He supplied his own answer: "Bring thy Appetite into Subjection to Reason." Of course, even Franklin's powerful reason couldn't bring his own appetite entirely under control. He could have stood to lose a few pounds himself.

Here's how you can shed some of that excess weight without the heartbreak of gaining it back.

Start Counting

"You can't lose weight consistently without eating fewer calories than you burn during the day," says Marcia Herrin, Ed.D., M.P.H., R.D., coordinator of the Nutrition Education Program at Dartmouth College and adjunct instructor of community and family medicine at Dartmouth Medical School in Hanover, New Hampshire. So what are those little measurement units that drive dieters nuts? "Calories are the measure of energy in food," Dr. Herrin explains. "Researchers literally burn food and measure the heat produced to determine the calorie content. A calorie is the amount of energy needed to heat one centiliter of water one degree."

And how many extra calories does it take to make you gain weight? "If you consume just 90 more calories a day than you burn, you can gain 10 pounds in a year," she says. Of course, the opposite is true as well—except for one thing: Fewer calories often mean a slower metabolism.

Get into the Fast Lane

The best way to jack up a slowing metabolism—making your body burn more food fuel—is to keep the body moving. "I see a lot of resistance when I prescribe exercise for overweight people," Dr. Herrin notes. "The very idea of exercise is such a turnoff for some people that they won't even try it. So I suggest that they do more vigorously what they like to do already: dance, walk, zip around the mall shopping, aerobic vacuuming, switching from an automatic to a push lawn mower. Once you start getting positive feedback from a slimmer body, you're inspired to do more serious exercise."

Medical research has shown that sustained activity can actually burn fat—not only during the exercise itself but for hours afterward as well. There's even some evidence that exercise can increase your preference for carbohydrates over fat, and a high-carbohydrate, low-fat diet can help you lose weight.

The Pot Called the Belly Fat

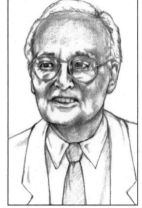

A PATIENT of mine named Frank came in for an insurance physical. I examined him on the same table I had used to deliver him 25 years earlier. He weighed 7 pounds 5 ounces the day he was born. During his insurance physical, he exceeded the limit of my scale, which went up only to 300 pounds.

I wrote "300-plus" on the insurance form without saying anything. Frank knew he was overweight. He'd been struggling with it for years, as many obese people do. It's an ailment that can be psychologically debilitating for some people. But not for Frank.

"Doc," he said to me when I had finished weighing him, "how much did you weigh the day you delivered me?"

"One hundred twenty-nine pounds," I replied.

"How much do you weigh now?"

"One hundred fifty-five."

"You've fleshed up a bit, haven't you?" he said.

BREWSTER MARTIN, M.D., *a retired family doctor in Chelsea, Vermont (population 1,166), and cofounder of the Chelsea Family Health Center. He was named Vermont Doctor of the Year in 1991.*

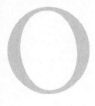

Join the Infantry

Once you start working some activity into your life, you're ready to step up to walking. "Walking is the most effective way of managing excess weight and keeping it off," says John Bland, M.D., a rheumatologist in Cambridge, Vermont. Dr. Bland notes that this is especially true for obese people, "whose extra weight may put them at some risk of muscle and joint injury." The ideal pace for losing weight, he says, is 3½ to 4 miles per hour, which will burn an average of 240 calories per hour. Walk three times a week for at least 20 minutes each time, he says.

Slosh to Weight Loss

"Water is the best diet drink around," Dr. Bland notes. "It gives you a feeling of fullness with zero calories." Before you hit the fridge, he suggests, down a glass of the clear stuff.

Stick to the Serving

When you dig into a box of low-calorie cookies, make sure you know just how many of those scanty calories you're getting. "Most people don't know what a serving size is, even if they look on the label to see the number of calories in a serving," says Patricia Edwards, M.D., a pediatrician in private practice in Concord, New Hampshire. "Don't just read how many calories and fat grams—see how much food is in a serving. For example, don't grab 10 crackers if a serving size is 4. Limit yourself to the 4."

Here, Kid, Go Buy Yourself a Mineral Water

"Sodas are the number one culprit in overweight children, and they're not so great for adults' weight either," Dr. Herrin says. "Limit both your kids and yourself to just one soda per week, and you'll save yourself useless sugar—sometimes more than 150 calories—for every soda you avoid." One alternative is bottled water. A water bottle has the feel of a soda bottle, allowing you to transfer your bottle habit to a healthy alternative.

Count the Calories in Other Bottles, Too

"Count the liquids as well as the other foods that are going into your and your child's bodies," says John C. Robinson,

M.D., a pediatrician in private practice in Quincy, Massachusetts. "There are a lot of calories in fruit juices, sodas, and even milk. And skim milk isn't necessarily a weight-loss drink—it packs 11 calories an ounce—while whole milk has 20 calories an ounce. That's 160 calories for an eight-ounce glass."

Chew a Lot

"It takes your stomach 20 minutes to tell your brain it's full," says Mary-Catherine Gennaro, D.O., a family osteopath in Warren, New Hampshire. "Eat slowly, and you can satisfy yourself with less."

Add Starch

Research by Australian biochemists shows that boiled potatoes fill you up faster than many other foods. So do what your mother told you to do: Eat your starch.

No Beer Is Less Filling

"Alcohol contains seven calories per gram," Dr. Herrin says. "When bagels were a bit smaller than they tend to be today, drinking one beer used to be equivalent in calories to eating one bagel." (Now a beer equals about three-quarters of a plump bagel, she says.) "I'd ask college students at a party whether they felt like eating three bagels. They'd always say no and then down three beers without thinking about it." While adding calories, alcohol also reduces inhibitions, she notes, making you more likely to eat excessively. So if you want to shed the pounds, shed the booze.

P

PHLEBITIS

*Ways to treat
those painful little blood clots*

That spot of pain on your leg could be a bruise. But if you can't for the life of you remember bumping into anything, take a closer look: One of your veins may be bright red and appear hard to the touch. Chances are good that the vein has become inflamed as a result of a blood clot that has caused blood to back up—a condition doctors call phlebitis.

"Phlebitis can be a darned nuisance," says Robert G. Page, M.D., a retired cardiologist in Londonderry, Vermont. "You usually get it in your legs because gravity makes your blood pool down there." But you can also get phlebitis in other places, such as your arm. And the condition isn't always painful. Your leg or arm may swell up mysteriously or feel strangely warm as the result of a clot in a vein deep under the skin. This is a more serious form of phlebitis, Dr. Page says, because the clot can cut loose and wander to your lungs or heart, damaging important tissue.

It's a good idea to have your doctor make sure which variety of phlebitis you have. If it's the superficial kind, you can treat it yourself with the remedies below. The deep variety requires special care.

Tilt Yourself

"Elevate your legs above the level of your heart when you're off your feet," says F. Daniel Golyan, M.D., a former New

Englander who is now an electrophysiologist in private practice on Long Island. "Put a pillow on the foot of a
recliner when you sit to read or watch
television."

Hose Them Up

"Try wearing support hose," Dr. Golyan
advises. "Your doctor can prescribe
hose that's right for you."

Pop Aspirin

"If the inflammation is mild, take aspirin
or ibuprofen," says Laurence Bouchard,
D.O., an osteopathic family physician in
Narragansett, Rhode Island.

Lighten Your Load

"People who are overweight have a
greater chance of getting phlebitis," says
Brewster Martin, M.D., a retired family
doctor in Chelsea, Vermont. "If you want to avoid clotting,
talk to your doctor about gradually losing weight."

Toast Your Leg

"Drink a glass of red wine at dinner every day if you have
phlebitis," says Mary-Catherine Gennaro, D.O., a family osteopath in Warren, New Hampshire. Research shows that
red wine, taken in moderation, can help improve your
circulation.

PINKEYE

Cures for gummy, itchy orbs

A dip in the pool or the onset of the sneezing season can make
your eyeballs look like your pet rabbit's—a bright, shocking
pink. Usually, a period of shut-eye will take care of the irritation. But sometimes the surface of your eye, the conjunc-
tiva, becomes inflamed. Your eyes itch and feel sore, and you
may see some goo on the edges. That's conjunctivitis, ap-
propriately nicknamed pinkeye.

P

The most common causes are viruses, bacteria, and allergies. The viral kind is usually nothing to worry about. "Viral pinkeye is usually associated with sore throat and colds and will run its course in about a week," says Eugene J. Bernal, O.D., an optometrist in private practice in White River Junction, Vermont. An allergic reaction—caused by pollen or other irritants—usually clears up when you deal with the allergies. But it's the bacterial kind that gives pinkeye a bad name.

If your eyes are crusty in the morning or they stick when you try to open them, chances are good that you have a bacterial infection. "If you have the gooey kind of pinkeye, you need to see a doctor for a prescription for an antibiotic," Dr. Bernal says. Unlike most viral or allergic kinds, bacterial conjunctivitis can cause permanent damage to eyes.

Kids tend to get pinkeye more than adults do. "The biggest spreaders are the toddler crowd—the 18- to 36-month-old children who are always touching things, putting things in their mouths, and putting their fingers in their eyes and noses," says Stephen Blair, M.D., a pediatrician in private practice in Claremont, New Hampshire. "Conjunctivitis can spread like wildfire through a day care center and on to the parents."

So what do you do if your own eyes have turned pink? Here are some solutions.

TIME TO SEE THE DOCTOR
If It Hurts, Don't Wait

IF YOUR eyes are pink or red and you feel pain or irritation in them as well, call your doctor," says Henry Kriegstein, M.D., an ophthalmologist in private practice in Hingham, Plymouth, and Sandwich, Massachusetts. "You need medical attention if it feels as though you have a foreign body in the eye or if your eyes ache or itch or are sensitive to light. Also be sure to see your doctor if you have pus or any other form of discharge from your eyes."

Steep Your Peepers

"Wet a clean washcloth in warm water, lie back, and drape the cloth over your eyes," says Susie Tann, R.N., an elementary school nurse in Bradford, Vermont. "The moist heat will help deal with the crust and make your eyes feel better in the short term."

Or Refresh Them

"Moisturizing drops will help make your eyes feel better until your doctor's cures take effect," says Dr. Bernal, who recommends Refresh, available over the counter at drugstores.

Keep Scrubbing

"If you have pinkeye or are around someone who does, the more you wash your hands the better," Dr. Bernal says. "People touch their eyes dozens of times in an hour without even realizing it. If you have pinkeye, you can get the virus or bacteria all over your hands. And if you've picked up the infection on your hands, failing to wash them will almost certainly mean you'll carry it to your eyes."

Store the Lenses

"If you wear contacts, you are at a higher risk of contracting pinkeye," Dr. Bernal says. "The lens holds things against the eye, including bacteria and viruses." Besides pinkeye, you also run the risk of getting an infection of the cornea—a serious ailment that can cause permanent damage to the eye. "So if you wear contacts, stop wearing them at the first sign of irritation and see your eye doctor," Dr. Bernal says.

POISON IVY AND OAK

Itching to deal with these irritating plants? Here's how

Poison ivy and oak are members of a plant family that includes poison wood (an itch-causing plant found in Florida) and poison sumac, according to W. Hardy Eshbaugh, Ph.D., a retired botanist in Oxford, Ohio. "Some other members of the same plant family can cause a rash in some people," Dr. Eshbaugh says. "The skin of a mango can be irritating to sensitive skin. And Chinese lacquerware boxes can cause a poison-ivy-like rash."

A
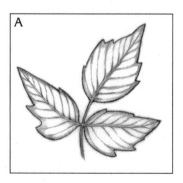

B
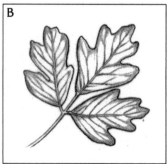

Members of an irritating family, both poison ivy (A) and poison oak (B) contain the itch-causing chemical urushiol.

P

"You can get the same kind of dermatitis from the shells of raw cashews," notes Kathryn A. Zug, M.D., a dermatologist at the Dartmouth-Hitchcock Medical Center in Lebanon, New Hampshire.

The culprit in all these plants is a potent chemical called urushiol. Seven out of 10 people are allergic to it, you can get a rash from just one-billionth gram of the stuff, and it remains potent on garden tools and other surfaces for up to five years. No wonder urushiol is the champion of all allergens—the cause of more allergies than any other known substance.

You needn't stay out of the fields and woods, though. Here are some remedies to deal with the itch.

Get the Poison Off Fast

"The best treatment for poison ivy or oak is to wash with soap in the shower within 5 to 15 minutes of exposure to the plant," Dr. Zug says. In other words, you need to wash off the urushiol long before you see a rash. This is possible, of course, only if you realize your mistake while you're in the woods. Rubbing alcohol also might work. "Rubbing alcohol is a solvent that, in order to be effective, must be applied and washed off with a washcloth soon after contact with the plant," Dr. Zug says.

Put Yourself in the Pink

"Calamine lotion is still one of the best treatments for moderate cases of poison ivy," says Robert Averill, M.D., a dermatologist in western Massachusetts and northern New Hampshire.

"It's the classic treatment for poison ivy," Dr. Zug agrees. "Calamine dries up blisters, it is soothing and cooling, and it relieves the itch."

Vinegar Works, Too

A vinegar compress is good for drying the rash and soothing the itching, says Robert Sommer, M.D., a dermatologist in Portland, Maine. "Use half a cup of white vinegar. Pour it into a pint container and add water up to the pint mark. Put it in the refrigerator; it works best cold." Dampen a cloth or gauze with the cold vinegar solution and apply it to the rash, Dr. Sommer says.

Use Milk to Shake the Itch

Dr. Sommer also recommends a cold milk compress, especially if you have poison ivy on your face, which can be irritated by vinegar. "You take a clean rag and soak it in whole milk. You need whole milk for the fat," he says. "Place the damp rag—damp, not runny—on the rash. Leave it on for 10 to 15 minutes. The cold stops the itch, while the fat lubricates the skin." Dr. Sommer says to rinse off the milk with warm water.

This Weed Is a Jewel

Corinne Martin, a certified clinical herbalist in Bridgton, Maine, likes to use jewelweed to soothe a poison ivy rash. A

P

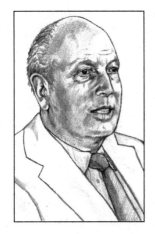

The Plant That Gets You from Its Grave

BEFORE I retired from practicing medicine, I used to see patients with poison ivy in the middle of winter. People would come tromping in through a foot of snow with itchy rashes all over their skin. I found it hard to convince them that poison ivy was their problem.

Here's what would happen: People often used firewood from trees that had been hauled out of the woods in summer before they were "bucked," or cut up. The trees got dragged through patches of poison ivy, picking up the irritating oil. The oil stayed active right into the winter, even after the plants were long past green. Then people put the logs into their fireplaces and woodstoves. They got the oil on their hands, touched the skin on the rest of their bodies, and came scratching to me convinced that it couldn't be poison ivy.

But it was. If you're especially sensitive to poison ivy, wear gloves when you stack firewood or feed your fireplace.

GERARD BOZUWA, M.D., *retired after 36 years as the sole family doctor for the town of Wakefield, New Hampshire.*

common plant found throughout the Northeast, jewelweed has a watery stem that contains juice good for stopping the itch. You can collect it in meadows during late summer. "Just crush the stems in your hands and rub the juice right on the rash," Martin says. She notes that Euell Gibbons, the famous natural food and remedy author, would process jewelweed stems and water in a blender and freeze the mixture in ice cube trays. "Jewelweed ice cubes are great against an itch because of the combination of the jewelweed and the cold," Martin says.

Listen to the Camp Nurse

"When the kids get poison ivy, I make a mixture of Domeboro and water and apply it to the rash with gauze pads," reports Tricia Barr, R.N., a nurse at Camp Walt Whitman in Pike, New Hampshire. Domeboro is an over-the-counter astringent that comes in tablet or powder form. "It's a good drying agent," Barr says.

Use the Ocean as a Lotion

Peter Brassard, M.D., a family doctor on Block Island, Rhode Island, says that a good sea bath can work. "Just the act of wading in the ocean will wash your sores," he says. "And the salt water will help dry them out."

Make Your Own Salty Sea

"Epsom salts dry things out," Dr. Zug says. "They are especially good for poison ivy and other oozy dermatitis. Just follow the directions on the box and sprinkle some into a lukewarm bath." You can get Epsom salts at your pharmacy or supermarket.

Feel Your Oats

"If you have itchy skin, try taking an oatmeal bath," says Donald Dickson, R.Ph., the owner of Dickson's Pharmacy in Colebrook, New Hampshire. Colloidal oatmeal, such as Aveeno, is made for bathing. You can buy Aveeno over the counter.

A Plant Man Picks Tecnu

As a botanist, Dr. Eshbaugh has spent years getting up close and personal with itch-causing plants. His favorite remedy?

Tecnu Oak-n-Ivy, available over the counter at drugstores. "Tecnu works on anything in the Anacardiaceae family—the family poison ivy and oak belong to," Dr. Eshbaugh says. "You can wash with Tecnu immediately after contact with poison ivy, or you can put it on before you go out into the field. You can even use it after you have already broken out with a rash. Each way seems to work."

Pump Up with Steroids

If other home remedies fail, a good fallback is a steroid such as over-the-counter 1 percent hydrocortisone cream, Dr. Brassard says.

POOR CIRCULATION

Jump-start your sluggish blood

Your shivering spouse may be the first person to complain that you have poor circulation when you shove those icy feet into bed at night. And it doesn't help when you reach over to comfort your bedmate with hands that feel as if they've been fished out of the Arctic Ocean.

Though your chilly extremities may raise a yelp from your lover, you probably don't have reason to be alarmed yourself. "Having cold hands and feet is just a variation within the normal range of blood circulation," says Mark Greenberg, M.D., a cardiologist at the Dartmouth-Hitchcock Medical Center in Lebanon, New Hampshire. "Some people move blood more slowly through their circulatory systems."

If just one or two of your fingers are cold and tend to turn white, your problem is probably not poor circulation but a condition called Raynaud's disease, Dr. Greenberg says. One in every 10 people has arteries that tend to constrict when confronted with cold or vibrations. Raynaud's is more annoying

> **TIME TO SEE THE DOCTOR**
>
> ### If It Hurts to Walk, Hop to a Checkup
>
> IF YOU feel an aching in your calves, thighs, or buttocks when you walk—and the pain stops when you do—call your doctor," says Mark Greenberg, M.D., a cardiologist at the Dartmouth-Hitchcock Medical Center in Lebanon, New Hampshire. "The aching is a sign of a possible blockage in an artery."
>
> A tingling in one arm, accompanied by a tight pain in the chest, is also reason to get medical help immediately. You could be having a heart attack.

Keep a Bit of Fat

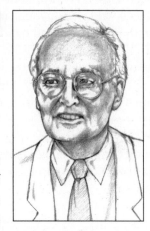

During the 40 years I was a family doctor, a lot of elderly ladies would come in to me complaining of poor circulation. "I'm cold all the time," they'd say.

One look at them would tell me that their problem wasn't circulation but fat—or the lack of it. The women complaining of feeling cold were skinny. They had no fat for insulation. I'd encourage them to add more good fat to their diet, such as food cooked in olive oil.

It's good to avoid being overweight, but you need a small layer of fat to protect you from the elements. Ask your doctor what your proper weight should be, and don't let your poundage drop too far below that level.

Brewster Martin, M.D., *a retired family doctor in Chelsea, Vermont (population 1,166), and cofounder of the Chelsea Family Health Center. He was named Vermont Doctor of the Year in 1991.*

than medically serious, but Dr. Greenberg says it's a good idea to get your tightening blood vessels checked to be sure your problem is Raynaud's and not a more serious circulatory ailment.

In the meantime, your partner will be glad to know that your relationship can be heated up with these hand- and foot-warming remedies.

Keep Rubbing

"If you have poor circulation, don't wait for your hands to get too chilly," says F. Daniel Golyan, M.D., a former New Englander who is now an electrophysiologist in private practice on Long Island. "Keep your hands moving against each other to stimulate circulation in them."

Be Forearmed

"Most people with poor circulation obsess over getting the warmest possible mittens and socks, and that's a good idea,"

Dr. Golyan says. "But you'd do even better making sure your arms and legs are warm. Wear long underwear made of silk or polypropylene. And wear a warm sweater even when you're inside."

Can the Smokes

"Smoking is the worst thing you can do if you have poor circulation," says Laurence Bouchard, D.O., an osteopathic family physician in Narragansett, Rhode Island. The smoke, Dr. Bouchard explains, causes blood vessels to go into spasm, shutting down like the faucet of your sink. "In medical school, we would stop the blood circulation in frogs by injecting them with nicotine, the drug that makes cigarettes addictive," he says. "The blood would stop flowing instantaneously, and the frogs would usually die—something to keep in mind when you light your next cigarette."

Dr. Bouchard adds that secondhand smoke can have the same effect on someone with poor circulation. "Stay away from smoke-filled rooms," he advises.

Sprinkle Your Bath

"If your hands and feet are often cold, get into the habit of taking baths with Epsom salts," says Jane Smolnik, owner of Crystal Garden Herbs in Springfield, Vermont. "Put three handfuls of salts into your bath as it begins to fill. Once the tub is full, add 5 to 10 drops of essential rosemary oil or juniper oil, available at health food stores and herb stores. Rosemary is good for stimulating blood flow, and it smells wonderful."

POSTNASAL DRIP
Ways to turn off your facial faucet

Here is a fact you may not want to tell your friends at dinnertime: You swallow a quart or two of mucus every day. "Most of us don't notice it," says Dudley Weider, M.D., an otolaryngologist at the Dartmouth-Hitchcock Medical Center in Lebanon, New Hampshire. Usually, the mucus is thin and watery, and it does a good job of keeping the membranes in your nose clean, moist, and free of infection. But

P

hay fever or a cold can kick the mucus-producing glands in your nose and sinuses into overdrive, allowing some mucus to drip into the back of your throat. Mucus that drips down the back of your nose is called postnasal drip.

Dry indoor air or a sinus infection can thicken the mucus, making it harder to swallow. Any of these causes can give you the feeling that a leaky faucet is sending mucus down your throat. Sometimes you can get that feeling because your glands produce *less* mucus—but it's thicker and therefore more noticeable. This sparse mucus production becomes more likely as you age. "Older people complain of postnasal drip much more often than younger people do," Dr. Weider says. "You hardly ever hear kids and teenagers talk about it."

Here's how to deal with that drippy feeling.

Drown the Drip

"Everyone has postnasal drip to some degree," Dr. Weider notes. "Some people are just more sensitive to it than others." The answer, he says, is to thin the mucus by drinking plenty of fluids. "If you increase your fluid intake, you are less likely to notice the mucus and to be bothered by it," Dr. Weider explains.

Humidify

"One chief cause of postnasal drip is a cold climate," says Robert Fagelson, M.D., an otolaryngologist in Brattleboro, Vermont. "The nose is the air conditioner for the body. Its job is to heat ingoing air to 98.6°F and to humidify that air to 100 percent. But the air inside an office or a house may be 72°F, and the humidity may be as low as 5 percent."

Outdoors in the winter, the opposite conditions may be in effect. "The temperature could be 5°F, and the humidity may be 75 percent," he says. "When you go in and out, back and forth between such extremes, the differences are hard on your nose, and it runs—sometimes backward into your throat." Your best bet is to keep room temperatures as cool as you can and to use a humidifier indoors, Dr. Fagelson says.

Dust Up

"Chronic postnasal drip is often due to an allergy from dust mites," says Richard Lee, M.D., an otolaryngologist in La-

Could It Be Your Septum?

A FREQUENT cause of postnasal drip is a deviated septum," says Dudley Weider, M.D., an otolaryngologist at the Dartmouth-Hitchcock Medical Center in Lebanon, New Hampshire. The septum is the wall inside your nose that divides it in two. A sharp blow or a birth defect can cause the septum to be twisted, or deviated, to one side. "A lot of people don't even know they have a deviated septum," Dr. Weider says. "But if there is a sharp spur on the deviated septum, mucus can get stuck there. It collects and drips down the back of the throat." Dr. Weider says that a simple surgical procedure can correct a deviated septum.

A normal septum (A) drips less, a deviated one (B) more.

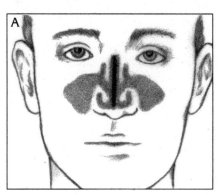 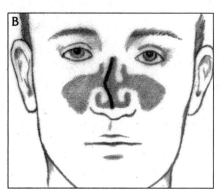

conia, New Hampshire. "Keep your house clean and talk to your doctor about the allergy."

Decongest

"The best thing for postnasal drip is Sudafed decongestant," Dr. Fagelson says. Sudafed is available over the counter at most drugstores. "Don't take it on a regular basis or if you have blood pressure or prostate problems," he warns.

Honey Your Cough

"For the tickly cough that sometimes comes with postnasal drip, try mixing equal portions of honey and lemon juice," says Elizabeth Lowry, M.D., who is retired after 38 years as a pediatrician in Guilford, Connecticut. "Take a spoonful as needed."

PREMENSTRUAL SYNDROME

*Cures for monthly episodes
that make you feel rotten, period*

You can see why our ancestors used to blame it on the moon. With lunatic monthly regularity, your hormones begin to change 7 to 10 days before menstruation. This chemical shift gives you any combination of a variety of ailments, physical and psychological. On the physical side, you can feel pain in your pelvic area, bloating, headache, or tenderness in your breasts. Your surging hormones also can mess with your head, giving you food cravings, irritability, anxiety, depression, or an inability to focus on anything for very long. "The symptoms are à la carte," says Thomas J. O'Connor III, M.D., an obstetrician-gynecologist in Rockport, Maine. "Every woman with premenstrual syndrome, or PMS, gets a customized set of problems."

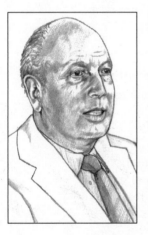

A WORD FROM DR. B.

It Finally Has a Name

W E DIDN'T have a name for PMS when I started in practice in New Hampshire more than 40 years ago. In fact, the term wasn't used commonly until fairly recently. What a thrill it was when we could find reasons for all those symptoms doctors had been seeing in women for centuries. Now we know that, besides focusing on individual symptoms, you can treat the syndrome with lots of exercise and reduced salt intake. Women also might want to ask their doctors about taking birth control pills, which can help change the hormonal levels in the body.

GERARD BOZUWA, M.D., *retired after 36 years as the sole family doctor for the town of Wakefield, New Hampshire.*

This unappetizing menu generally goes away within a few days after you begin menstruating, thank goodness. And PMS usually eases off later in life, disappearing altogether after menopause.

Although the menstrual cycle and the hormonal changes that go with it are clearly behind PMS, "researchers still don't understand why some women suffer from it more than others, or why you'll suffer more one month than another," Dr. O'Connor says. "Women suffering from PMS have no apparent hormonal or chemical abnormalities. PMS is a highly individual ailment." Remedies for your monthly symptoms need to be individual as well, he explains. "Experiment a little, targeting the symptoms that are most bothersome, and see what works for you."

What's the most important part of your cure? "A supportive partner," Dr. O'Connor replies. "PMS isn't all in a woman's head. It's a physical problem that needs help and sympathy."

Along with a host of more down-to-earth remedies to choose from. We offer some below.

Cut the Vices

"We don't know why, but alcohol, caffeine, and nicotine all can make PMS worse," Dr. O'Connor says. "If you suffer a lot from PMS, cut out coffee and cocktails for the week before your period. And cut out smoking, period."

Can the Salt

"Salt increases your body's tendency to store water," Dr. O'Connor says. "If swelling and bloating are part of your PMS, cut down on your salt intake all month. That reduces the bloat."

Have a Good Evening

"Evening primrose oil, taken in capsule form, is helpful for relieving PMS," Dr. O'Connor notes. "You can buy it at health food stores and drugstores. Take one capsule twice a day during the premenstrual phase of your cycle."

Leave the House

"Women with premenstrual syndrome should exercise for an hour a day," says Eric A. Sailer, M.D., an obstetrician-gynecologist at the Dartmouth-Hitchcock Medical Center in Lebanon, New Hampshire. "Take a long walk, run, swim, or bike each day throughout the month, but especially during PMS time. You need to do something active, not just house-cleaning or mowing the lawn." Exercise increases your endorphins—natural painkillers in your body that also help stabilize your premenstrual mood swings.

Even Out the Sugar

"Research seems to show that it is helpful to keep blood glucose levels steady, maintaining the amount of natural sugar in your body so it doesn't fluctuate too much during the day," says Teri Pearlstein, M.D., a psychiatrist who is chief of women's programs at Butler Hospital in Providence, Rhode Island. "Eat four or five small meals a day, rather than two or three big ones."

Try a Great Escape

"An over-the-counter tea called PMS Escape is helpful for relieving the symptoms of premenstrual syndrome," says Hope Ricciotti, M.D., an obstetrician-gynecologist at the Beth Israel Deaconess Medical Center in Boston. Containing a cocktail of simple and complex carbohydrates, along with dietary additions such as calcium, magnesium, and vitamins C and B_6, it comes in lemon, strawberry-kiwi, and raspberry-lime flavors. Mix it in an eight-ounce glass of water and take it once or twice a day.

PUFFY EYES

Remedies to try when your baby blues have had too swell a time

You look in the mirror after a night on the town or a day in front of a computer screen, and the skin around your eyes looks as if it's on steroids. How'd it get so puffed up?

"The puffiness is nothing more than increased blood flow to the skin around your eyes," says Gary Venman-Clay, M.D., a family doctor in Bellows Falls, Vermont. "The tissue around your eyes tends to swell up easily." An allergy could be the cause, or an injury such as an errant baseball or overuse of the eyes at a double feature or a late-night work session. A good cry can get your eyes puffed up, as blood rushes in to your teary orbs. So can any illness that causes swelling elsewhere in the body. "If your ankles swell first, and then your legs, hands, and eyes, you probably have an illness that should be checked out by a doctor," Dr. Venman-Clay says.

But for that short-term puffiness, turn those swollen headlights on to these remedies.

Get Seepy

"Lie back, place a warm tea bag on each eye, and rest for 10 minutes," says Julia Foote, R.N., a retired nurse living in Norwell, Massachusetts. "The tannic acid in tea bags is an astringent that relieves the swelling in tissue." Foote warns that the acid also can temporarily stain your skin, so you might skip this remedy if you have a big date coming up.

Clothe Them

"Put a washcloth soaked in cold water against your eyes," Dr. Venman-Clay advises. "The cold will reduce the blood flow to the area around your eyes and thereby reduce the swelling."

TIME TO SEE THE DOCTOR

When the Puff Won't Let Up

IF YOUR eyes stay puffy for more than a week, have a doctor look at them, says Laurence Bouchard, D.O., an osteopathic family physician in private practice in Narragansett, Rhode Island. "Puffy eyes may be a sign of something more serious than a lack of sleep or allergies. You could have a urinary tract infection, hypothyroidism, or some other serious but treatable illness."

PUNCTURE WOUNDS

Keep yourself whole by treating accidental holes

"Ah, it's nothing," you might say bravely after poking yourself with a screwdriver. "There's hardly even any blood." Actually, the lack of visible gore may not be such a good thing, according to Douglas Deaett, M.D., an emergency room physician at Alice Peck Day Memorial Hospital in Lebanon, New Hampshire. Blood helps cleanse a wound, carrying germs out of the puncture site. "The real problem with puncture wounds is that they are so difficult to clean from the outside," Dr. Deaett says.

A puncture can introduce germs from a variety of sources into the skin. "For example, if a child steps on a nail while wearing sneakers, bacteria from the sneaker can be introduced into the wound, as well as germs from the floor or ground and from the nail itself," Dr. Deaett explains. Toxins created by the bacteria are a serious cause for concern. "If it has been close to five years since you had a tetanus booster, you should get another tetanus shot after a puncture wound." Also see your doctor if you notice any red streaks radiating through the skin from the wound.

A WORD FROM DR. B.

The Boy Who Stood Very Still

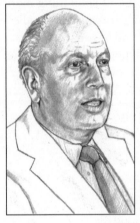

WHEN I was still a young doctor, I thought I was having an especially busy day in my home office—I was seeing one patient and had two more in the waiting room—when a woman called saying that her 12-year-old son had just stepped on a nail. Would I please come over? she asked. Although I did make house calls, I didn't want to give my other patients short shrift. So I inquired about the boy's tetanus immunization and told the mother to bring him in.

"No," she said. "Please come here!" Something in her voice made me decide that I had better go. I jumped in my car and drove to the family's nearby lakeside cottage. Well, standing on the dock was her boy, and he had a big, fat, two- or three-inch-long nail with its point sticking up right through his foot. He just stood there, unable to move. The sight of him froze me.

After the initial horror went away, I opened my black bag and filled a syringe with Novocain. The boy took one look at the needle and yanked his foot right off the nail.

Sometimes a puncture wound doesn't seem so bad. But as long as you're not nailed to something, go see your doctor if the wound is more than superficial.

GERARD BOZUWA, M.D., *retired after 36 years as the sole family doctor for the town of Wakefield, New Hampshire.*

Dr. Deaett sees his share of punctured patients. "The more common puncture cases I see are screwdriver jabs to the hand, kitchen knife accidents, the crosslike puncture marks of nail guns, and—most common of all—nails in feet," he says.

"Any puncture wound that's more than a nick in the skin should be seen by a doctor," Dr. Deaett says. And don't let the lack of blood fool you. "I once had a fellow come in complaining of pain in his jaw," Dr. Deaett recalls. "He'd been working with a nail gun and assumed that his pain was caused by the kickback from the gun hitting him in the jaw. He was talking kind of funny, not really opening his mouth. So we took x-rays. There was a six-inch nail jammed straight into his jaw. Somehow it had missed his tongue and teeth." Dr. Deaett reports that the man laughed when he saw the x-ray, saying, "If only my mother could see me now. She always said that if I didn't shut up, she'd nail my mouth shut."

You don't have to grin and bear it when you get a puncture wound. Here's what you can do at home if the wound is shallow.

Get the Stuff Out

"First, be sure that nothing is still in the wound," says John Dunn, M.D., an emergency room physician at the Northwestern Medical Center in St. Albans, Vermont. "Check for a thorn, glass, or even a piece of rust from a nail. If anything is blocking the hole—such as a small flap of skin—trim it off and get it out of the way so the wound can drain."

Get Soaked

"Soak the wound for 15 minutes in warm, soapy water," Dr. Dunn says. "This will keep the wound open and allow it to drain. Repeat the soaking three or four times a day for several days."

Give the Wound a Raise

"Particularly if the puncture wound is in the foot, elevate the wound," Dr. Dunn advises. "Elevation will lessen swelling. And swelling impairs good drainage."

R

RASHES

Seek these remedies
for trouble with your hide

Rashes, like beauty, are not always skin-deep. Red eruptions on your skin can warn of something serious underneath. "Most rashes are harmless," says John C. Robinson, M.D., a pediatrician in private practice in Quincy, Massachusetts. "But some aren't." Lyme disease, a bacterial infection spread by deer ticks, causes a tiny bull's-eye rash that gradually gets bigger and can be accompanied by serious illness and even paralysis. A bacterial disease called meningococcemia, which can result in the life-threatening brain swelling of meningitis, can start out as a bruiselike rash. The fiery red rash that's the hallmark of measles comes in the fifth or sixth day of this spotty illness.

"Any rash that occurs with bruising or that doesn't disappear when you stretch the skin around it is reason to call your doctor immediately, especially when it's associated with a fever," Dr. Robinson says. A rash that doesn't blanch when you stretch the skin could be a sign of petechia, a leaking of the tiny blood vessels just under the skin. Petechia can be a sign of a serious underlying disorder, he explains.

In most cases, though, a rash is the only symptom you'll have—which can be symptom enough. And there are plenty of possible causes: an allergy to something you ate; a reaction to chemicals in your clothing, sunscreen, or cosmetics; a fungal or yeast infection such as athlete's foot; scabies, a contagious condition caused by tiny parasitic mites; or just plain dry skin.

If you know what's causing your rash, the best cure is to remove the culprit, Dr. Robinson says. In addition, here are some soothing remedies.

Try a Rash Solution

"A fast-acting remedy for most rashes is over-the-counter hydrocortisone cream in a 1 percent solution," says Laurence Bouchard, D.O., an osteopathic family physician in Narragansett, Rhode Island. You can find several brands of hydrocortisone remedies at most drugstores. Dr. Bouchard suggests that if you've never used hydrocortisone cream, it's wise to test yourself to make sure the cream doesn't cause a rash on its own. "Dab a bit inside your arm and wait two hours to see if your skin reacts," he says. "A few people are allergic to hydrocortisone, and they shouldn't use it. Putting it on their rashes is like spreading kerosene on a fire."

Scrap the Whole Thing

If you tend to get rashes where your skin folds rub against each other, "try putting a strip of cotton cloth between the folds," says Kathryn A. Zug, M.D., a dermatologist at the

R

TIME TO SEE THE DOCTOR

Don't Connect the Dots Yourself

IF YOU have any question about what caused your rash, don't play detective by yourself, advises John C. Robinson, M.D., a pediatrician in Quincy, Massachusetts. "A rash could be the surface sign of a serious disease," he says. "The itchy bumps you got after walking bare-legged through poison ivy can be treated at home. But anything mysterious should be looked at by your doctor."

Any one of the following warning signs should quickly prompt a call to your doctor's office, according to Dr. Robinson.

- Your rash consists of a single, painful, red spot with a circle of pink around it.
- The rash doesn't disappear when you stretch the skin.
- You also have a fever or sore throat.
- You also have a headache.
- You developed the rash after taking medication.
- Your rash burns or stings.

Her Past Was Behind Her

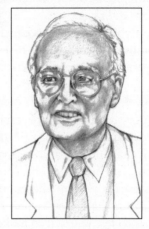

An ELDERLY Vermonter named Gail was a patient of mine. She kept a journal her entire life, from childhood on. She never came to see me. I always went to her house to care for her, and when I arrived she would share passages from her journal with me. I took care of her during the last two decades of her life, so I ended up reading a fair amount of that journal.

I learned that when Gail was a young woman, her family regularly had the high and mighty over for dinner. Gail's diary entry for one day read, "During the course of the evening, both Mark Twain and Teddy Roosevelt tried to pinch my bottom."

Some time after I read this passage, I visited Gail to treat a slight skin rash on her derriere. "I now have my claim to fame," I said to her after I finished. "I have now touched the buttocks that were touched by Mark Twain and Teddy Roosevelt."

I do love being a doctor.

BREWSTER MARTIN, M.D., *a retired family doctor in Chelsea, Vermont (population 1,166), and cofounder of the Chelsea Family Health Center. He was named Vermont Doctor of the Year in 1991.*

Dartmouth-Hitchcock Medical Center in Lebanon, New Hampshire. "This is an easy trick. The cotton helps absorb the moisture and decreases the friction of the folds rubbing against each other."

Dr. Zug also suggests using over-the-counter talcum powder in your skin folds after you've stepped out of the shower and patted yourself dry. "And avoid tight clothing," she says. A final piece of advice: "Weight loss may help in some cases."

Soak Your Oats

An oatmeal bath is one of the best ways to soothe irritated, rashy skin. "A special kind of finely ground oats, called colloidal oatmeal, is made for baths," Dr. Zug says. "You can buy a common brand, Aveeno, at drugstores and supermarkets. Follow the instructions on the label."

Skip the Wipes

"To avoid causing rashes on your infant's skin or making existing rashes worse, avoid baby wipes when you change your child's diaper," Dr. Zug says. "Use a clean cloth or moist toilet paper instead. Baby wipes are highly perfumed and full of preservatives, which is asking for trouble with sensitive baby skin."

Dress Up Your Hands

"If you tend to get rashes on your hands after using latex gloves, throw them away and get hypoallergenic gloves from your drugstore or medical supply store," says Daniel Caloras, M.D., a family doctor in private practice in Charlestown, New Hampshire. Five to 10 percent of the population is allergic to latex, which causes rashes on their skin. If you're one of this unlucky group, alert your doctor to your allergy before any surgery—you don't want latex surgical gloves touching your innards.

Run Your Own Tests

Medical researchers suspect that people with latex allergies may also be allergic to certain foods, such as bananas, avocados, chestnuts, and melons, which are in the same plant family. If you find yourself getting frequent rashes after meals, consider cutting out these foods one by one to see if your problem clears up.

Watch Your Neck

If you get a rash on your neck, arms, or legs, you might want to switch laundry detergents. "Sometimes detergent will accumulate on just one sleeve, causing a rash on one arm and not the other," Dr. Caloras says. "When I see a patient like that, I ask if anything has changed in his habits. Often the person will say, 'Well, I got this detergent on sale . . .'"

Don't Doctor with Pepper

If you use ointments containing capsaicin, a chemical found in red peppers, watch for rashes, Dr. Caloras says. "Lots of people use rubs such as Zostrix for sore muscles or arthritis," he explains. "In sensitive skin, the lotion can cause a rash like a burn." You don't have to give up rubs altogether, "just use a lotion with a lower concentration of capsaicin."

Or Have a Friend Lend a Hand with the Cooking

If you react to rubs, be careful when you cook with red peppers. Some cooks get a rash called Hunan hand, named after the irritating reaction to cooking spicy Chinese food. The solution: latex gloves—unless, of course, you're allergic to latex.

RECEDING GUMS
A bit long in the tooth?
Sink into these cures

Know where the expression *long in the tooth*—meaning a person who's getting on in years—comes from? Before this century—back in the days before toothbrushing—gum disease was even more common than it is today. "Lengthening teeth" were an optical illusion. It's not that the teeth were getting longer; the gums were pulling back, revealing more of a smile. (Actually, the term originally applied to horses—which also explains why people looked gift horses in the mouth: to see how old and decrepit they were.)

We now know that receding gums (in humans, at least) are a symptom not of old age but of gum disease, according to Peter Lodge, D.M.D., a dentist in Narragansett, Rhode Island. Your gums become inflamed when food mixed with saliva gets deposited at the line where your gums meet your teeth. After 24 hours, this gooey mixture, called plaque, hardens and becomes a cementlike substance called tartar, which generally can be removed only with special dental tools. Tartar is a friendly environment for bacteria, which cause a long-lasting infection in the gums—breaking down tissue and, eventually, even bone.

"Once your gums recede, you can't regrow them," Dr. Lodge notes. "But you can avoid the worst stages of bone and tooth loss by taking care of the gums that are left." Here's how.

Stimulate

"Buy packets of Stim-U-Dents at your drug-store," says Robert Keene, D.M.D., a dentist in Hanover, New Hampshire. Stim-U-Dents are special toothpicks made of orangewood, which softens with use in your mouth. "Get in the habit of using Stim-U-Dents or round toothpicks after every meal," he says. "That will clean your teeth and stimulate your gums, increasing the blood supply to help fight off bacterial infection."

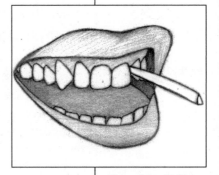

Use a Stim-U-Dent to get the food out and perk up your gums.

Get Sandy

"To detoxify the bacteria surrounding your teeth, mix baking soda and hydrogen peroxide until you get a paste the consistency of wet sand," Dr. Keene says. "Use this mixture on your toothbrush, massaging it in and around the neck of each tooth—the part where tooth and gum meet. Do this daily."

Arm with Powder

"One of the most effective over-the-counter products for taking care of your teeth and preventing receding gums is Arm & Hammer Tooth Powder," Dr. Keene says. "The powder has extra baking soda, which is great in fighting gum disease." Use it instead of toothpaste, he says.

Floss Your Kids

Good gum care should start young. That means flossing your kids' teeth before they're old enough to do it themselves. "Until children are at least seven or eight, they don't have the coordination to floss their teeth well," Dr. Keene notes. As soon as your child has baby teeth big enough to be in tight contact with one another, floss the teeth every night. "Have your child lie flat on the floor or on a bed or couch," Dr. Keene says. "Put her head in your lap and tilt the head back. That way, you can clean the teeth well." He cautions that the procedure may take two parents if the child resists.

REPETITIVE MOTION INJURY
Marshal your defenses against the force of habit

It can happen from stacking firewood or writing memos on a computer. You start getting a tingling or numb feeling in the overworked joints, pain or a loss of strength in the stressed-out area, or any combination of these symptoms. If you keep doing what caused the feeling in the first place, those sensations can get progressively worse.

The most common repetitive motion injury is carpal tunnel syndrome, an inflammation and compression of nerves in the wrist. Caused by typing on computer keyboards, by repetitive use of a screwdriver on an assembly line, or by some other repeated task, carpal tunnel syndrome usually first causes you to feel numb in your thumb, index finger, and middle finger, especially when you flex your wrist. "Sometimes the first sign is an achy feeling in your shoulder or arm," says Peter Mason, M.D., a family doctor in Lebanon, New Hampshire. The condition can be painful, and if it's not recognized and treated early, it may result in permanent loss of strength in the hand.

If you're starting to feel pain or numbness from your work or play, here's how to get back to normal once more, with feeling.

Break Every 30

"The most important thing to remember in preventing repetitive motion injury is to avoid doing the same small motion for more than 30 to 40 minutes at a time," says John Bland, M.D., a rheumatologist in Cambridge, Vermont. "Make a phone call or go to the bathroom—anything to give yourself a break."

Hold Still

"If you find yourself with a repetitive motion injury, splint or immobilize the injured part," says Hugh P. Hermann, M.D., a family doctor in Woodstock, Vermont. "Ask your doctor for splints that are appropriate for your injury. Most of the time, they'll just hold your wrists in the proper position and still allow you to work."

Fight the Fire

"An anti-inflammatory drug such as ibuprofen can help reduce the pain and inflammation of a repetitive motion injury," Dr. Hermann says.

Get a Temp Worker

"Ice can help reduce the swelling and inflammation of a repetitive motion injury, reducing pressure on the nerve," Dr. Mason says. "If your wrists are hurting, rest them on an ice pack with a cloth draped over it," he says. Keep the ice in place for about 15 minutes at a time.

Change Positions

"If you find yourself suffering frequently from repetitive motion injuries, you need to redesign your workstation," Dr. Hermann says. "When you type on a keyboard, your wrists should be supported, and your hands should be at right angles to your elbows." If you can't afford a specially made workstation, try putting a book in your desk's top, middle drawer to support your wrists in front of the keyboard. Or you can buy a special wrist pad at a computer supply store.

Or Change Habits

"I have tennis elbow, but I didn't get it from playing tennis," Dr. Mason says. "I got it from the bad habit of stacking wood with one hand. I would pick up a log by the butt end and then flex my wrist to lift the log into place on the pile. That's a bad idea. Use two hands to stack wood."

R

TIME TO SEE THE DOCTOR

Take a Tingle In

IF YOU show signs of carpal tunnel syndrome—a feeling of numbness in the thumb, index finger, and middle finger, as well as half of the fourth finger—get medical attention, says Peter Mason, M.D., a family doctor in Lebanon, New Hampshire. "If carpal tunnel syndrome isn't treated early, you may get irreversible damage."

Try the stiff-arm technique with a folded magazine. If it helps, ask your doctor about a fancier treatment.

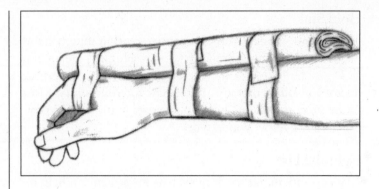

Brace Yourself for Sleep

"You can get symptoms of carpal tunnel syndrome while you're sleeping," Dr. Mason notes. "When you fall asleep, your hand can flop down in a relaxed manner, which compresses the carpal tunnel and may produce numbness in your fingers or aching in your arm or shoulder." To fight the flopping, take a magazine, fold it in half lengthwise, and tape it over the back of your hand and wrist to keep the joint from bending. If you get a good night's sleep with this homemade splint, Dr. Mason says, "that is good evidence that you have carpal tunnel. You may benefit from more sophisticated splinting or other treatment."

Try This, Honey

"Ask your doctor about using bee venom for a repetitive motion injury such as carpal tunnel syndrome," says Bradford Weeks, M.D., a former New Englander who is now a family physician and nutritional biochemist in Clinton, Washington. And just how do you get hold of bee venom? By getting hold of the bee. But first, Dr. Weeks says, it's wise to see your doctor or allergist to be tested for any allergies against bee stings. If you're allergic to the venom, he says, skip this cure.

Once you get the okay from your doctor, make sure he gives you a bee sting kit, which allows you to treat yourself immediately in case (despite what your tests showed) you get a bad reaction to a sting. Now ask a local beekeeper for a few healthy honeybees. Hold some ice against the affected area to numb it. Then, with a pair of tweezers, carefully pick up a bee and press its rear end against your achy area. Ouch! "The stinger will remain in your skin with the venom sac and will continue pulsating after you remove the bee," Dr. Weeks says. "This is a sterile and efficient delivery system for a potent medicine."

Leave the stinger in for 10 to 30 minutes, until a red mark appears around the sting. The spot should be itchy and a bit swollen for as long as 24 hours. If you find yourself swelling up or getting itchy elsewhere in your body after you've stung yourself, "see a physician immediately," Dr. Weeks says. Most of the time, though, "bee venom is great stuff. It contains anti-inflammatory peptides that can reduce the pain and inflammation of an injury."

R

RESTLESS LEGS

*Get some peace
when the joints are jumpin'*

It tends to happen when you go to bed and start to get settled: The rest of you feels sleepy, but your legs feel wide-awake. You have a maddening creepy-crawly sensation down there, along with a terrible urge to get up and walk around. Some people with restless legs also find that their leg muscles jerk involuntarily. A few sufferers get the same crazy-legs feeling in their arms as well.

There doesn't seem to be any one explanation for restless legs. Any of a variety of causes might be triggering the late-night urge—including such widely ranging problems as diabetes, back trouble, varicose veins, and an imbalance in your brain's chemistry. Pregnant women often get restless legs. An iron deficiency can give you the same symptoms, as can rheumatoid arthritis or drugs prescribed to relieve depression.

Whatever the cause, restless legs tend to run (so to speak) in families. Kids frequently start feeling the discomfort in their legs before age 10—a jumpiness that's often wrongly attributed to "growing pains." The feeling usually gets more intense in middle age and beyond. And it can drive you ab-

> ### TIME TO SEE THE DOCTOR
> ## *Walk Your Legs to Help*
>
> IF YOUR restless legs become unbearable, ask your doctor to examine you," says Lawrence H. Bernstein, M.D., a former family doctor who is the medical director at Jewish Geriatric Services in Longmeadow, Massachusetts. "A prescription medication for seizures has been known to work for restless legs."

solutely crazy. "People with restless legs simply can't hold them still," says Richard Nordgren, M.D., a pediatric neurologist at the Dartmouth-Hitchcock Medical Center in Lebanon, New Hampshire. "This is a major problem because they can't sleep—they have to walk."

Here's how to tone down that wanderlust.

Take a Fizz

"Try drinking 6 to 12 ounces of tonic water before bedtime," Dr. Nordgren says. "The quinine seems to help relieve restless legs in some people." He cautions, though, that you shouldn't use quinine while you're pregnant.

Drown Your Sorrows

"A warm bath can be very helpful for restless legs," says Michael Sateia, M.D., director of the Sleep Disorders Clinic at the Dartmouth-Hitchcock Medical Center in Lebanon, New Hampshire.

Put Yourself at "E's"

"A vitamin E pill, taken daily, may help with restless legs," Dr. Nordgren says. But don't take more than 800 milligrams per day, he cautions.

Say Good Night to Joe

"Avoid any stimulants, such as coffee," Dr. Nordgren advises. They only make the problem worse.

Give Your Legs a Hand

"A bedtime massage of the legs may lessen the symptoms of restless legs," Dr. Nordgren says.

S

SCARRING

Minimizing the remains of scrapes, burns, and gashes

"Scarring is an ordinary part of the healing process," says Gerard Bozuwa, M.D., a retired family doctor in Wakefield, New Hampshire. Most scars on the skin are harmless, Dr. Bozuwa adds. Some may even be attractive. In nineteenth-century Germany, young gentlemen actually picked fights in the hope of getting a good-looking dueling scar.

Most visible scars fade after a couple of years, according to Kathryn A. Zug, M.D., a dermatologist at the Dartmouth-Hitchcock Medical Center in Lebanon, New Hampshire. "You can make them less noticeable in the first place if you take good care of a wound," Dr. Zug says. Here's how.

Get It Clean

"First, carefully wash any wound with soap and water to prevent infection. If the area gets infected, you'll have a bigger scar," says Charles Hammer, M.D., a dermatologist with the North Country Outreach Program of the Lahey Hitchcock Clinic in St. Johnsbury, Vermont.

Make Ends Meet

"To minimize a scar, bring the skin together," says Lawrence H. Bernstein, M.D., a former family doctor who is the medical director at Jewish Geriatric Services in Longmeadow, Massachusetts. "Doctors use suturing—stitches—to bring the skin together. If you're out hiking in the woods, you can do the same thing with a butterfly bandage." That's an adhesive bandage with flaring ends like a butterfly's wings to grip the skin. "If you aren't carrying a butterfly bandage," Dr. Bernstein says, "use a regular Band-Aid by putting the adhesive part on the wound, not the little square gauze pad. Don't change the bandage for 10 days. When you do remove it, do so gently."

Moist Is Good

"The old wives' tale was that you had to keep a wound dry," Dr. Hammer says. "That's turned out not to be true. A dry wound actually heals more slowly. Keep any cut moist with petroleum jelly, and add a sterile bandage bought from your drugstore."

An Antibiotic Helps

"The best thing to do for a healing laceration is to keep it soft," Dr. Bozuwa says. "Put Bacitracin on it. It's what all the plastic surgeons use, but you can buy it over the counter at your drugstore." Bacitracin, an antibiotic formula in petroleum jelly, helps prevent scabs, which often lead to scars, he explains.

Glue Yourself Back Together

To prevent scarring from a small cut, Dr. Bernstein recommends superglue. "Get a little tube at a hardware store and carry it in your backpack," he says. "Superglue will glue anything, even skin. It is nontoxic, and you can reapply it as necessary. It may sting a bit, but superglue is essentially what surgeons use in hip replacements." First, clean the wound with soap and water. Then bring the edges of the skin together and put a single bead of glue on the middle to seal it shut, Dr. Bernstein says.

SHINGLES

Ways to get through chickenpox: part II

Just when you thought you were safe from childhood diseases—you're an adult, after all—your past comes back to haunt you. That nasty bout of chickenpox can return like gangbusters, causing you to itch all over, just like old times. You feel a sharp, burning pain in nerves all over your body, and blisters break out in a line up one side of your body. You have shingles, a disease caused by the varicella virus, the same bug that gave you chickenpox way back when.

Aren't you supposed to develop immunities to childhood diseases after you get them? Often, yes, but varicella works differently. "Once you've had chickenpox, the virus lives in your nerves as long as you live," says Kathryn A. Zug, M.D., a dermatologist at the Dartmouth-Hitchcock Medical Center in Lebanon, New Hampshire. Illness, lowered immunity from a medication such as the steroid prednisone, or the weakened immune system that can come with getting older can awaken the virus, causing it to inflame a sensory nerve (and sometimes two or three) in the skin.

The pain and itching usually last from three to six weeks, although the blisters tend to scab over within two to three weeks. People over the age of 50 often experience lingering aftereffects of shingles, in the form of long-lasting pain called postherpetic neuralgia. You may start feeling pain again a

---

TIME TO SEE THE DOCTOR

Make Sure It's Really Shingles

IN GENERAL, it's a good idea to get any case of shingles checked out by a professional, says Kathryn A. Zug, M.D., a dermatologist at the Dartmouth-Hitchcock Medical Center in Lebanon, New Hampshire. You could have a serious illness that predisposes you to shingles. And though you can treat a mild case yourself with home remedies, "be sure to get medical help if you're in severe pain," Dr. Zug advises.

Here are some other reasons to return to the doctor for your shingles, according to Dr. Zug.

- You're having trouble controlling your muscles.
- Your shingles are accompanied by a high fever.
- You're having problems with urination or bowel movements.
- Shingles blisters appear on your face. "They need to be evaluated by a physician," Dr. Zug says. "The virus can affect the nerves going to the eyes and cause blindness."

And Don't Get Your Hopes Up for a Telephone Either

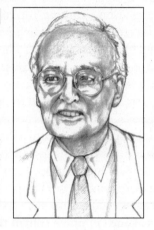

UP IN my neck of the woods, old-time New Englanders have raised their frown-and-bear-it attitude to an art form. For some of them, it's a point of pride never to complain—an admirable trait that sometimes makes diagnosing illnesses a little tricky.

A perfect illustration of this refusal to gripe was a man I met during one of my long walks in the high hills above my Vermont home. I came across a house I'd never seen before. It seemed, well, pretty rural, with aged clapboards that looked as if they'd never seen paint.

An old man was outside the house, chopping wood. I went up and asked him if he had electricity.

"Nope," he said. "I signed up for it, and they told me it would take 8 months." He paused and thought a bit. "That was 18 years ago."

BREWSTER MARTIN, M.D., *a retired family doctor in Chelsea, Vermont (population 1,166), and cofounder of the Chelsea Family Health Center. He was named Vermont Doctor of the Year in 1991.*

month or more after the shingles go away, and it can last for years. Fortunately, doctors can treat postherpetic neuralgia with medications used to cure depression.

If the shingles are not too severe, you can usually deal with them at home. Your mother doctored your chickenpox; now it's your turn to doctor yourself, using the remedies below.

Give It the Ivy Cure

"You can treat the itchiness and blistering of shingles the same way you treat poison ivy," Dr. Zug says. "Mix up some over-the-counter Burow's solution, spread it on a clean cloth, and drape the cloth on the blisters. The wet compress should feel soothing. Use this compress three or four times a day for five days."

Smear with Pink

"Early on in the course of shingles, calamine lotion may provide some relief to the affected areas," says Richard Nordgren, M.D., a pediatric neurologist who practices at the Dartmouth-Hitchcock Medical Center in Lebanon, New Hampshire.

Try the Allergy Stuff

"An oral antihistamine such as Benadryl can help with the itching," Dr. Nordgren says.

Or Try the Hot Stuff

Medical researchers have had some success in treating the burning pain of shingles with a lotion made of capsaicin, an extract of the same red peppers that are used in hot sauce. You can buy topical capsaicin over the counter as Capzasin or Zostrix. Put it directly along the nerve that's affected by the shingles. The hot stuff interferes with the transmission of pain stimuli to the brain.

SHINSPLINTS
*Ease the pain
of those aching gams*

Just when you thought you were getting yourself back in shape with a regular jog around the neighborhood, your shins start telling you they've had enough. You feel a sharp pain next to your shinbone, especially when you run or walk briskly.

Congratulations: You've reached that state of athleticism (or other leg-abusing habit) in which you've acquired shinsplints. In most shinsplints, the sheath that attaches to your muscles and shinbone has become inflamed. But that might not be your problem. "*Shinsplints* is a catchall term covering any number of problems in the lower leg, from a serious stress fracture of the shinbone to tendinitis to a muscle strain," says Raymond Rocco Monto, M.D., an orthopedic surgeon at Martha's Vineyard Orthopedic Surgery and Sports Medicine in Oak Bluffs, Massachusetts.

Ill-fitting shoes are a common cause of the pain. So is a sudden increase in activity, according to Dr. Monto. Here's how you can get those shins back in running trim.

Run Right (and Left)

"Buy proper running shoes and break them in slowly," Dr. Monto says. "Buy shoes with a wide-based heel called a lateral flare. That will help prevent your feet from turning in when you run, which can cause shinsplints. Run only on smooth surfaces, and don't make a sudden switch to a different running course. If you train on grass, keep running on grass, or switch to asphalt gradually. And whether you run on a track or around the block, run the opposite way every other time."

Take a Paddle

"If you have shinsplints from running, give your legs a break for a couple of weeks," says Hugh P. Hermann, M.D., a family doctor in Woodstock, Vermont. "Instead of running, try another exercise, such as swimming. And in addition to buying new running shoes, buy new going-to-work shoes at least once a year."

Keep your shin under wraps if the pain makes you limp.

Rub On Comfort

"Pick up some over-the-counter Iodex at your drugstore and rub it on your sore shin," says Gerard Bozuwa, M.D., a retired family doctor in Wakefield, New Hampshire. "It'll really help ease the splints."

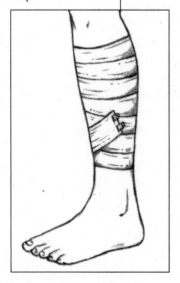

Lay On Warmth

"A warm compress, such as a hot-water bottle or a towel soaked in hot water, can be soothing to shinsplints," Dr. Bozuwa says. "Apply the compress for 10 minutes three times a day until your leg feels better."

Acquire a Means of Support

"If your shinsplints are severe enough to make you limp, support the leg with a bandage wrap such as an over-the-counter elastic bandage," says Randal Schaetzke, D.C., a chiropractor at the Wholistic Health Center in Quechee, Vermont.

Get a Lift

"An inexpensive cure for your shinsplints might be to buy an over-the-counter orthotic heel lift, such as Dr. Scholl's," Dr. Monto says. "You place the lift inside your shoe on the outer edge of the heel. It can ease some of the stress on the shin."

S

SHOULDER PAIN
Relief for when your shoulders
want to socket to you

With your shoulders packing 3 bones, more than 15 muscles, and an overall range of motion that's greater than that in any other part of your body, it's a wonder that they don't have more problems than they do.

There is certainly a lot of equipment that can malfunction there. The tendons holding your shoulder in place can deteriorate from wear and tear. Calcium can build up in the joints and irritate the area. The bursae—tiny fluid-filled sacs that provide lubrication—can become inflamed, a painful condition known as bursitis. Your shoulders also can suffer from impingement, in which muscles and tendons get pinched between bones and ligaments. And then there's frozen shoulder, which makes it hard to move your arms without pain.

Fortunately, frozen shoulder usually goes away—eventually. A dislocated shoulder stays dislocated, though, until you seek medical help. Dislocation is what happens when an accident such as a fall yanks your arm out of its socket. You need a doctor to put the bone back in place.

For less traumatic shoulder problems, here's what you can do on your own.

> ### TIME TO SEE THE DOCTOR
> ## *Don't Ignore*
> ## *That Detached Feeling*
>
> SEE your doctor if the pain in your shoulder doesn't improve after three days, you can't lift your arm above your head, your shoulder is frozen, or it feels as though it's detached from its socket.

Get Pilled

"Shoulder pain responds well to over-the-counter pain relievers," says Sarah Johansen, M.D., medical director of emergency services at New London Hospital in New London, New Hampshire. Effective choices include aspirin, ibuprofen, and acetaminophen. Avoid giving aspirin to children, however, because of the risk of Reye's syndrome.

Give Pain the Cold Shoulder

"Ice the shoulder right after any injury or strain," Dr. Johansen advises. "You don't need anything fancy from a store—just a plastic bag with ice cubes and a towel wrapped around it. Or try holding a bag of frozen peas or corn against your shoulder." Frozen vegetables conform better than ice to the shape of your shoulder, she explains. Hold the ice pack on for about 15 minutes at a time.

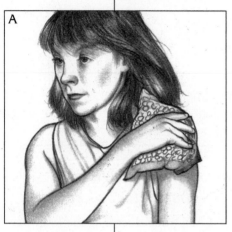

Then Use Heat

"If the sore area isn't warm to the touch, apply heat to relieve the soreness," says Randal Schaetzke, D.C., a chiropractor at the Wholistic Health Center in Quechee, Vermont. "Use a warm, moist towel or hot-water bottle." If your joint feels hot, use ice instead of heat, he says.

Hey, Stretch

"Slowly stretching a shoulder often can make it feel better," Dr. Schaetzke says. "Working on the side with the sore shoulder, hold an unopened soup can in your hand, with your arm down at your side. Bend over and make gentle figure eights with your hand. Do between 10 and 20." If you feel any numbness, tingling, or pain in your arm, stop, says Dr. Schaetzke.

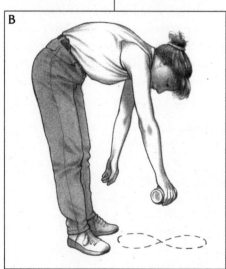

Hold frozen peas on the shoulder (A). Or stretch, making figure eights with soup can in hand (B).

Hang It All

"A sore shoulder needs rest for a couple of days," Dr. Johansen says. "Take a large, clean fabric scrap, tie it in a circle, and drape it over your neck to form a sling. Then stick your

SHOULDER PAIN

arm in it to take its weight off your shoulder." Most shoulder injuries improve after two or three days if you've immobilized your joint. "If you don't feel better after three days with a sling, see your doctor," Dr. Johansen says.

SIDE STITCHES
Trot out these remedies for the jogger's cramp

You've finally made yourself get outside and start jogging again. Moving briskly in your new white running shoes, you think to yourself, "Hey, I'm not in such bad shape after all!" That's when the side stitch hits—a sharp pain in your side that hurts even more when you breathe deeply. Runners aren't the only people who get stitched; aerobic exercisers, weekend football players, anyone who moves his legs rapidly and breathes fast is susceptible.

Most side stitches are a spasm in the diaphragm, the muscle that works your lungs. The organs below the diaphragm get bounced around when you exercise, pushing against that hardworking muscle and yanking it out of sync. Most side stitches occur on your right side—a result of your liver playing havoc with your diaphragm. Running in cold weather can trigger a spasm. So can exercising on a full stomach.

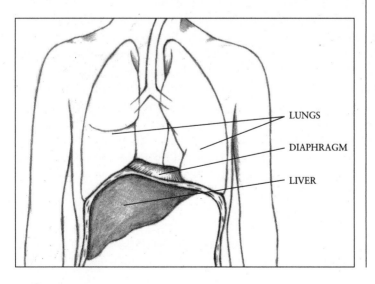

LUNGS

DIAPHRAGM

LIVER

An out-of-sync diaphragm can cause the one-sided pain called a stitch.

S

"If you get a side stitch while exercising, slow down or stop running," says Robert F. Wilson, M.D., a pediatrician who is retired from his practice in Dover, New Hampshire. "You'll probably feel better within a few minutes."

If that quick breather doesn't work, try these cures.

Press the Pain

"To get rid of a side stitch, stop what you're doing and apply pressure to the spot where it hurts," says Sarah Johansen, M.D., medical director of emergency services at New London Hospital in New London, New Hampshire. "Press your hands into the spot and rub gently. It sometimes helps to bend over while doing this." Such gentle massage can stop the spasm and help get rid of lactic acid in your diaphragm. "That acid builds up while you exercise, and it can cause a side stitch," she says.

Sound Manly

If you feel a side stitch coming on while you're running, try grunting with every step. "That helps relax the diaphragm," Dr. Johansen says.

Don't Run in Thirst Place

"You can help avoid cramps of all kinds, including side stitches, if you keep yourself from getting dehydrated," says Laurence Bouchard, D.O., an osteopathic family physician in private practice in Narragansett, Rhode Island. "Drink plenty of water at least an hour and a half before you go out running."

Hit the Gas

"Some side stitches are caused by a buildup of gas in the stomach," Dr. Bouchard says. "You can ease a gas-caused stitch by taking an antacid such as Pepto-Bismol."

Lay on the Heat

"For a side stitch, apply a heating pad right where you feel the cramp," says Daniel Caloras, M.D., a family doctor in private

---

TIME TO SEE THE DOCTOR

When the Stitch Continues in Time

SEE your doctor if your side stitch isn't your only symptom," says Sarah Johansen, M.D., medical director of emergency services at New London Hospital in New London, New Hampshire. "If your stitch is accompanied by vomiting, fever, or blood in your stool, get checked out." She adds that you should see your doctor if your side stitch lasts more than a few hours. "And you need immediate attention if the pain in your side spreads to your chest, shoulder, or back. That could be a sign of a heart attack."

practice in Charlestown, New Hampshire. "Put a towel between your skin and the pad to keep from burning yourself."

SINUS PROBLEMS
The solutions you seek for trouble behind your beak

Need pain like a hole in the head? Well, sinuses (the areas shaded here) are actually hollow places in the nose, face, and forehead.

The pain you feel in the front of your face is very likely caused by hollow parts of your head. Now, don't feel insulted. Everyone has these hollows, called sinuses—air pockets that fill the space inside the nose, face, and forehead. "No one knows exactly what sinuses are for," says Robert Fagelson, M.D., an otolaryngologist in Brattleboro, Vermont. "Some think the sinuses lighten the skull, the way a bird's bones are hollow to make them weigh less. Or the sinuses could serve as resonators for speech, although mammals that don't speak still have sinuses."

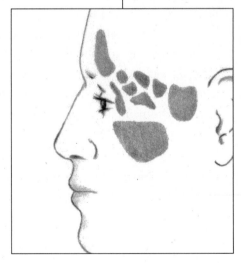

S

Whatever their purpose, the sinuses sometimes get plugged up. Reasons can include a bacterial or viral infection, irritating smoke or chemicals in the air, allergies, or a physical blockage such as a nasal polyp. A head cold is the most common cause. The irritation caused by a respiratory virus swells up sinus membranes and shuts off the sinuses' openings into the nose. An inflammation called sinusitis can result. Most sinus pain that results from a head cold eventually takes care of itself. But you can get some relief in the meantime, especially if you can open things up. Here's how.

Hey, Squirt

"Over-the-counter nasal sprays contain mild vasoconstrictors that help shrink the swollen passages inside the nose," Dr. Fagelson says. "But you have to be very, very careful using them. They are addictive, and you should follow the

---

A WORD FROM DR. MARTIN

Here's a Method to Snort At

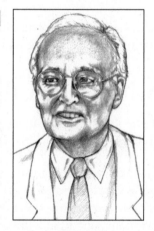

As a family practitioner, I never told my patients what to do without listening to them first. I found out what remedies they had already used on themselves and what their parents or grandparents did before them. Unless I knew the practice was detrimental, I wouldn't say anything. If you think it helps and it doesn't hurt, then you should do it.

But one thing you shouldn't do is to blow your nose the way most people do. A big honk forces bacteria up higher into your nasal passages, causing infections. You should blow your nose gently. Actually, I recommend not blowing at all. A snort and swallow does less damage than blowing hard. Plus you eliminate the problem of dealing with a dirty handkerchief or tissue.

BREWSTER MARTIN, M.D., *a retired family doctor in Chelsea, Vermont (population 1,166), and cofounder of the Chelsea Family Health Center. He was named Vermont Doctor of the Year in 1991.*

---

instructions very closely." Don't use nasal sprays for more than three days in a row, he says. And beware of the rebound effect: "No matter how long you use them, you'll be stuffier when you stop."

Tap the Hot-Cold Cure

"Use hot packs on your congested sinuses as often as possible during the day for as long as possible," Dr. Fagelson says. A warm washcloth will do, he adds, as will a hot-water bottle.

Do a Steamy Scene

"Taking a hot shower and breathing in the steam really helps," says Julia Foote, R.N., a retired nurse living in Norwell, Massachusetts. "I know, because I've done it myself."

Vicks Does the Trick

"My wife likes to use Vicks VapoRub in a pot," says Paul Lena, M.D., a retired physician of internal medicine in Concord, New Hampshire. "It works for her." A tablespoon of Vicks in near-boiling water does the trick, Dr. Lena says. You can also use Vicks in a vaporizer, as long as you keep the vaporizer scrupulously clean with regular scrubbings of vinegar. But "a regular kitchen pot is cheaper and easier to keep clean," Dr. Lena notes. Heat the water and Vicks in the pot until the water is steaming, then remove the pan from the heat and "just stand over the pot with a towel draped over your head for 10 minutes or so, until you feel better."

Sudafed Is Suitable

"A couple of the old prescription standbys for sinus problems are now available over the counter: Sudafed and Tavist-D," Dr. Lena says. "As decongestants, they are very effective in reducing the swelling in your nasal passages."

And Spice Is Nice

As a Korean-American, otolaryngologist Richard Lee of Laconia, New Hampshire, likes to take friends to dinner at a

---

Korean restaurant. "Some people tell me that the spicy Korean food really opens the sinuses," Dr. Lee says. "If you like to eat spicy, you might try it when your sinuses are giving you trouble."

SKIN FUNGUS
Relief from problems that grow on you

It's not pleasant to think of yourself as a habitat, but if you have itchy, scaly patches on your skin, you may be providing fertile ground for any one of a variety of fungi.

The most common of these trespassers is the tinea fungus, which is known by a variety of aliases. When tinea takes up residence between your toes or on the sole of your foot, it's called athlete's foot. On your scalp or face, it's called ringworm, even though it isn't a worm at all. "Dairy farmers often get ringworm on their cheeks when they rest their faces against infected cows while milking them," says Owen Reynolds, M.D., a dermatologist in private practice in North Andover, Massachusetts. Tinea also can lodge in the skin on your hands, stomach, or derriere.

But that's not the only unwelcome visitor that can take up residence on your skin. You can pick up a nasty skin fungus called *Microsporum canis* from a cat or dog, for example. And babies get a form of fungal diaper rash called moniliasis.

Doctors aren't sure why some people seem to suffer more than others from fungal infections. Heredity may be one factor—some people's immune systems just seem better than others' at fighting off skin invaders. Hygiene and weight control affect the skin's environment, too. Like most other fungi, the kind that lodges on your skin likes nothing better than damp darkness. Skin that's irritated from rubbing against clothing or other skin can provide a fungal beachhead. And

---

Ward Off Fungi and Friends in One Fell Swoop

A TRADITIONAL remedy for skin fungus is to rub raw garlic or onion on the nasty spots. Now medical researchers in India and Egypt say there may be something to that old cure. Garlic oil and onion oil have been effective in killing skin fungi in the laboratory.

---

an illness such as diabetes can make your skin more inviting to fungi.

Here's how to show those unwelcome visitors the door.

Cream It

"Over-the-counter Clotrimazole cream is good for treating ringworm," says Charles Hammer, M.D., a dermatologist with the North Country Outreach Program of the Lahey Hitchcock Clinic in St. Johnsbury, Vermont. Use it twice a day for 10 days, he says.

Pick Your Litter

"Cats are particularly common carriers of skin fungi," Dr. Reynolds says. "Most commonly infected are stray cats and those that come from crowded pet stores. If you want a pet cat, go to a reputable breeder."

Treat Your Pet

"If you think you picked up ringworm from your pet, get treatment for the pet first," says Daniel Caloras, M.D., a family doctor in private practice in Charlestown, New Hampshire. Get a prescription for your pet so that the animal won't reinfect you. Then use Clotrimazole cream on yourself.

TIME TO SEE THE DOCTOR
When a "Fungus" Isn't

OTHER problems are sometimes misdiagnosed as ringworm, according to John C. Robinson, M.D., a pediatrician in private practice in Quincy, Massachusetts. "It's much more likely that you have impetigo, a staph or strep infection of the skin," he says. "If you have a round sore with a yellow crust on it, see your doctor, who'll probably prescribe an antibiotic. Don't leave it alone. Certain kinds of strep can result in kidney disease."

Some skin problems that appear to be fungal infections are actually the result of a different life-form altogether: yeast. A form of yeast called candida can lodge in your armpits, groin, or skin folds; between your toes; or on your private parts. It often takes a doctor to tell the difference between a fungal and a yeast infection.

SLEEPWALKING

*Try these remedies to keep
your snoozer from taking a hike*

You're watching the late news when you see your kid strolling by, oblivious to the fact that she was sent to bed a couple of hours ago. You ask what she's doing up, and she answers in total gibberish, with a blank look on her face. You have a sleepwalker on your hands.

"Sleepwalking is technically called partial arousal disorder," says Michael Sateia, M.D., director of the Sleep Disorders Clinic at the Dartmouth-Hitchcock Medical Center in Lebanon, New Hampshire. "It's a close cousin of night terrors." Sleepwalkers often do their wandering in the first three hours of sleep, and the trek can last anywhere from half a minute to half an hour, during which the child will often seem twitchy.

Nighttime meandering is not very common in adults, "and it becomes increasingly uncommon as the years go by," Dr. Sateia says. "This is because sleepwalking comes from a partial arousal from deep sleep, and the deepest stages of sleep tend to drop out as we age," he explains.

What exactly happens in that restless period? "The brain is trapped midway between sleep and wakefulness during a sleepwalking episode," Dr. Sateia says. "That's why the sleepwalker may act as if she has some sort of purpose in mind." But she's still asleep. "She won't respond well to your efforts to get her to go where you want," Dr. Sateia says. "One father of a strapping 17-year-old patient of mine tried to get his son back to bed. Dad got in the kid's face and told him to go back to bed. The boy swung at him and broke his jaw. The poor kid was really sorry about that the next day— the punch had been entirely unconscious."

TIME TO SEE THE DOCTOR

A Teenage Walker Should Get Checked

IF SLEEPWALKING disrupts your family or affects the sleepwalker's health, see your doctor or head to a sleep disorders clinic, says Patricia Edwards, M.D., a pediatrician in private practice in Concord, New Hampshire. "A child who continues to sleepwalk after the age of 14 should get checked out by a doctor as well," she says. "Sleepwalking is less common in teenagers and adults. There may be physical or psychological problems that need a doctor's cure."

The moral of the story: Don't get rough with sleepwalkers. Here are the alternatives.

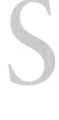

Steer Gently

"Don't wake a sleepwalker," says Patricia Edwards, M.D., a pediatrician in private practice in Concord, New Hampshire. "Just gently guide him back to bed."

Block the Wandering

"The most important thing you need to do is to protect sleepwalkers," says Mark Harris, M.D., a pediatrician in Bradford, Vermont. "To prevent a small child from falling down the stairs, keep a baby gate across the top of the stairway. If your child tries to leave the house, you may need to install locks that can't be opened easily from inside at night." Childproof doorknob covers are available at many hardware stores. They keep sleepwalkers from getting some unintended night air. If your sleepwalker is old enough to drive, says Dr. Harris, "don't leave the car keys handy. One patient of mine came to and found herself sitting in her car in the driveway at her sister's house, eight miles from home."

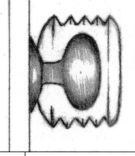

A childproof doorknob cover just spins in a child's hand. When an adult squeezes it, the knob turns.

Break the Pattern

"Some children tend to sleepwalk at the same time every night," Dr. Edwards says. "Try waking the child each night a half hour before sleepwalking time. For example, if the kid sleepwalks every night at 11:00, wake him up at 10:30. Do this for a week. That should stop the problem."

Check the Ritalin

Ritalin, the medication often prescribed by doctors to control hyperactivity in children, can cause sleepwalking after the child reaches puberty. "If your teenager is on Ritalin and sleepwalks, ask your doctor if you need to change the drug or the dosage," Dr. Edwards says.

AN OUNCE OF PREVENTION

Be in the Zone

THE temperature of the bedroom can affect sleepwalking," says Kathleen Kovner-Kline, M.D., a child psychiatrist at the Dartmouth-Hitchcock Medical Center in Lebanon, New Hampshire. "A room that's too warm or too cool can make people arouse more easily, and half arousal can result in a sleepwalk. Don't let the temperature fall below 54°F or get above 75°F if you can help it."

SNAKEBITE
What to do when your personal Garden of Eden is invaded

If you've been bitten by a snake, chances are about one in six that there was poison involved. Even poisonous snakes often don't inject much venom with a bite. And nonpoisonous bites rarely transfer the sorts of diseases spread by biting mammals, according to Scott Jackson, a herpetologist and conservation specialist at the University of Massachusetts Extension service in Amherst. "The worst thing most people get is an allergic reaction to the snake's saliva," Jackson says.

Still, unless you can identify the species, it's safest to assume that a bite is poisonous. "The best treatment for a poisonous snakebite is a set of car keys," Jackson says. "You want to get the victim to a hospital as fast as possible."

Here are some other things you can do.

Relax

"The first rule if you are bitten by a poisonous snake—or by one that may or may not be poisonous—is to stay calm," Jackson says. "Don't run around and scream. Avoid any physical exertion that can help spread any poison faster."

AN OUNCE OF PREVENTION
Avoid Six-Pack Venom

OF THE hundred or so snakebite calls that come into the Arizona Poison and Drug Information Center in Tucson every year, the majority involve 15- to 25-year-old males who were teasing poisonous snakes, says Nancy Mellor, R.Ph., a poison information specialist at the center. Most of the victims are under the influence of alcohol when they are bitten, leading the workers at the center to quip that "snakes are attracted to alcohol." The obvious answer: To keep from getting bitten, avoid getting drunk around dangerous snakes.

When walking through snake territory, wear ankle-high boots and long pants, advises Mary Droege, a steward for the Vermont Chapter of The Nature Conservancy. "Carry a walking stick with you and use it to part tall grasses or low shrubs," Droege says. "If you come upon a snake, back off and leave it alone."

Skip the Movie Cure

"The old cut-and-suck method, the cure you see actors using in movie westerns, has been discredited," Jackson says. "You can cause more damage with the cutting than the snake did. Save the wound for the physician."

Clean the Wound

Most of the snakebites seen by John Dunn, M.D., an emergency room physician at the Northwestern Medical Center in St. Albans, Vermont, are caused by poison-free garter snakes.

"In most snakebites, the important thing is care of the wound," Dr. Dunn says. "You want to wash the bite carefully with plenty of water. Then you can apply an over-the-counter antibiotic such as Bacitracin." If the bite is poisonous, Dr. Dunn says, the physician will want to judge the severity of the bite before prescribing antivenin to counter the poison. "Some people can get a dangerous allergic reaction to the medicine, so antivenin isn't administered at the drop of a hat," he explains.

SNEEZING
How to eschew
what makes you go ah-choo

Bless you! Before this century, people used to take sneezing very seriously. Early Europeans believed that a sneeze could accidentally eject the soul from the body. That's why it's traditional to bless a sneezer—just in case the soul needs a good quick cleansing.

We still bless people after a big sneeze, but it's no longer a major cause for alarm. It can be annoying, though, especially if you don't make it to a handkerchief in time. How do you stop the explosions? First, you have to figure out the cause, says Stephen Blair, M.D., a pediatrician in private practice in Claremont, New Hampshire. "Be a detective," he says. "If you sneeze just a few times during the day and feel achy all over, you probably have a cold."

By contrast, rapid-fire, uncontrollable sneezing is probably an allergy. "You need to hunt down the cause of the al-

Slergy and figure out how to avoid it," Dr. Blair says. "Have you just mowed the lawn, or sat next to someone smoking a cigar, or stood in an elevator next to someone wearing heavy perfume?" Some allergens are harder to track down. You may be allergic to cats, for example, and suffer from the allergy even if you don't own a cat. "Your best friend may have one. You hug your friend, who's covered with cat dander without even knowing it, and you start sneezing like crazy."

Some sneezing fits aren't due to allergies. "Some things are irritating to your nose, such as pepper or milkweed fluff," Dr. Blair says. "And if there's enough tree pollen in the air, it might make you sneeze even if you're not allergic to it." A change in temperature, such as getting into an air-conditioned car, can make some people sneeze. Bright light can raise a sneeze. And the hormonal changes of pregnancy can irritate the sinuses and cause sneezing.

So what do you do when your honker starts honking? Follow your nose to these remedies.

Strike Early

"It's often too late to do much once the sneezing starts," says Lawrence H. Bernstein, M.D., a former family doctor who is the medical director at Jewish Geriatric Services in Longmeadow, Massachusetts. "Your best bet is to take an over-the-counter antihistamine such as Benadryl one to two hours before you go someplace where you know you'll be exposed to an allergen. For example, before you visit your neighbor's cat, give yourself a dose against the dander."

Wear Shades

"Some patients who are sensitive to light have sneezing attacks from the bright lights that dentists and orthodontists shine in their faces," says Gregory L. Baker, D.D.S., an orthodontist in private practice in Woodstock, Vermont, and West Lebanon and New London, New Hampshire. "I keep

---

Don't Seal Yourself Up

DESPITE what your mother told you, it's not harmful to suppress a sneeze, says David Goodman, M.D., a pediatric allergist in Lebanon, New Hampshire. "Just don't hold your nose or mouth shut. You could injure your eardrums by forcing air up your eustachian tubes." Instead, Dr. Goodman says you can try to swallow hard just before sneezing. And don't look at bright light when you feel an attack coming on.

---

a drawer full of sunglasses for these patients. If you're sensitive to light, you might bring your own dark glasses with you to the dentist."

Stiff the Stuffed Ones

"If your child has allergies or asthma and tends to sneeze a lot, you may have to find a new home for the stuffed animals," says David Goodman, M.D., a pediatric allergist in Lebanon, New Hampshire. "Stuffed animals collect dust mites, which tend to cause allergies. Make them a bed across the room from your child's bed." That doesn't mean your child has to sleep friendless, however. "Pick a favorite stuffed animal that can be washed and then dried in a hot dryer. Your child can sleep with that animal if it is washed weekly."

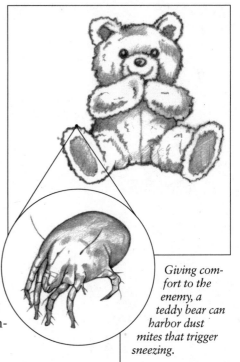

Giving comfort to the enemy, a teddy bear can harbor dust mites that trigger sneezing.

SNORING

Do you saw in your sleep? Here are some tools to stop it

"The tunable serenade of that wakeful nightingale, his nose." Well, that's one somewhat overblown description of snoring—from George Farquhar in the second act of *The Beaux' Stratagem.*

If snoring's not your idea of making beautiful music in bed, join the crowd. Some 45 percent of adults snore; one-quarter of the adult population makes a habit of it. Twenty of the first 32 U.S. presidents snored, including Washington, Lincoln, both Adamses, and both Roosevelts (snoring tends to run in families). Pity their first ladies. Scientists have recorded snoring levels in excess of 80 decibels, equivalent to the sound of a motorcycle revving up at close range.

How can so much noise roar out of just one throat? Snoring begins when the air you're breathing rushes past the

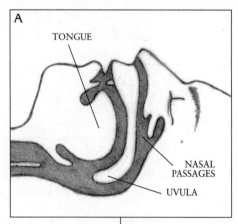

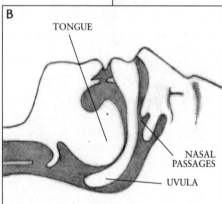

A wide-open air passage (A) allows quiet breathing. But when the muscles relax, the passage gets smaller (B). Then the walls can vibrate tunefully.

soft palate at the back of your throat and your uvula—the pink, pear-shaped hunks of flesh that dangle from the back of your mouth. When you sleep, the muscles in your air passages relax, coming closer together or allowing the tongue to fall back toward the throat. The restricted passage starts vibrating when your breath hits all that muscle and flesh, stirring up sound—the same way a reed on a clarinet's mouthpiece vibrates and sings.

Snoring may sound funny, but it can be medically serious. Habitual snorers tend to suffer more than most people from high blood pressure, heart disease, and stroke. Some snorers also have sleep apnea, a condition in which they occasionally stop breathing for 10 seconds or more during the night. Some 4 percent of men and 2 percent of women have sleep apnea, with breath-stopping periods numbering from 10 to hundreds of times per night. The disruptions can prevent a good night's sleep, leaving you groggy the next day. People with sleep apnea are more likely than the general population to be involved in car and workplace accidents.

And we haven't even mentioned the suffering that the families of chronic snorers go through. Here are ways to turn down the volume and let everyone—including you—enjoy all 40 winks.

Lose the Fat

"Adults who are 50 pounds overweight tend to be snorers," notes Dudley Weider, M.D., an otolaryngologist in Lebanon, New Hampshire. "The more overweight you are, the more you'll snore. That's because your airway gets smaller as fat encroaches on it, increasing the vibrations in the airway." But that works the other way as well: "Lose weight, and the snoring may stop."

Tennis Ball, Anyone?

"If you sleep on your side or stomach, you will probably snore less," Dr. Weider says. "To keep yourself from rolling onto your back, try this old remedy: Sew a tennis ball into the back of your pajamas."

Richard Lee, M.D., an otolaryngologist in private practice in Laconia, New Hampshire, explains that when a snorer lies on her back, the tongue falls back into the throat, partly blocking an already limited airway. "Sleeping on the tummy or side helps keep the airway open," Dr. Lee says.

Skip the Cocktails

"Drinking alcohol before bed will make snoring worse," Dr. Weider says. "It decreases muscle tone in the airway, increasing the vibrations that constitute snoring." Dr. Weider suggests that you avoid sleeping pills for the same reason.

Put a Damper on the Smoke

"If you are a snorer, you need to maximize breathing function," Dr. Lee says. "Smoking puts you at a disadvantage as a breather. It irritates and causes swelling of an already narrowed airway." Researchers have found a link between patients with sleep disturbance problems and smoking. "So if you're a snorer who smokes, cut out the cigarettes," Dr. Lee says.

Think Dee-fense

Robert Fagelson, M.D., an otolaryngologist in Brattleboro, Vermont, suggests using Breathe Right, a small, disposable adhesive strip of plastic that some pro football players wear in the belief that it helps them take in more air. "It opens the nostrils," Dr. Fagelson says. "That alone can cure snoring." You can buy Breathe Right strips at the drugstore.

TIME TO SEE THE DOCTOR
Are You Still Sleepy?

IF YOU are a snorer, ask your spouse or roommate if you stop breathing when you sleep," says Robert Fagelson, M.D., an otolaryngologist in Brattleboro, Vermont. "The gaps may last just a couple of seconds and increase in length to 10 seconds or more. See a doctor immediately if you stop breathing between snores, even for short periods."

Dr. Fagelson also recommends getting medical attention if you are chronically fatigued even after being in bed for at least eight hours every night. "You may think you're sleeping during all that time, but you're actually waking up each time you stop breathing," he says. "You're being deprived of sleep. Some snorers tend to fall asleep at work or at a stoplight. The condition could be dangerous."

Beat the Snorer

No, we don't mean smack him. Instead, go to bed before your snoring mate. "That way, you'll be asleep before the snoring begins," Dr. Fagelson says.

Rise Above Your Snoring

Use a cervical pillow, a wedge-shaped piece of foam available from most medical supply stores and home health catalogs, to raise your head and open your airway. "Or you can put bricks under the bedposts at the head of your bed," Dr. Fagelson says.

SNOW BLINDNESS
Fixing a glaring exception to the fun of winter

You're having a lovely time schussing down perfect powder on a dazzlingly brilliant early-spring day. What could possibly go wrong?

The dazzling part, that's what. Suddenly everything is tinted a weird pink or white, or—if you're really suffering—you can't see a thing. You feel a sharp, penetrating pain in your eyes, as if they're burning.

Actually, they are. "Snow blindness comes from too much reflected ultraviolet light," says William Lavin, M.D., an ophthalmologist in private practice in Waterville, Maine. "The brilliant rays burn the surface of the eye, destroying the outside layer of cells. The effect is the same as if your cornea were scratched."

You don't have to be in snow to suffer the symptoms associated with snow blindness. "A very similar eye injury is welding flash," Dr. Lavin says. "This happens when a welder fails to protect himself from the bright ultraviolet light of a welding torch." You can get the same burning pain from a day at the beach, where ultraviolet light bounces off the water.

Whether your burning eyes result from sun on the slopes or welding at work, here's how to cool things down and let your sight heal.

Look for the Dark Side

"Ordinary ski goggles are not dark enough to protect against snow blindness," says Dudley Weider, M.D., an otolaryngologist at the Dartmouth-Hitchcock Medical Center in Lebanon, New Hampshire. Dr. Weider is also a founding member of the Geriatric Adventure Society, a group of older outdoorsmen who venture north of the Arctic Circle every year. "You should wear glacier goggles underneath your ski goggles," he says. Glacier goggles are dark glasses with flaps on the sides to keep out glare. "In the Swiss Alps, you aren't allowed out on organized expeditions without them." Glacier goggles, available at outdoor-equipment stores, are a good idea for cutting harmful glare even if you're just hitting the slopes for a day, Dr. Weider says.

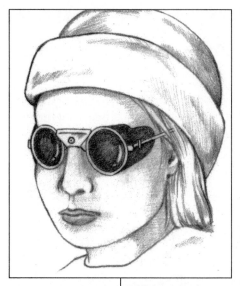

Glacier goggles have side flaps to block the glare that comes with snow.

Protect Totally

"Toy sunglasses for children are not a good idea," says Eugene J. Bernal, O.D., an optometrist in private practice in White River Junction, Vermont. "You need 99 percent protection against ultraviolet rays for your kids—and for yourself as well." You can't tell whether a pair of sunglasses have total UV protection by looking at them, unless they have a tag noting the degree. "You'll have to pay more to get all 99 percent," Dr. Bernal says, but he adds that it's worth the money.

Have a Cool Bedtime

"Put a wet, cool washcloth on your injured eyes and go to bed for a few hours," recommends Mary-Catherine Gennaro, D.O., a family osteopath in Warren, New Hampshire. "The cool compress will lessen the pain by reducing the inflammation in your eyes."

Darken Your Specs

"You can have UV protection added to your glasses and contact lenses by an optometrist," says Stephen Moore, M.D., an ophthalmologist in Great Barrington, Massachusetts.

SORE MUSCLES
Cures for times when your workout doesn't quite work out

Sure, you felt great during that extra-long jog or weight lifting bout, but that was yesterday. Today you feel as though somebody was working out on top of you. Your muscles also can ache from the flu or from your prescription medication, especially blood pressure medicine. Arthritis or a thyroid problem can bring on muscle pain. But most achiness is caused by garden-variety gardening—or heavy lifting, a weekend fun run, or any other muscle workout.

"Actually, a little muscle soreness isn't such a bad thing," says Raymond Rocco Monto, M.D., an orthopedic surgeon at Martha's Vineyard Orthopedic Surgery and Sports Medicine in Oak Bluffs, Massachusetts. "Every time you work out, you cause microscopic tears in your muscles. In other words, exercise is a form of controlled injury. Your body repairs that injury by inflaming the site slightly and replacing the damaged tissue with more muscle tissue. The end result is a stronger muscle, but you can be sore for a couple of days in the meantime."

Here's how to beat the soreness while your muscles recover.

TIME TO SEE THE DOCTOR

Does the Ache Keep on Aching?

IF YOUR muscles have been hurting constantly for more than three months, get a doctor to look at them. You could have fibromyalgia, a chronic pain that can be caused by inadequate sleep, injury, physical or emotional stress, or illness. The most painful points: the neck, shoulders, chest, back, and buttocks. Your doctor can search out the cause and give you the best solution.

Heat Them Up

"I like moist heat for muscle soreness," says Daniel Caloras, M.D., a family doctor in private practice in Charlestown, New Hampshire. "Buy a hot-water bottle at your drugstore or discount store, fill it with hot water, drape a towel around it, and apply it directly to the sore muscle." An even simpler remedy: "Just use a warm, damp bath towel by itself."

Cool Them Down

John Morton recommends jumping into a bath of cold water or hosing down your legs after a long run. Morton should know: He was on the U.S. biathlon team in the 1972 and 1976 Olympics and the team leader in the 1988, 1992, and 1996 Olympics. "A world-class over-40 marathoner from Australia introduced me to this remedy," Morton reports. "He says if it's good enough for racehorses, it's good enough for him."

Dr. Monto confirms that cool water can help reduce the inflammation right after a workout. "After an hour or so, switch to heat for the soreness," he says. A heating pad will do the trick at that point.

Pull Out the Pillbox

"To reduce the inflammation that comes with microscopic muscle damage, take a nonsteroidal anti-inflammatory medicine," Dr. Monto advises. "Ibuprofen and aspirin are both effective in dealing with the achiness." Do not give aspirin to children, however, because of the risk of Reye's syndrome.

There's the Rub

"In many a Pain which vexes us, it would be good Advice . . . to Say, Beat it," wrote Cotton Mather, a Puritan minister and medic. Mather's prescription: "A continued Beating on the Place, with a Fist, or Some other Instrument." Today we'd call a more sophisticated version a vigorous massage.

The gentle, rubbing kind works even better to soothe aching muscles, according to Morton. "At most big marathons, there are massage therapists at the finish line," Morton notes. "The first 100 or so finishers get a massage as soon as they cross the line. It works wonders."

Couples can learn to massage each other, adds Randal Schaetzke, D.C., a chiropractor in Quechee, Vermont. "Take a class in massage. It works to get lactic acid out of the muscles after a workout or strain. The lactic acid contributes to soreness."

ANNALS OF MEDICINE

And the Smell Makes You Forget the Pain

COTTON Mather, the famous Puritan clergyman and part-time doctor, prescribed onions for muscle pain. Boil them, drain away the water, beat them to a pulp, and apply them as a poultice "as hott as the Patient can bear," he said.

"Although I wouldn't recommend onions myself, a hot poultice can be very soothing to sore muscles," says Sarah Johansen, M.D., medical director of emergency services at New London Hospital in New London, New Hampshire. "Skip the vegetables and use a towel soaked in warm water. Put it right on your muscles."

Make Sure You're Pasta Prime

"Get a well-balanced diet if you want to exercise without overly sore muscles," Dr. Monto says. "Make sure you get plenty of carbohydrates for fuel. The night before a major workout such as a big run, have spaghetti and bread for dinner."

SORE THROAT
When gulping gets you down, try these simple soothers

Lots of things can cause a sore throat—from cold and flu viruses to streptococcus bacteria, which cause strep throat. You can get a sore, froggy feeling from an infected voice box, from hay fever, or from the dry heat in your home during the winter. Some morning throats get sore from nighttime reflux, in which acid comes up into the throat from the stomach during the night. You usually feel better later in the day. Your throat can give a painful protest if you've been around tobacco smoke or irritating chemicals, had a few too many cocktails, eaten hot and spicy food, or hollered at a football game.

If your sore throat is caused by a bacterial infection, such as strep, your doctor can identify the problem with a throat culture and clear it up with an antibiotic. Treatments haven't always been so simple, or so successful. Medical historians say that George Washington died from an infected, severely swollen throat—and from the rough treatments the doctors provided, such as bleeding him. Sore throat medicine is much more benign these days—including the cures below.

Play Misty for Your Throat

"Dry nighttime air in your bedroom can cause you to wake up with a sore throat," says Robert Fagelson, M.D., an oto-

Don't Put Up With It When You Have a Fever

Any sore throat that lasts for more than a week should be seen by a doctor," says Robert Fagelson, M.D., an otolaryngologist in private practice in Brattleboro, Vermont. "See the doctor even before that if your sore throat is accompanied by a fever. That could be a sign of strep throat."

Other signs of strep: "The throat will look fiery red and may have a whitish exudate, like pus, on it. If you have more than one case of strep throat a year, that could mean your tonsils are harboring the strepto-coccus bacterium and may have to be removed by surgery."

See your doctor if you have any of these other symptoms with a sore throat.

- Trouble breathing
- Difficulty swallowing
- Problems opening your mouth wide
- Joint pain
- Earache
- A rash over even a small part of your body
- Blood in your mouth
- A lump in your neck

laryngologist in Brattleboro, Vermont. "It will usually go away within an hour in the morning. But you can prevent it from happening in the first place by placing a cold-water humidifier in your bedroom."

Hose Down the Fire

"If the sore throat is the beginning of a cold, drink plenty of fluids to keep your throat moist and comfortable," Dr. Fagelson says.

This Potion's Like the Ocean

"A saltwater gargle can help a sore throat that accompanies the beginning of a cold," Dr. Fagelson says.

Swallow Some Help

"Acetaminophen is a good pain reliever when your sore throat is part of a cold," says Richard Lee, M.D., an otolaryngologist in Laconia, New Hampshire. Don't substitute aspirin if the patient is a child, because aspirin can cause Reye's syndrome in youngsters.

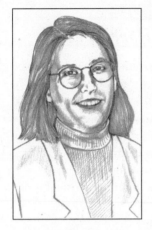

The Case of the Poisonous Pie

ONE Thanksgiving, an anxious couple from Korea came in with their five-year-old boy, saying he had eaten a "poisonous pumpkin pie." They reported that, after eating dessert, he kept turning blue and passing out. They could revive him only by using the old Korean remedy of sticking pins under his nails.

I looked down the boy's throat: His tonsils were so swollen that they touched each other. When he lay down, the tonsils blocked his breathing. That's why he was turning blue. The pumpkin pie had nothing to do with it. As for the old Korean remedy, the pins stirred him only because they hurt so much.

I sent the boy to the hospital. He had his tonsils out, and his "pumpkin" problem was cured.

MARY-CATHERINE GENNARO, D.O., *a family osteopath who makes house calls in Warren, New Hampshire.*

Stop the Pain with Lidocaine

Dr. Lee recommends Xylocaine lozenges to deaden the pain of a sore throat. Available over the counter in drugstores, Xylocaine contains the anesthetic lidocaine.

A Suggestion: Fight the Congestion

"Some sore throats are caused by postnasal drainage and swelling," Dr. Fagelson notes. "Taking an over-the-counter decongestant such as Sudafed will help."

Say Hi to Herb

Some old-time herbal remedies are tried-and-true soothers. "Wild indigo, echinacea, licorice, bitter orange, and slippery elm are all good for sore throats," says Maureen Williams, N.D., a naturopath in Hanover, New Hampshire. All are available at health food stores. (Skip the echinacea if you're allergic to ragweed. The two plants are closely related.) Dr.

Williams notes that just a few drops of bitter orange will numb the throat and that "licorice fights viruses, supports the immune system, and feels very soothing going down." She suggests buying comforting slippery elm in the form of lozenges that also contain zinc, which has been found in some studies to shorten the span and severity of colds.

Give Your Toothpaste the Brush-Off

A study by Finnish researchers shows that many brands of toothpaste contain substances that can cause allergic reactions, including sore throats, in some people. The worst culprits are cinnamon oil, peppermint, and some preservatives. If you suffer from a persistent sore throat and your doctor hasn't pinpointed any other cause, consider switching toothpastes.

SPLINTERS

Country cures for when wood wreaks its revenge

Not all splinters are created equal, as professional woodworkers will tell you. Some are bigger and deeper than others. "I use mahogany and spruce in my boats," says Dana Whipple, owner of D. L. Whipple Boatworks in Georges Mills, New Hampshire. "I try to get any splinters right out with tweezers." Which isn't always easy. Spruce splinters tend to have little barbs on the end of them, making them tough to remove.

> **TIME TO SEE THE DOCTOR**
> ### Is It In Too Deep?
> GET a doctor to help you out if the splinter is deep under your skin or close to an eye.

Not all splinters are made of wood, of course. You also can pick up a sliver or two while working with steel wool in your shop or kitchen.

Here's how you can unhand that foreign object.

Needle It

The best way to remove a splinter, according to Robert F. Wilson, M.D., a pediatrician who is retired from his practice in Dover, New Hampshire, is to heat up a needle and use it to retrieve the splinter. "Take a sewing needle or a sharp needle of just about any variety," he says. "Hold a match to it until it glows red. Let it cool for about a minute before using it." Don't dig into the flesh with the needle, Dr. Wilson says. "Instead, use the needle to get hold of the 'handle'— the bit of the splinter that's sticking out of the skin." And if there is no handle? "Take your splinter to a doctor."

Clamp It

"Maple and oak splinters are hard enough to be pulled out with tweezers," says Hugh P. Hermann, M.D., a family doctor in Woodstock, Vermont. "Other woods will simply break off—unless you use forceps. That's the kind of tiny vise that fly fishermen use to extract a hook from a fish." You can buy forceps from a bait and tackle shop or sporting goods store that carries fishing supplies. Use them to squeeze the splinter site. Then try the tweezers, he says.

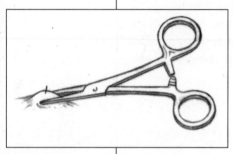

Fishermen's forceps let you squeeze the skin around the splinter. Then you can bring on the tweezers.

Soak It

"Soak the splinter for 15 minutes several times a day until it comes out," says John Dunn, M.D., an emergency room physician at the Northwestern Medical Center in St. Albans, Vermont. "The moisture will keep the track, or the splinter's pathway, open, and make it easier for your flesh to drive the foreign object out. This open track also will allow for drainage if the splinter site gets infected."

Cover It

"One thing that seems to work is covering the splinter with a piece of adhesive tape," says Susie Tann, R.N., an elementary school nurse in Bradford, Vermont. Clean the area with soap and water before applying the tape. "After two days, the splinter is often loose enough to come out when the adhesive tape is pulled off," she says. "Kids sometimes prefer the wait to having their parents go after the splinter. Some parents dig down to China trying to get a splinter out."

Leave It

"You should wear gloves when you work with steel wool— particularly fine steel wool, which can give you some nasty splinters," Dr. Hermann says. "These splinters tend to be very brittle and to break off when you try to remove them. If it's a major splinter, have your doctor remove it. Otherwise, you can wait for the splinter to work itself out or to rust away. For some reason, steel wool splinters usually don't get infected."

STOMACHACHE
Belly up to these
gut-soothing remedies

Back in the old days when water supplies were chancy, and in the days before refrigeration was developed to keep nasty bacteria out of food, there was a lot of bellyaching going on. Doctors in colonial times believed that most stomachaches were caused by cold innards. A prescription for warming up cold guts: a hot compress on the navel, or hot peppered milk. Yikes!

These days, you're more likely to blame an overdose of pepperoni pizza than a chilly belly for your ache. A big or spicy meal can double you over. So can the gas of food that's being digested, or just the air you swallowed while gulping your Big Mac. But there are lots of other reasons for what old-time doctors called "the gripe." An ulcer could be one cause. A sore inside your digestive tract, it's a pain that can last until you get treated by a doctor. And if your child has a stomachache and scratches his anus at night, he might have intestinal worms—a problem that needs to be treated by a doctor.

Too much aspirin can cause stomach problems. So can food poisoning, caused by bacteria picked up from improperly stored or prepared food. And any one of a variety of diseases of the digestive tract can cause terrific pain in the abdomen.

A sharp pain should send you right to the doctor, says Lawrence H. Bernstein, M.D., a former family doctor who is the medical director at Jewish Geriatric Services in Longmeadow, Massachusetts. "It could be appendicitis," he says. "In a child, it'll start with a pain near the belly button, followed by nausea, vomiting, and loss of appetite." You don't want to wait if a child or adult has these symptoms. "Get medical attention right away," he says. "You don't mess with appendicitis."

For the run-of-the-mill sore gut, here's how to restore the good feeling.

Make the Acid Placid

"An over-the-counter antacid such as Mylanta or Maalox will help if acid indigestion is the cause of your stomachache," says Sarah Johansen, M.D., medical director of emergency services at New London Hospital in New London, New Hampshire. But don't get into the habit of downing antacids if you get stomachaches frequently, she cautions. "You might very well have something other than acid indigestion, and your stomach could come to rely on the antacids for its chemical balance." If your stomachaches are frequent enough to cause an antacid habit, see your doctor, she says.

Treat Yourself Gingerly

"Anything with ginger in it, such as ginger ale or ginger tea, is good for a stomachache," Dr. Johansen says.

Or Make a Mint (Tea)

"Peppermint tea contains a mild antispasmodic that soothes the walls of the stomach," says Jane Smolnik, the owner of Crystal Garden Herbs in Springfield, Vermont. Try it to counteract a mild stomachache.

Sleep through the Midnight Snack

"The peak time for acid secretion in your stomach is in the middle of the night, around 2:00 A.M.," Dr. Johansen says. "You can make an acid stomach worse if you eat a late-night meal, a spicy snack, or something fatty like ice cream before bed. You may find yourself waking up with a stomachache."

But Chow Down Early

"Often a stomachache is caused by an empty stomach," says Susie Tann, R.N., an elementary school nurse in Bradford, Vermont. "Make sure everyone in your family eats breakfast before going to work or school."

Don't Trouble Your Stomach

"If a stomachache is chronic and not associated with any other symptom, such as diarrhea, vomiting, or weight loss, the most common underlying cause is anxiety," says John C. Robinson, M.D., a pediatrician in private practice in Quincy, Massachusetts. "This is especially common in children. Most anxious adults get headaches, but children often feel it in their stomachs."

Dr. Robinson recalls an 11-year-old boy who came in with chronic stomachaches. "I ran a number of tests on him and then sent him to a psychologist, who cured him in one visit. It turns out the boy didn't want to play football, and the father was coaching the team. The father laid off, the boy quit the team, and his stomachaches went away." The moral of that story, according to Dr. Robinson: "Treat the underlying anxiety. Try to find out what's troubling you or your child and deal with the cause."

STRESS
Hang loose with these cures when you're feeling uptight

Your alarm clock fails you, and you get up late. Your teenage kid refuses to get out of bed, then won't tell you where he hid the cereal. Your favorite pair of pants has a ketchup stain. Some jerk cuts you off on the highway to work while you

S

listen to a gloomy forecast for the weekend weather. You get to work and realize you've forgotten to bring lunch.

No big deal, right? The sky isn't falling, right? You still have your health—right?

Not necessarily, according to Kathleen Kovner-Kline, M.D., a child psychiatrist at the Dartmouth-Hitchcock Medical Center in Lebanon, New Hampshire. "Your body reacts to stress along with your mind. The first symptom of stress is irritability, but that quickly moves on to weight gain or loss, sleeplessness, or some other form of sleep disturbance. You also might start biting your nails, grinding your teeth, or pulling on your hair. You can get aches and pains in your muscles, along with headaches and stomachaches."

If you could just get everyone to drive politely, your household equipment to work right, your kids to be perfect . . . Well, okay, it's just about impossible to remove the little frustrations that add up to stress. "If one big part of your life is causing you stress, such as a job you hate or a marriage that needs serious fixing, you need to deal with the basic problem, not the symptoms," Dr. Kovner-Kline says. "But in most cases, your stress is caused by cumulative frustrations, not one big one. The secret is to learn to react to stress so that it doesn't make you sick."

Here's how.

Have a Cup of Cheer

"Drink a glass of wine in the evening to help reduce your stressful feelings," Dr. Kovner-Kline suggests. "Alcohol has a mood-altering effect similar to that of major tranquilizers, which cost a lot more and require a doctor's prescription." Aside from alleviating stress, moderate alcohol consumption—a beer or a glass of wine a day—can bring a whole range of health benefits, including lowering the risk of heart disease, she says. "A professor in medical school liked to say, 'Skinny women who jog between bars will live forever.' He meant that women tend to live longer than men generally, but that both men and women live even longer if they exercise, maintain a healthy weight, and consume alcohol in moderation." Dr. Kovner-Kline cautions that you should avoid alcohol if you or anyone in your immediate family has an addiction problem.

Lap Stress Up

"Regular exercise causes your body to release endorphins, which are natural stress relievers," says Mary-Catherine Gennaro, D.O., a family osteopath in Warren, New Hampshire. "I think of *exorcising* when I exercise—getting rid of the little demons inside me," she says. "Sometimes, if I'm really in a bad mood, I'll yell underwater when I swim. When I come out, I may be a little hoarse, but I'm not stressed out anymore."

Or Yuck It Up

"Laughter is wonderful for relieving stress," Dr. Gennaro says. "When I was 11, I had to stay in the hospital with a broken leg. I remember lying there, laughing my head off

---

Choose Your Exercise Carefully

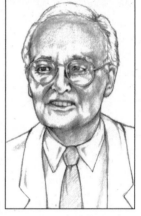

Early in our marriage, when I was still in medical school and my wife, Clara, was working to help support us, we were enjoying an evening at home. I was studying, and she was reading. At one point, I glanced over at Clara and was surprised to see tears streaming down her face.

"What's the matter?" I asked. She responded by throwing her book smack in my chest. I picked it up. It was the story of a woman who works to put her husband through medical school. The man becomes a successful doctor, joins a country club, and runs off with a younger woman he meets playing golf. "If you ever do that to me, I'll murder you," Clara said.

I never did join a country club.

Exercise can be a great stress reliever—for you. Make sure it doesn't increase the stress on your spouse.

Brewster Martin, M.D., *a retired family doctor in Chelsea, Vermont (population 1,166), and cofounder of the Chelsea Family Health Center. He was named Vermont Doctor of the Year in 1991.*

Kids React Differently

"STRESS in children is not always manifested the same ways it is in adults," says John C. Robinson, M.D., a pediatrician in private practice in Quincy, Massachusetts. Kids show a variety of signs when they're under stress. "They may become depressed or excessively demanding, act out, or behave aggressively toward their younger siblings."

Children tend to think they're responsible for everything that happens around them. "Presumed guilt is a major cause of stress," Dr. Robinson says. "They may tell a brother or sister in anger, 'I hate you. I wish you were dead.' If that sibling becomes ill, the child thinks she caused it." In a child's mind, just thinking about something can make it happen. "This is true of divorce," Dr. Robinson says. "Children hold themselves responsible for the failure of the marriage."

Teenagers aren't immune to this guilt either. "In adolescents, stress often results from an attempt to help a friend out of the dumps," Dr. Robinson explains. "If the child fails to rescue the friend, he may become stressed."

If your child shows serious signs of stress, take her to a qualified therapist, Dr. Robinson advises. "We are all under stress in one form or another," he says. "Kids have to learn to adapt to a certain amount of it."

---

watching the Smothers Brothers on TV. I wanted to write those guys a thank-you note for making me forget where I was for an hour." Want a quick stress reliever? Rent a funny video, she says.

Smell Vacation

"I have a friend who wears sunblock all winter, even if she doesn't plan to go outside," Dr. Kovner-Kline says. "Although it's good to screen the sun's rays, even in winter, my friend does it because the sunblock reminds her of summer. For a great stress reliever, smell something that has pleasant associations for you—your favorite flower, a special perfume, an ingredient that recalls a romantic dinner. The smell receptors in your brain are powerfully linked with emotions."

Dog Your Worries

"The most stressful time for me is when my husband is away on business for the night," Dr. Gennaro says. "I just can't sleep well without the company. Now I have a dog named Charlie, who makes me feel much safer and less stressed-out. Not that he's that great a watchdog—he'd probably open the door for a burglar and give him a beer. But at least he'd make a lot of noise doing it, and I find it much less stressful to go to sleep in a house with a dog in it." Feeling stressed yourself? "I'll write you a prescription for a dog!" Dr. Gennaro says. Besides providing some measure of security, "a pet provides something to snuggle with and feel connected to."

Try the Jewel of Denial

"It doesn't always help to face your stress head-on," Dr. Gennaro notes. "My husband, an orthopedic osteopath, served in Saudi Arabia during the Persian Gulf War. I saw no point in getting all stressed-out by being hooked up to CNN every minute of the day, so I called our cable TV company and had my service switched to the Disney Channel." Dr. Gennaro says that if a source of stress is beyond your control, "don't butt your head against it. Try to go around it."

Get Hounded

"The first part of your body that tends to show tension is the forehead," says Randal Schaetzke, D.C., a chiropractor at the Wholistic Health Center in Quechee, Vermont. To soothe your beaten brow when you're feeling stressed, "imitate a basset hound." Relax your forehead and drop your jaw. "Have you ever seen a tense basset hound?" Dr. Schaetzke asks.

Eat Calmly

Your moods march on your stomach, Dr. Schaetzke says. "Don't overeat, and don't skip meals either. Poor eating habits add to stress."

Soak Your Head

"The common doctor's recommendation for stress is 'Learn to relax,'" Dr. Schaetzke notes. "Just hearing that advice tends to make people nervous. 'I don't know how!' is what patients say to me." Dr. Schaetzke's prescription: a bathtub filled with hot water, along with Epsom salts or bathing herbs. "Dim the lights and put on some soothing instrumental music. Get in

The Thankful Rider

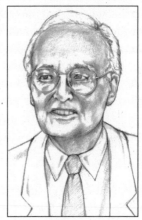

A NUMBER of years ago, I took care of a young man who had been shot in the ankle during a hunting accident. I had to call his parents in Boston and tell them not to come to my office but to a large hospital an hour away. The young man had suffered a lot of damage. He spent six months in the hospital and still wears all kinds of braces.

One Saturday morning several years later, I was out in front of the Congregational church in town watching the filming of the movie *Stranger in the Kingdom*. As I stood there, two elegantly dressed horseback riders came down the mountain into town to watch the filming. We got to talking, and then I introduced myself. "I knew I recognized that voice," the woman said. It was the mother of the young man who had been shot four years before. We'd talked only that once on the phone, but she hopped right off her horse and gave me a big hug.

On the whole, it wasn't so bad being a country doctor.

BREWSTER MARTIN, M.D., *a retired family doctor in Chelsea, Vermont (population 1,166), and cofounder of the Chelsea Family Health Center. He was named Vermont Doctor of the Year in 1991.*

the tub and breathe deeply and slowly. In 10 or 15 minutes, you'll sense that your heart rate has slowed. Note that sensation. Get enough practice with hot baths, and you'll learn to get the same feeling sitting in a chair."

STUTTERING

Eloquent solutions to short-circuited speech

If your three-year-old trips over some words now and then, it could be that his mouth hasn't yet caught up with his brain. "Stuttering comes at the beginning of a sentence or a word," says Barry Guitar, Ph.D., a speech language pathologist and chairman of the department of communication sciences at the University of Vermont in Burlington. "No one is sure why this is, but it could be that the child is so busy planning what to say that the thinking process gets overloaded. The stutterer repeats sounds, syllables, or words, prolongs sounds, or has a block—an inability to get a sound out."

About 1 out of 20 children go through a period of stuttering, Dr. Guitar says. "Most outgrow it," he notes. But some don't; about 1 percent of adults are stutterers.

Four out of five of them are males. Why's that? "The preponderance of adult male stutterers may have a problem with the way language is centered in the brain," Dr. Guitar says. "Typical males have language in their left brain hemisphere. Males who stutter appear to have language switched to the right hemisphere." In females, language is usually found in both hemispheres, "which may make women's brains more resilient to problems," he says.

No one expects a toddler, male or female, to speak perfectly right off the bat. How can you tell if your novice speaker is turning into a stutterer? "It's hard for parents to know if stuttering is beginning," Dr. Guitar says. One indication of a potential problem is that your child stutters with all kinds of sounds, not just the ones that usually trip up toddlers. "The s and r sounds come later in development, so three-year-olds often have trouble with them," Dr. Guitar says. "But in stutterers, any sound can cause trouble." Other warning signs of serious stuttering include the following, according to Dr. Guitar.

- The child tends to repeat the same word or sound three times or more.
- His face shows dismay when he tries to talk, or he seems to be physically struggling to get a word out.
- He tells you he can't say a particular word.
- He quits talking altogether.

In most cases, your kid will be talking a blue (and unimpeded) streak within a few months, even without any cures. Here's how to smooth the way.

Listen Up

"The most helpful thing you can do for a stuttering child is to be the best listener possible," Dr. Guitar says. "Parents should refrain from making specific suggestions. Do not ask

S

a stuttering child to slow down. That only increases the pressure on the child, which can make the problem worse."

Table the Interruptions

"One of the hardest times for a stutterer is the time around the family dinner table," Dr. Guitar says. "Make some rules: No interrupting, and everyone gets a turn. And provide some parental guidance for the discussion, such as 'Let's let Joey have some time to tell us about his day.'" To make sure everyone knows who has the dinner table podium, "place a particular item, such as a saltshaker, in front of the person whose turn it is to talk."

Be a Good Neighbor

"A powerful way to help a stuttering child is to slow your own rate of speech," Dr. Guitar advises. "The speech rate of Mr. Rogers, who welcomes children to *Mister Rogers' Neighborhood* on public television, is ideal." It's not easy to slow to a drawl all day, Dr. Guitar concedes. "If you think your child is beginning to stutter, set aside 5 to 10 minutes each day of relaxed one-on-one time with your child. Concentrate on speaking slowly. This will help calm a stuttering child."

Go to Bat

"You need to be an advocate for your stuttering child," Dr. Guitar says. "If your school has a speech pathologist, have that person evaluate your child and work with the teachers. Make sure the teachers don't tolerate teasing in class."

Teach the Teasers

Your kid will probably be teased at some point, notes Dr. Guitar. "It may help to work with the child, helping him to

---

TIME TO SEE THE DOCTOR

If the Stuttering Lasts a Season, See a Specialist

IF YOUR child's stuttering continues for more than three months, have her professionally examined, says Barry Guitar, Ph.D., a speech language pathologist and chairman of the department of communication sciences at the University of Vermont in Burlington.

"A stutterer should see a speech-language pathologist who is experienced in treating stuttering," Dr. Guitar says. "Not all speech pathologists are." To find a specialist near you, he suggests calling the Stuttering Foundation of America. (Get the number for the foundation by calling toll-free directory assistance at 800-555-1212.) The foundation also has low-cost videos and books for children, teenagers, parents, and adult stutterers.

---

come up with responses to teasing so he doesn't feel so passive about it," he says. If your stutterer feels up to it, he might even teach his class about stuttering. "I go with my patients to class. They teach their schoolmates how to stutter themselves. The child who stutters critiques their technique, which gives him the chance to feel like an expert."

Take Your Time

If you're an adult stutterer, try to smooth the flow of your speech by making yourself speak slowly and deliberately, Dr. Guitar says.

Practice, Practice

"Turn avoidances into approaches if you're still stuttering as an adult," Dr. Guitar suggests. "Make a list of situations that are hard for you, and try to practice them often."

STY
Eye these remedies
to put a lid on your problem

Quicker than you can bat an eye, an obstacle can get into an oil gland behind your eyelashes and cause a sty. "Usually, it's an oil gland on the lower lid that gets plugged," says Gerard Bozuwa, M.D., a retired family doctor in Wakefield, New Hampshire. A piece of dandruff, dirt, or oil from the gland itself can block the gland, creating a cyst. "When the cyst is on your eyelid, we call it a sty," Dr. Bozuwa explains. Some-

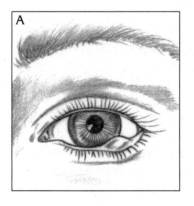

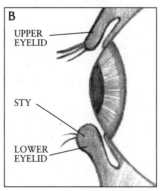

UPPER EYELID

STY

LOWER EYELID

That lump next to your eye (A) is usually caused by a plugged oil gland (B).

times a sty gets infected with bacteria and becomes red, swollen, and extremely painful. But it's not that harmful. "A sty is a lot like a pimple," Dr. Bozuwa says. Don't squeeze it, just as you wouldn't squeeze a pimple, he notes.

Rural Yankees used to recommend rubbing a sty with a gold ring—a remedy that country doctors don't endorse today. Instead, they suggest these cures.

Juggle Balls

"If you have a sty, put fairly warm water—about 100°F—in a small bowl," Dr. Bozuwa says. "Put a cotton ball in each hand. Dip one into the warm water. Hold it against the sty while dipping the other ball into the water. Keep alternating cotton balls for five minutes." He recommends doing this ball-juggling technique several times a day for three or four days. "Almost always, the sty will drain," he says.

Take It to Tea

"A warm tea bag applied to the eye is a good idea for a sty," says Henry Kriegstein, M.D., an ophthalmologist in private practice in Hingham, Plymouth, and Sandwich, Massachusetts. "A tea bag has its own little reservoir of hot water, which helps it stay warm longer. A warm compress increases the blood flow to the sty and helps open it up."

Here's Egg in Your Face

"A warm hard-boiled egg wrapped in a washcloth will stay warm for five minutes," Dr. Kriegstein says. "That's just how long you need to keep something warm against your eye."

Hands Off!

Keep your dirty fingers away from your eyelids, and you're less likely to get a sty, advises Brewster Martin, M.D., a retired family doctor in Chelsea, Vermont.

Save Face

"Change your entire eye makeup kit every few months if you want to help avoid sties," says Eugene J. Bernal, O.D., an optometrist in private practice in White River Junction, Vermont. "Brushes and tubes can become contaminated with bacteria, causing the sort of infections that make for sties."

SUNBURN
How to deal with the dark side of a bright day

Back in the prebikini era, when modesty forced people to cover up and a pale complexion was a sign of beauty, sunburns were less common than they are today. Now, near nudity on the beach and a gaping hole in the ozone layer redden unprecedented acres of skin nationwide.

And that means more than just the immediate pain and embarrassment of the burn. By exposing ourselves to the sun, we've managed to double the incidence of skin cancer in the United States in the past decade alone. More than 1 million new tumors now show up on Americans' skin annually, making skin the most common site of cancer in this country. People who burn easily are at the greatest risk.

The answer, doctors say, is to make your skin less burnable by covering up with clothing or sunblock. These precautions are especially important for children, according to Jorge Crespo, M.D., a dermatologist who left New England to work with the Clark & Daughtrey Medical Group in Lakeland, Florida.

But even the best-laid plans to stay protected go astray once in a while. What do you do if you get scorched?

Go Bayer

"Any inflammation to the skin, including sunburn, can be blocked by taking aspirin every three to four hours," Dr. Crespo says. Take aspirin immediately if you know you've overdone it on the beach, he advises. By reducing the inflammation, Dr. Crespo says, aspirin "can minimize the ultimate damage." Avoid giving aspirin to children; it can cause a serious illness called Reye's syndrome. Substitute nonsteroidal anti-inflammatory medicine such as pediatric ibuprofen.

Bring Some Lotion to the Ocean

"Prevention is key," says Gerard Bozuwa, M.D., who is retired after 36 years as a family doctor in Wakefield, New Hampshire. "But once you've let the sunburn horse out of

S

the barn, corticosteroid ointments are the most soothing."
A popular corticosteroid ointment, Cortaid, is available at
drugstores. Dr. Bozuwa recommends using it or another corticosteroid ointment for only a few weeks at a time. "Prolonged use can cause atrophy of the skin," he says.

Reduce the Wrath with a Cold Bath

"A cold bath is particularly soothing for sunburned children,
whose skin tends to be especially sensitive," Dr. Bozuwa says.

Or Try This Version of Immersion

"A cold shower followed by a cream moisturizer will help
alleviate the hot feeling," says Charles Hammer, M.D., a dermatologist with the North Country Outreach Program of the
Lahey Hitchcock Clinic in St. Johnsbury, Vermont. Avoid
moisturizers containing fragrances, though, as "they could
be irritating to the skin."

Remember, the Sun Likes Water

"Watch your back when you're spending time in the water,"
Dr. Bozuwa warns. "Sunburn is common in people who
snorkel. They tend to be unaware that their backs are exposed. Wear a shirt when snorkeling." You might wear a shirt
that's been around the block a couple of times. Researchers in
Australia discovered that a pure cotton T-shirt gives twice the
protection after it has been washed daily for ten weeks.

Screen Out the Problem

"There is no such thing as a healthy tan," says Susan Silverman, coordinator of the Skin Cancer Prevention Program
for the Massachusetts Division of the American Cancer Society in Framingham. To avoid getting that not-so-healthy
color in the first place, Silverman says the American Cancer
Society recommends always using a sunscreen with a sun protection factor of 15 or higher if you plan to be outside.

Apply Again

Silverman notes that one application of sunscreen is not
enough. Reapply the lotion after swimming or excessive
sweating, she advises, even if the label says the product is wa-
terproof. And give yourself another dose every two to four
hours in any case.

Block That Sun

"WANT to see what the sun does to skin?" asks Jorge Crespo, M.D., a dermatologist who left New England to work with the Clark & Daughtrey Medical Group in Lakeland, Florida. "Take a good look at your grandfather's face. Then ask him to pull down his pants." Assuming that you have an amazingly cooperative grandfather, Dr. Crespo says that you'll probably discover young-looking, wrinkle-free skin where the sun don't shine. "And yet your grandfather's bottom is just as old as his face," he points out. "The best way to prevent wrinkles is to prevent exposure to the sun." And how do you do that? Three ways, according to Dr. Crespo.

1. Sunblock, of course, but not just any sunblock. "Read the label to make sure your lotion blocks both UVB and UVA rays," Dr. Crespo says. One of the least expensive of the effective sunblocks is No-Ad, available at drugstores. It's called that because the company doesn't advertise.

2. Cover your neck as well as your head. "The Australians wear hats in the style of the French legionnaires," he says. "The hats cover the neck and ears. When my patients say they're afraid they'll look silly, I tell them they'll look like real nerds with a piece of an ear or nose missing from skin cancer."

3. Ease into the sun. "The worst thing you can do for your skin is get a binge sunburn," Dr. Crespo says. "That's when you launch yourself into a winter vacation down South without tanning gradually." Instead, he says, you should work your way into a tan for the first few days of vacation by using maximum sunscreen, avoiding the peak sun hours of 10:00 A.M. to 2:00 P.M., and wearing a hat. "You'll still end up getting a tan, which will protect your skin," he adds.

"The Australians are light-years ahead of us in dealing with the sun," Dr. Crespo notes. "They have education programs in the schools aimed at the youngest children. The motto they teach is 'Slip, slap, slop': Slip on a shirt, slap on a hat, and slop on the sunscreen."

Don't Stow the Sunscreen Come Fall

Even in midwinter, the sun can seek you out, scorching exposed parts of your skin from the sky and from rays reflected off the snow. "Dope up heavily when you're outdoors in the snow," advises Nick Yardley, former director of the International Mountain Climbing School in North Conway, New Hampshire. "If you're in snow, put sunblock under your chin. And don't open your mouth too much. You can burn the roof of your mouth."

Dr. Hammer agrees. "You can get sunburned any time of year," he says.

In warm but snowy areas, avoid the temptation to strip down to a T-shirt, Yardley warns. "Consider wearing a white, long-sleeved, cotton dress shirt," he says. "It reflects the ultraviolet light and covers you to the max."

SWIMMER'S EAR

Immerse yourself in these pain-stopping remedies

"Swimmer's ear is an infection of the outer ear canal—the part of your ear that extends from the eardrum to the visible part of the ear," says Robert Fagelson, M.D., an otolaryngologist in Brattleboro, Vermont. Contrary to popular belief, you don't have to swim in dirty water to get a case of swimmer's ear. "Swimmer's ear has nothing to do with where you swim or what kind of water you are in," Dr. Fagelson says. "You can get it without swimming at all."

Dr. Fagelson explains that excess water in the ear—caused by swimming, taking a bath, even getting doused in a rainstorm—can penetrate the layer of wax that usually waterproofs the skin of the ear canal. "If the water remains, it can soften the skin in the canal," he says. "The bacteria that are naturally in your ear can get a foothold in the skin, leading to infection. It isn't necessarily a bad infection, but it can be very, very painful." Dr. Fagelson notes that frequent bouts of swimmer's ear can damage your ear's wax-producing

---

AN OUNCE OF PREVENTION

Don't Let the Water Get to You

YOU can prevent swimmer's ear by putting a few drops of rubbing alcohol in each ear after you come out of the water," says Robert Fagelson, M.D., an otolaryngologist in Brattleboro, Vermont. The alcohol eliminates the water and therefore helps fight infections.

If you get ear infections frequently, "wear form-fitting earplugs when you go swimming," Dr. Fagelson says. "The best kind of plugs are made of silicone. You can get them at drugstores."

glands. With less wax in your ears, the skin in the outer canal is even more susceptible to infections.

If you find yourself getting swimmer's ear repeatedly, here are remedies to dive into.

Get Some Vinegar Down There

"You can treat swimmer's ear at home by using a mixture of equal parts vinegar and water," Dr. Fagelson says. "Put a few drops in the infected ear several times a day for several days. If it isn't better within three days, or if the pain gets worse, see a doctor. The ear canal can actually swell shut, keeping antibiotic eardrops out."

Give Your Ear Some Warmth

"Heat will help relieve the pain of swimmer's ear," Dr. Fagelson says. "Just put a heating pad, set on Low, or a hot-water bottle against the sore ear."

SWOLLEN GLANDS
Choose not to take your lumps? Here's how to reduce them

What we call glands, doctors call lymph glands and lymph nodes. Almost 600 glands are located throughout the body.

AN OUNCE OF PREVENTION
When Bugs Do the Bump

TODDLERS are especially susceptible to swollen glands behind the ears or on the back of the neck during "bug season." This is when biting insects are at their hungriest and most numerous, according to Elizabeth Lowry, M.D., who is retired after 38 years as a pediatrician in Guilford, Connecticut. "The bites themselves tend to heal fairly quickly, but the glands go down gradually," Dr. Lowry says. She recommends protecting a young child from bites with a long-sleeved T-shirt that has a hood on it. "Those little caps with neck flaps on them also are effective against insects," she says. "Either kind of clothing will protect the especially tender, and tasty, back of a child's neck."

Those Glands Need Your Doctor's Glance

IN MOST cases, swollen glands are a reason for a visit to the doctor. Be especially sure to get checked out if any of the following situations also exist.

- You have glands that stay swollen for more than two weeks after an infection is over.
- You have swollen spots throughout your body.
- You can't explain why your glands are swollen. The swelling hasn't been triggered by a cold or an infection.
- Your gland feels hard.
- You also have trouble breathing or swallowing.
- You have a fever.
- One of your neck glands is more swollen than the others.

The lymph glands are staging grounds for the immune system. It's in the lymph glands that white blood cells gather to fight off invading bacteria. The lymph glands also serve as waste disposal sites, storing the debris of that war on infection and then passing it along to the bloodstream, allowing efficient disposal—usually. But during an infection, glands and nodes can get overloaded, swelling up as white cells gather and as waste products get dumped into the nodes.

"Swollen lymph nodes in the neck tend to be caused by a throat infection or a viral sore throat," says Robert Fagelson, M.D., an otolaryngologist in private practice in Brattleboro, Vermont. "Usually, you can feel a swollen gland there. There will be a sensation of fullness in the neck, and the neck will feel tender." You also can get swollen glands in your neck from a dental infection, from a viral disease such as the measles, or even from an insect bite. It's a good idea to have your doctor check out swollen neck glands, Dr. Fagelson says. "It could be strep throat, and there can be dire complications if you leave strep untreated."

On your way to the doctor, here's how to make yourself more comfortable.

Drink Some Heat

"If you have swollen glands that started as the sore throat of a cold or the flu, stay in bed for two or three days and drink plenty of hot liquids," says Lawrence H. Bernstein, M.D., medical director at Jewish Geriatric Services in Longmeadow, Massachusetts. Rest will help your system recover more quickly, he says, and fluids will help flush out those lymph nodes.

Or Raise the External Temperature

A warm washcloth or heating pad applied to a painfully swollen gland for 15 minutes at a time, several times a day, can bring some relief, Dr. Bernstein says.

Watch Out for That Stone Building

"Sometimes a duct in your salivary, or spit, gland can be blocked by a salivary stone," says Richard Lee, M.D., an oto-laryngologist in private practice in Laconia, New Hampshire. "A stone is a mineral buildup in the gland. When you eat, saliva builds up inside the gland but can't get out, causing painful swelling in the gland behind your jaw." As a temporary measure, Dr. Lee says you can massage the swollen gland to work out some of the saliva. But eventually you'll have to see a doctor to take out the stone or the gland, he says.

T

TEETH GRINDING
*Follow these tips
and stop wearing yourself down*

If you clench your teeth during the day or grind them at night, you have a habit that dentists call bruxism. Stress is a common cause. So is a problem with your jaw joint; the uncomfortable fit of your upper and lower teeth has you instinctively gnashing around for a better bite.

"Bruxism can be damaging because it tends to chip the tooth enamel," says Gregory L. Baker, D.D.S., an orthodontist in private practice in Woodstock, Vermont, and West Lebanon and New London, New Hampshire. "When you clench or grind your teeth, even one tiny movement can put as much as 1,200 pounds of pressure on the enamel. Grinding also can wear down the jaw joint." And that's not all. Bruxism and its accompanying jaw problems can cause headaches as well as pain in your face and jaw.

Here's how you can eschew the habit and get some relief from the daily grind.

Rest Your Neck

Dr. Baker recommends buying a contoured pillow at a medical supply store. This wedge-shaped pillow "helps hold

---

TIME TO SEE THE DOCTOR
*Could Something
Be Bugging You?*

SOME cases of teeth grinding aren't caused by stress but by something else inside you: a parasite, according to Bradford Weeks, M.D., a family doctor who moved from New Hampshire to Clinton, Washington. "If home remedies don't cure your bruxism within a couple of months, ask your doctor to check you for parasites," he says.

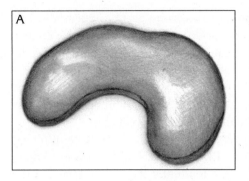

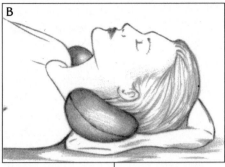

the cervical collar—the bones between your shoulders and chest—in the correct position," which can prevent teeth grinding, he says.

A contoured pillow (A) holds your cervical collar in place (B), making you less likely to grind your teeth.

Guard Your Mouth

Wearing a mouth guard at night may not stop the grinding, but it will protect your teeth, says Robert Keene, D.M.D., a dentist in Hanover, New Hampshire. "If you wear a mouth guard, you're grinding plastic, not your teeth's enamel," Dr. Keene says. He recommends asking your dentist for the guard that's best for you.

Stop Grinding Your Coffee

"Avoid stimulants such as caffeine and chocolate," says Bradford Weeks, M.D., a family doctor who moved from New Hampshire to Clinton, Washington. "Stimulants only make a teeth-grinding habit worse."

Float Your Stress Away

"Dehydration is a form of stress that can cause teeth grinding," Dr. Weeks says. "Make sure you're getting plenty of liquids."

TENDINITIS
How to calm your angry attachments

Your tendons are tough customers. These cords that attach your muscles to your bones can take a lot of abuse—but eventually they may let you know about it, in the form of pain every time you move a certain part of your body. And that can include just about any part that you move a lot. Tennis elbow, which can flare up not only after time on the court but also from other repeated motions such as hammering, is a form of tendinitis. Writers can get serious tendinitis in their wrists, and so can knitters and quilters. Joggers can get tendinitis behind the heel or in the hip.

"Just about any repeated motion can cause tendinitis," says Gerard Bozuwa, M.D., a retired family doctor in Wakefield, New Hampshire. "Tendinitis occurs in the part of the tendon where it runs through the tendon sheath. When the tendon is injured or irritated, it swells and won't fit properly in its sheath. If you try to force your motion, you can cause more pain and swelling."

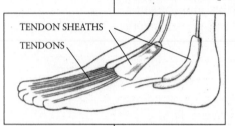

TENDON SHEATHS

TENDONS

If tendons don't fit properly in their sheaths, you can feel the pain.

Hmmm. Pain and swelling: Sounds like a pulled muscle, doesn't it? Not really, Dr. Bozuwa says. "It's easy to tell the difference between a pulled muscle and tendinitis. A pulled muscle is in spasm, meaning it will hurt constantly, and the pain is felt deep in the muscle. Tendinitis will not hurt at all if you immobilize the tendon that's affected—for example, if you put an inflamed wrist in a splint."

Because it hurts to move an inflamed tendon, most people are inclined to give it what Dr. Bozuwa calls "the ideal treatment": rest. But that's not all you can do for a tender tendon. Read on.

Give It a Break

"A week is the minimum amount of time to rest an inflamed tendon," says Lawrence H. Bernstein, M.D., medical director at Jewish Geriatric Services in Longmeadow, Massachusetts. "Two weeks is better. Lay off the activity that caused the problem in the first place—whether it was typing, jogging, running up stairs, or whatever."

Ice the -Itis

"Apply ice to tendinitis when you can feel heat in the skin over the tendon," says Randal Schaetzke, D.C., a chiropractor at the Wholistic Health Center in Quechee, Vermont.

"Apply a cloth-covered bag of ice to the tendon for 20 minutes every hour until the inflammation has subsided. Then make sure you've cooled down the tendon by applying ice for 20 minutes every couple of hours for the rest of the day."

Add Heat

"Sometimes contrast therapy works for tendinitis," says Dr. Schaetzke. "Apply ice for 20 minutes, take a break for 20 minutes, then apply heat—in the form of a hot-water bottle, heating pad, or hot, moist towel—for 20 minutes. Rest for another 20 minutes, then repeat the whole routine. The ice slows the pain messages to your brain while reducing swelling, and the heat increases blood flow, which speeds up nutrient exchange and the removal of waste from the injured

---

A WORD FROM DR. LARRY

Physician, Heel Thyself

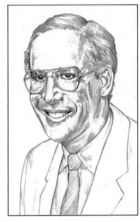

IF YOU have Achilles tendinitis—an inflammation of the tendon that runs up the back of your leg above your heel—you need to ease off your activities for a while. Don't ignore your Achilles tendon. If it's inflamed, it's more likely to rupture, and that hurts like crazy. I should know: My own Achilles tendon snapped recently.

Like everyone else with a ruptured Achilles tendon, I had a choice. It will usually heal on its own eventually, but the resulting scar tissue won't stretch, and it can restrict your activity. That's fine if you don't mind switching from, say, tennis or basketball (activities that need a good, flexible Achilles tendon) to sports such as swimming and biking, where your feet and heels don't bear your weight.

Well, I like tennis too much. I had a surgeon repair my tendon. It's doing just fine.

LAWRENCE H. BERNSTEIN, M.D., *a family doctor who made house calls in Storrs, Connecticut, for 22 years. He now works at Jewish Geriatric Services in Longmeadow, Massachusetts.*

---

cells. Taken together, both techniques promote healing." In general, if the area feels warm to the touch, "ice is the priority," he says. If the area is painful but not warm or reddish, "heat is the priority."

Send It a Massage

"Gentle massage often helps tendinitis, because it helps increase circulation, aiding the body's natural capacity to make inflammation go away on its own," Dr. Bozuwa says. "If you can reach the tendon yourself, do your own massage. That way, you know just how much pressure to apply before it hurts too much."

Iodine Out

"A very good treatment for tendinitis is Iodex, an iodine ointment that you can buy over the counter at drugstores," Dr. Bozuwa says. "Just rub it on your sore tendon. It's very soothing."

THUMB SUCKING

*Is the little nipper acquiring
a taste for himself? Read on*

Kids have been growing attached to their thumbs for ages, and parents have worried about the habit for just as long. "In the old days, doctors used to fit thumb suckers' mouths with special forks that fit on the palate with the tongs facing forward," says Everett Orbeton, M.D., a retired pediatrician who practiced in Portland, Maine. "A kid would stab his thumb if he tried to stick it in his mouth. It was a kind of torture machine."

Actually, some dentists still use the device, according to Gregory L. Baker, D.D.S., an orthodontist in private practice in Woodstock, Vermont, and West Lebanon and New London, New Hampshire. But he is vehemently opposed to it. "It's right out of the Middle Ages," he says.

Dentists now say there's no need for such dramatic measures—or cures of any kind—while children are still little. Thumb sucking is a natural instinct. Fetuses can be seen to do it in the womb, and almost half of all kids continue to do it once they're out in the cruel world. And, hey, there are worse uses for a little kid's thumb—hitchhiking, for example.

On the other, um, hand, the sucking habit can cause trouble when your child reaches the age of six or seven and begins to grow adult incisors. A thumb can steer these adult teeth in the wrong direction. "Thumb sucking in an older child can lead to an incorrect bite," says Gregory Colpitts, D.M.D., a dentist in private practice in Franklin, New Hampshire. "The habit also can lead to a tendency toward mouth breathing, which can cause plaque to accumulate on the teeth and decay them."

If your child needs a nudge away from the habit, try these remedies.

Switch Digits

"If your child is sucking so vigorously that the thumb makes a popping sound when you pull it out, that means the thumb is pushing on the roof of the mouth," says Patricia Edwards, M.D., a pediatrician in private practice in Concord, New

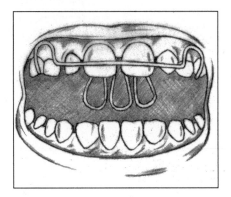

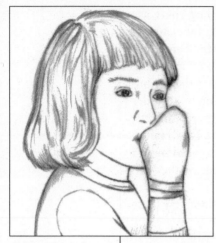

Held with masking tape, a sock is a suck stopper.

A deer tick in nymph stage (A) can look no bigger than a grain of pepper. The adult female deer tick (B) will triple in size when engorged (C). Before feeding, an adult female dog tick (D) is roughly twice the size of a deer tick.

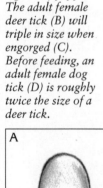

Hampshire. "That isn't good. Encourage your child to suck on a finger instead."

Stick a Sock on It

"I once had a thirteen-and-a-half-year-old girl whose teeth had been badly deformed from years of sucking," Dr. Colpitts says. "She really wanted to stop. I put her hand in a sock and wrapped it with masking tape. She finally broke the habit."

Decorate

"Thumb suckers will sometimes stop sucking if you paint their nails with nail polish," Dr. Edwards says. "They won't want to ruin the pretty look. You also can buy little nail stickers at discount stores, which can have the same effect. Some kids will stop sucking in order to keep the stickers on."

TICKS
Removing critters that dig in for a meal

It's no fun finding a tick crawling on you. But if it's crawling, you have nothing to worry about—just get rid of it. "A lot of people get freaked out when they find a tick on themselves, but it takes hours for a tick to dig in and transmit diseases," says Peter Mason, M.D., a family doctor in Lebanon, New Hampshire. Still, once a tick settles in, it can spread any of a variety of nasty ailments, including Rocky Mountain spotted

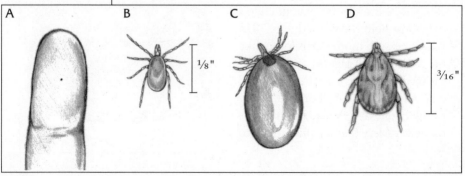

A   B   C   D

1/8"   3/16"

Wear Tick-Unfriendly Fashions

To keep ticks off, wear light-colored cotton pants when you go out in the woods or walk through grassy spots in tick-infested areas," says Peter Mason, M.D., a family doctor in Lebanon, New Hampshire. "Ticks are more attracted to dark-colored creatures." He adds that long socks, pants, and shirt sleeves are a good idea for keeping ticks off your skin when you head out into the wild.

If you really want to protect yourself, try a repellent called Permanone, which is found in garden and hardware stores. "You spray it on your clothing, not on your skin, to keep ticks off," says Peter Brassard, M.D., a family doctor on tick-infested Block Island, Rhode Island. "It's the best tick repellent there is."

fever, Colorado tick fever, tularemia, and, most common of all serious tick-borne illnesses, Lyme disease.

It's primarily the tiny deer tick, barely bigger than the point of a pin, that spreads Lyme disease. But you don't want the deer tick's bigger cousin on you either. The dog tick, about three-sixteenths inch long, is a more widely spread species that finds humans tasty. It can cause a skin infection and some nastier problems.

If you develop flulike symptoms within a few days of having a tick embedded in you, get yourself to the doctor. You could have Lyme disease, which needs medical attention as soon as possible.

To prevent disease in the first place, you need to get the tick off. Here's how to get rid of the stubborn ones that are embedded.

Unscrew It

"Take a pair of tweezers and gently unscrew the tick in a counterclockwise direction," says John Dunn, M.D., an emergency room physician at the Northwestern Medical Center in St. Albans, Vermont. You can also try simply tugging the tick with the tweezers, he says. "I don't think you need to be too concerned about leaving the tick's head embedded in you," Dr. Dunn adds. "The head will eventually work its way out, like a splinter. There's a possibility of a slight infection, but that can be cured with hot compresses."

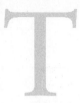

Meet Its Match

"Light a kitchen match—the big wooden kind—blow it out, and immediately touch the match to the tick's body," says Harry Rowe, M.D., a family doctor in Wells River, Vermont. "The tick will usually let go."

Use the Hard Stuff

"A dab of rubbing alcohol, applied to the back of the tick, can make it back out of your skin," says Sarah Johansen, M.D., medical director of emergency services at New London Hospital in New London, New Hampshire. The alcohol suffocates the tick, Dr. Johansen explains.

TOENAIL FUNGUS

Treating an irritant that creeps up on you

You notice a little yellowish or greenish tinge in the corner of your toenail, along with some sawdustlike powder under the nail. After some weeks, that color spreads, heading inward. Chances are, you've got a fungus growing there—a condition doctors call onychomycosis. "You get toenail fungus the same way you get athlete's foot," says Nicholas Vachon, D.P.M., a podiatrist in private practice in Ellsworth, Maine. "If you like to go barefoot in public places such as swimming pools and locker rooms, you are more likely to get infected. Any injury to your toenail can provide a way for fungal spores to get in." And how do the spores get there in the first place? "You usually pick them up with your bare feet—then they hang around inside your sneakers, waiting for the opportunity to get into your nails."

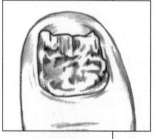

A regular garden of fungus: the toenail.

If some sneaky fungus has already gained entry, it can be extremely hard to shake, he says. But if you have to live with an alien invader, at least this one is fairly benign. Toenail fungus rarely hurts, and it often can be hidden with nail polish.

Stay Dry

"Manage toenail fungus the same way you would athlete's foot," says Brewster Martin, M.D., a retired family doctor in Chelsea, Vermont. "Keep your feet dry, and change your shoes and socks daily."

Switch Shoes

Don't wear the same pair of shoes all day long, Dr. Martin suggests. Moisture can build up, providing the ideal environment for a nasty toenail fungus. Bringing an extra pair of shoes to work is a good way to keep those toes dry, he says.

Get a Drop on the Fungus

"When the area affected by the fungus is still small, buy some over-the-counter Clotrimazole liquid at your drugstore," says Charles Hammer, M.D., a dermatologist with the North Country Outreach Program of the Lahey Hitchcock Clinic in St. Johnsbury, Vermont. "Place a drop at the edge of the nail and let it get drawn in. Don't use a toothpick to push the medicine in, though—you'll only make more room for the fungus."

Give Your Toes the Old One-Two

If you injure your toenail, you need to apply both an antifungal and an antibiotic ointment," Dr. Vachon says. "The combination of these over-the-counter remedies will prevent most kinds of infection, including toenail fungus."

TIME TO SEE THE DOCTOR

Does the Fungus Have More Than a Toehold?

You can stop a toenail fungus with home remedies as long as it's not yet fully entrenched," says Charles Hammer, M.D., a dermatologist with the North Country Outreach Program of the Lahey Hitchcock Clinic in St. Johnsbury, Vermont. "But if the fungus has invaded more than an eighth of an inch into your nail, see your doctor." You may be given a prescription that kills the fungus.

TONGUE AND CHEEK BITES
Making up for poorly aimed teeth

Chomp! Nothing spoils a good meal more than when your teeth mistake your tongue or the inside of your cheek for food. Besides the excruciating pain, a nasty bite can cut through the soft tissue, giving entry to the slew of bacteria that inhabit your mouth. Fortunately, "the inside of your

T mouth—the gums and the tongue—tend to heal rapidly," says Gregory Colpitts, D.M.D., a dentist in Franklin, New Hampshire. "The cells there have a rapid turnover rate, getting replaced in a day or less."

Still, if you find yourself biting your tongue or cheek frequently, "see a dentist," Dr. Colpitts says. "Those bites probably mean your teeth aren't meeting properly."

For those mercifully rare misaimed bites, try these healers.

Do the Ocean Potion

"The best thing for a tongue or cheek bite is a warm saltwater rinse," Dr. Colpitts says. Stir 1 teaspoon salt into 1 cup warm water. Take a mouthful and swish it until your wound starts to feel better—"a minute is as long as most people can stand to do it," Dr. Colpitts says. Then spit it out.

Use Ice in a Trice

"Wrap an ice cube in a clean cloth and apply it to the sore," says Elizabeth Lowry, M.D., who is retired after 38 years as a pediatrician in Guilford, Connecticut. "An uncovered ice cube might be too cold and sloppy. A covered cube is just enough to slow the bleeding."

Drink Something Cold

"Drinking some ice water slows the bleeding," says Gregory L. Baker, D.D.S., an orthodontist in private practice in Woodstock, Vermont, and West Lebanon and New London, New Hampshire.

Lick the Pain

"A bitten tongue can be a scary thing for a parent and child," says Ann Bracken, M.D., a pediatrician at the Dartmouth-Hitchcock Medical Center in Lebanon, New Hampshire. "The tongue has a profuse blood supply, so it bleeds a lot. But the best thing to do is to give the child a hug and a frozen ice pop. The combination of cold and comfort constitutes a great cure."

TONGUE FROZEN ON COLD METAL

Cures for an unspeakable predicament

Do people really get their tongues frozen on pump handles? Well, pumps are pretty scarce these days, but kids on a dare seem perfectly willing to find a substitute. "My friends and I would lick the metal tips of our skis when we were kids," admits Betsy Storrs, a farmer, schoolteacher, and lifelong resident of Etna, New Hampshire. "Sure, our tongues would stick to the metal—our parents had warned us that that would happen—but we'd do it anyway." And what was the cure? "We'd just pull the skis off, along with a layer of our tongues. It hurt like heck, but our tongues didn't bleed."

Injury from touching cold metal is not just a childhood hazard. "My rule is, don't touch bare metal—it will touch you back," says Murray Hamlet, D.V.M., chief of the Research Support Division at the U.S. Army Research Institute of Environmental Medicine in Natick, Massachusetts, and an expert on coping with cold-weather conditions. "A combination of cold and moisture causes the problem. When you take your hand out of a glove or a mitten, your skin is moist. Then when you touch cold metal, the moisture freezes, bonding your skin to the metal."

The answer? "Keep your gloves on when you touch metal in the winter," Dr. Hamlet says. "That's one reason I recommend that you wear polypropylene glove liners under your mittens. The liners keep your fingers free while offering some protection."

And what do you do if your tongue—or any other part of your body—is stuck to metal?

Pour Some Warmth

"When I was growing up in North Dakota," Dr. Hamlet says, "we'd tempt kids to taste our sled runners. We told them the runners were salty, which wasn't really true. Some kids would get their tongues stuck that way. *Really* stupid kids would lick fire hydrants." To get unstuck, "the best

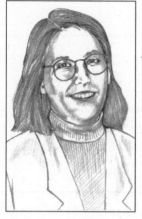
treatment is to pour anything warm where the skin is stuck—warm water, coffee, whatever comes to hand."

"Warm water will melt the body part off the metal," agrees Dudley Weider, M.D., an otolaryngologist in Lebanon, New Hampshire. "Usually, the injury isn't too bad. It just hurts a lot." He notes that the liquid should be at room temperature to avoid sudden thawing that can damage flesh.

TOOTH STAINS
Restoring the gleam to your grin

If your teeth are taking on the color of an old undershirt, you have a stain problem. "Anything that can stain your clothes can stain your teeth," says Peter Lodge, D.M.D., a dentist in Narragansett, Rhode Island. The biggest culprits are nicotine and caffeine—tobacco, coffee, tea, and cola. Frequent swimming in chlorinated pools can create brown tooth stains.

But even the most tooth-friendly lifestyle may not lead to a dazzling smile. "Age alone can darken teeth," says Gregory Colpitts, D.M.D., a Franklin, New Hampshire, dentist. "As we age, the enamel gradually gets thinner. This makes sense when you consider that we get our grown-up front teeth at age six or seven. As the years go by, the thinning enamel lets the darker layer, called dentin, show through."

Then there are the kinds of stains dentists call "intrinsic"—coloration that comes from within the tooth itself. Some drugs, such as antibiotics or gum inflammation medicines, can stain teeth from within. Teeth can be stained even before you're born. Drugs such as some antibiotics taken by a woman when she's pregnant can permanently stain the teeth of the child developing in the womb.

Too much fluoride—from taking fluoride tablets, say, while drinking water that contains fluoride—can discolor your teeth or pit the enamel. "This pitting looks like white stripes," Dr. Colpitts says. "If I see a little bit of this in a child, it doesn't bother me a bit. It means that someone is making sure the kid's teeth are protected." Dr. Colpitts suggests that if you drink well water and are considering giving fluoride tablets to your children, you might hold off on the tablets until you have the water tested for fluoride. "Ninety percent of wells have little or no fluoride in the water," he says. "But the town of Epsom, New Hampshire, near where I live, has high levels of fluoride in its wells." In most cases, if your drinking water is fluoridated, your kids don't need fluoride pills. (If your drinking water is from a town supply, ask your town office for information on fluoridation.)

TIME TO SEE THE DOCTOR
Are Your Pearlies Still Not White?

IF YOU want dramatic results and have the cash, ask your dentist about professional bleaching, says Gregory Colpitts, D.M.D., a Franklin, New Hampshire, dentist. It's an expensive process, but this approach might actually be cheaper than some over-the-counter bleaches by the time your teeth are whitened to your satisfaction, Dr. Colpitts says. "Professional whitening is faster and safer, and the bleaching is monitored by experts," he explains.

T

If your teeth are already stained, take heart: Not all stains are hopeless. Your dentist can remove many of them, and you can do some things for yourself at home.

Get Clean

"The plaque on your teeth is what collects the stains that form on the outside," says Gregory L. Baker, D.D.S., an orthodontist in private practice in Woodstock, Vermont, and West Lebanon and New London, New Hampshire. Plaque is the bacteria-filled gunk that collects on improperly brushed teeth. "Keep it off, and your teeth will stain less," Dr. Baker says.

Buy a Machine

Studies by dental researchers show that electric toothbrushes work significantly better than ordinary brushes in removing stains. The most effective electric toothbrushes are of the oscillating/rotating variety—the kind that rapidly imitates the motion of a zealous human toothbrusher. Among the best is the Braun Oral-B Plaque Remover, available at department stores.

Swish and Swallow

"After you've had staining substances such as coffee, tea, or nicotine, try the swish-and-swallow method," Dr. Baker advises. "Swish a mouthful of water around your mouth, then spit it out or swallow it."

Soda Up

"Baking soda is good for stains on teeth," says Corinne Martin, a certified clinical herbalist in Bridgton, Maine. "Use it as a toothpaste occasionally, and it will brighten things up. Or you can achieve much the same effect by fraying the end of a witch hazel stem and chewing it." Avoid using baking soda if you're on a low-salt diet, though.

Hit the Bleach

Hydrogen peroxide, available over the counter at drugstores, can help whiten teeth. "It's a weak bleaching agent that won't hurt your teeth," Dr. Colpitts says. "Just be sure you don't swallow it. Swish a little in your mouth and then spit it out."

ULCERS

*Take these cures when your gut
tells you it hurts*

Not so long ago, doctors believed that ulcers—open sores in
the lining of the stomach or intestines—were caused by stress
and bad habits. And doctors still believe that, in some cases,
nerves, overeating, alcohol, spicy food, smoking, and too
much coffee or aspirin can destroy the tissue in your innards.
But research now shows that most ulcers are triggered by a
bacterial infection. The guilty bug is *Helicobacter pylori,*
a bacterium that appears to weaken mucous tissue and ren-
der it less able to fend off assaults from digestive acids and
other tissue eaters. Doctors aren't sure how the bacterium is
spread, though they've noticed that it tends to appear among
family members, suggesting that it can be spread within a
household.

The first sign that you have an ulcer may be a pain in your
stomach—it can be a deep, burning feeling or a dull ache—
especially in the morning or between meals. "You might feel
nauseous or lose your appetite for days on end," says Laurie
Duncan, M.D., an internist who moved from Cooperstown,
New York, to Washington, D.C. "Or you may not have any
symptoms at all. Some ulcers show up only during regular
physical exams or are discovered because the patient is mysteriously losing weight."

Once found, any ulcer should be checked out by a doctor.
"The most common kind, the one caused by bacterial infec-

tion, can be cleared up with prescription antibiotics," Dr. Duncan says. But ulcers of all kinds can be relieved at home. Here are some ways to soothe those deep-down sores.

Stuff the Puffs

"If you have ulcers, don't smoke," says Peter Mason, M.D., a family doctor in Lebanon, New Hampshire. "Nicotine irritates the lining of the stomach." Medical data show that smokers are twice as likely as nonsmokers to have ulcers.

Stop the Aspirin

"Not all ulcers are associated with bacterial infection," Dr. Duncan notes. "A number are caused by excessive use of aspirin or ibuprofen and other nonsteroidal anti-inflammatory drugs, or NSAIDs. Your doctor will need to prescribe acid-blocking medication to heal an NSAID-caused ulcer. In the meantime, you need to stop taking the NSAID." Some other painkillers, such as acetaminophen, are much less harsh on your stomach, she notes.

Cut the Cocktails

"Alcohol can harm the mucus that protects the lining of your digestive tract," Dr. Duncan says. "If you have ulcers, you need to eliminate all drinking."

Let Your Hair Down

Although the frustrations of daily life don't cause most ulcers, "stress is a major factor in their severity," Dr. Duncan says. "An important element in long-term management of ulcers is to deal with matters in your life that are causing stress. Consider getting psychological counseling if stress is making your ulcers worse."

Skip the Milk Cure

"The old ulcer diet, which doctors prescribed up through the 1960s, called for lots of milk," Dr. Mason says. "But we now know that calcium produces what doctors call rebound hy-

TIME TO SEE THE DOCTOR

Signs of Blood Should Send You In

THE first sign of an ulcer may not be pain but blood in your vomit or stools," says Laurie Duncan, M.D., an internist who moved from Cooperstown, New York, to Washington, D.C. "If you are throwing up what looks like coffee grounds, call your doctor immediately. Also get help if your stool is unusually dark and tarry."

The Secret to Harmonious Living: A Barn

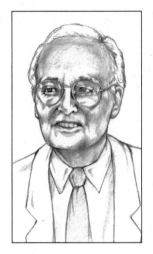

Two patients of mine, Arthur and Edna, went to a party thrown for their 75th anniversary. That night, Arthur called. "Come over," he said. "Edna's sick."

The couple lived a very simple life, including eating simply. I examined Edna and told her that she had become ill from eating too much rich food. I gave her something to soothe her stomach.

As I was leaving, I asked Arthur the secret to being married for 75 years. He thought for a moment and said, "Well, sometimes the best thing is to put on your frock and go out to the barn." Arthur definitely knew one secret to a good marriage: When you're angry, take it outside.

BREWSTER MARTIN, M.D., *a retired family doctor in Chelsea, Vermont (population 1,166), and cofounder of the Chelsea Family Health Center. He was named Vermont Doctor of the Year in 1991.*

peracidity. Your stomach counteracts the milk by actually producing more acid. You feel better for the first 10 to 15 minutes after drinking a glass of milk, but ultimately you feel worse." Milk is okay in moderate amounts, but Dr. Mason says not to overdo it.

Safely Graze

"Eat small meals frequently," Dr. Mason advises. "When you keep a bit of food in your stomach, you produce smaller amounts of acid to deal with it, which helps keep your ulcers from being irritated."

Plant Your Digestion

"A digestive plant enzyme—such as maltase, lactase, sucrase, papain, bromelain, or pepsin—can help ease your digestion, relieving your ulcers," says Lawrence Bronstein, D.C., a chiropractor and certified nutrition specialist in Great Bar-

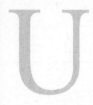

rington, Massachusetts. All are sold over the counter under a variety of brand names.

Sip This Remedy

"To soothe an ulcer, try marshmallow root tea, available at health food stores," says Corinne Martin, a certified clinical herbalist in Bridgton, Maine.

Or Try Chamomile

"Chamomile tea is soothing to the nervous system, and it reduces inflammation in mucous tissue," Martin says. "That makes it wonderful for treating ulcers."

URINARY TRACT INFECTIONS
*Getting your disposal system
back in gear*

If you feel a burning sensation when you urinate, find yourself making frequent trips to the bathroom, and happen to be a woman, chances are you have a urinary tract infection (UTI), caused by out-of-control bacteria inflaming your plumbing. Women are 25 times more likely than men to suffer from a UTI. By age 25, one-quarter of all women have felt the all-too-familiar burn. And once you've had a UTI, you're much more likely to get an unwelcome repeat performance.

Why do UTIs pick on women? "The reason is that the urethra—the tube that carries urine from the bladder and out

A woman's short urethra offers bacteria easy entry to the bladder.

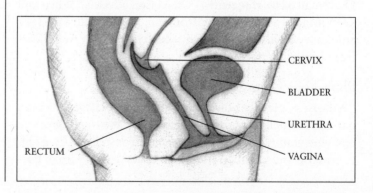

CERVIX

BLADDER

URETHRA

RECTUM

VAGINA

of the body—is extremely short in a woman," says Stephen Rous, M.D., chief of urology at the Veterans Administration Medical Center in White River Junction, Vermont, and author of *Urology: A Core Textbook.* "Stray bacteria from the outside don't have far to go to the bladder, where bacteria can cause infections. A man's urethra is long enough to keep bacteria out of the bladder." While most women are free of UTIs all their lives, "bacteria stick to some women more readily than to others," Dr. Rous says. Sex can sometimes push bacteria into the vagina, where it can spread to the urethra, he adds.

Not all men get off scot-free. "Men who do get infections may have chronic bacterial prostatitis—an uncommon disease of the prostate," Dr. Rous says. "And some older men who have trouble completely emptying their bladders may

---

AN OUNCE OF PREVENTION

Fight Infections Habitually

You can lessen your chances of getting a urinary tract infection by adopting these helpful habits, according to Stephen Rous, M.D., chief of urology at the Veterans Administration Medical Center in White River Junction, Vermont.

- It would be ideal if you could shower after every bowel movement, says Dr. Rous. Since that's impractical, however, "a woman may also want to use Betadine sponges to wash her perineum—the area between the anus and the vagina—after moving her bowels. This will help prevent bacteria from traveling up through the urethra to the bladder," Dr. Rous explains. You can buy these antibacterial sponges at most drugstores.

- "Empty the bladder every couple of hours during the day if you know you are going to have intercourse during the evening," Dr. Rous says. "If the bladder isn't emptied often enough, urine can press against the side of the bladder, depriving it of its normal supply of blood. This sets up the lining for an infection if there is intercourse."

- Urinate both before and after intercourse to wash away any harmful bacteria.

- Take two grams of vitamin C per day or drink two quarts of cranberry juice to acidify the urine, making it an unfriendly place for bacteria. Cut back on your vitamin C intake if you develop diarrhea.

URINARY TRACT INFECTIONS

Go In if the Burn Concerns

IF YOUR urinary tract infection gets worse over the course of a week, see your doctor, says Stephen Rous, M.D., chief of urology at the Veterans Administration Medical Center in White River Junction, Vermont.

set the stage for infections." By age 65, men are as likely as women of the same age to suffer from UTIs.

The burning may feel awful while it lasts, but our country contacts offer ways to catch it early and avoid a visit to the doctor.

Guzzle the "C"

"Any drink with vitamin C in it will help when you have a urinary tract infection," says Hope Ricciotti, M.D., a Boston obstetrician-gynecologist and coauthor of *The Pregnancy Cookbook*. "If you start drinking early and often, you can usually avoid having to ask your doctor to prescribe an antibiotic."

And Just Plain Guzzle

"You should drink two quarts of fluid a day, especially if you feel a urinary tract infection coming on," says Brewster Martin, M.D., a retired family doctor in Chelsea, Vermont. "Your urine should be dilute."

Bog Yourself Down

"Cranberry juice has proven to be very effective in acidifying the urine and relieving cystitis," says Paul Lena, M.D., a retired physician of internal medicine in Concord, New Hampshire. "The acid prevents bacteria from multiplying. Drink a lot—as much as two quarts a day—to really flush the kidneys when you feel the burning coming on."

V

VAGINAL PROBLEMS
*Private remedies for the most
personal of discomforts*

If you were a bacterium or a yeast culture, your idea of heaven would be a dark, warm, moist environment where you could spread out and live in comfort—like, say, a vagina. With the sort of amenities available there, you have to wonder why you don't suffer even more from the itching, burning, and discharge that signal a bacterial or yeast infection.

In fact, yeast is a normal inhabitant of your vagina. And so are bacteria. Most of the time, the pH balance—the amount of acidity—inside keeps the yeast under control. But illness, a skewed diet, medication, hormonal changes during the menstrual cycle, or sexual intercourse can knock things out of whack, causing an explosion in the yeast population or a proliferation of harmful bacteria. The result: vaginal problems.

A reaction to chemical irritants, such as the perfume in your douche, can make your vagina itch. So can an allergic reaction to the same perfume,

---

AN OUNCE OF PREVENTION

Don't Give Yeast a Chance

WANT to keep your vagina healthy? Follow these steps.
- Avoid eating sugary sweets, which can encourage the growth of yeast in your vagina.
- Don't wear deodorant tampons.
- Change immediately out of your wet bathing suit or sweaty leotard.
- Wear cotton underpants, which "breathe" better than nylon.
- Don't use douches. They can cause vaginal problems.

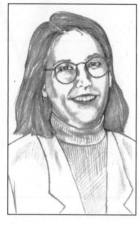
when your immune system raises an objection to substances in the formula.

An irritated vagina can become dry or swollen, making intercourse painful—a condition that doctors call dyspareunia. As many as 60 percent of all women suffer from this pain at some point in their lives.

Fortunately, there are plenty of home remedies to deal with these problems. Here are some of the best.

Cream the Yeast

"If your vagina is producing a cottage-cheese-like discharge, you probably have a yeast infection," says Eric A. Sailer, M.D., an obstetrician-gynecologist at the Dartmouth-Hitchcock Medical Center in Lebanon, New Hampshire. "Yeast infections often go away on their own, but you can speed things up with over-the-counter remedies such as Monistat and Gyne-Lotrimin. These medications have saved women a lot of office visits and a whole lot of money." If they don't work after two weeks, see your physician. "You might have trichomonas, an organism that can be stopped only with prescription antibiotics," Dr. Sailer says.

Fight Yeast with Yeast

"Eat yogurt daily if you're getting a yeast infection," Dr. Sailer says. "Read the label to make sure the yogurt has live yeast cultures, especially acidophilus," he says, explaining that an infusion of this "good" yeast can help balance a vagina that's out of whack.

Wear Protection

"Couples can pass a yeast infection back and forth," notes Brewster Martin, M.D., a retired family doctor in Chelsea, Vermont. "When a woman is being treated for a yeast infection, her partner ought to wear a condom during intercourse." Although a man usually won't feel the effects of yeast, he can reinfect his mate later, Dr. Martin explains.

Go Light on the Tissue

"Some women tend to wipe a bit too hard, lodging tiny pieces of toilet paper in the vagina, which causes irritation," says Robert F. Wilson, M.D., a pediatrician who is retired from his practice in Dover, New Hampshire. "Be gentle when you go to the bathroom."

Sacrifice Your Breath

"Eating garlic as part of your diet can help restore the natural balance in your vagina and fight the overgrowth of bacteria," says Hope Ricciotti, M.D., an obstetrician-gynecologist at the Beth Israel Deaconess Medical Center in Boston. You can also apply garlic directly to your problems, she says. Peel a clove of garlic, wrap it in a small piece of cotton gauze, and insert it into your vagina overnight. Remove it in the morning.

ANNALS OF MEDICINE

"You May Feel a Little Burning..."

DURING the 1800s, doctors blamed most "female problems"—from headaches to emotional distress to cancer—on their sexual organs. The uterus and vagina were thought to be the center of a woman's health, both physical and mental.

A common doctor's cure for a vaginal infection in those days was zapping it with a hot iron or caustic chemicals. This "local" treatment, as doctors called it, often caused permanent damage—but it may well have cured women of complaining about vaginal infections.

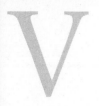

VARICOSE VEINS
The best ways to deal with spidery legs

Those intricate designs your veins have started making are harmless, but they're not altogether flattering. And you sure don't remember having them when you were 16.

That's because your skin doesn't hold up your veins as well as it used to. As your skin becomes less elastic, the veins close to the surface get less help from the leg muscles in pumping the blood back up to the heart. The backlog screws up the valves that keep the blood from going in reverse, and blood starts to pool up—causing the veins to swell and become more prominent. The result: varicose veins.

Women are four times as likely as men to have the problem. Heredity seems to be a factor. If your mother had varicose veins, you're more likely to have them yourself. During pregnancy, the baby can put pressure on the veins that hang down into your legs, causing them to swell with blood and stay dilated. Other forms of pressure in your abdomen—such as the strain of lifting heavy objects or of trying to have a bowel movement—can fill up veins and make them stand out. Standing for long periods—while, say, staffing the cosmetics counter in a department store—also can give you varicose veins.

"It used to be common practice to operate on the big ones," says Laurence Bouchard, D.O., an osteopathic family physician in private practice in Narragansett, Rhode Island. "But fewer doctors operate these days unless the veins are especially swollen or painful. Varicose veins usually look worse than they are. Beware of charlatans who want to inject veins with chemicals to shrink them. The practice is rarely effective and could cause harmful side effects."

Instead, try these home remedies.

Hose Your Veins Up

"Support hose is a good way to help your skin support your veins," says Robert G. Page, M.D., a retired cardiologist in Londonderry, Vermont. "You can buy all kinds from your drugstore, a medical supply store, or a catalog. But your best bet is to ask your doctor to measure the amount of pressure you need. You can have him prescribe graduated-pressure hose, which puts the most pressure down low at the ankles, where it's needed the most."

Sit!

"Try taking a load off your legs," says Thomas Roy, M.D., a former New England cardiologist who moved to Minocqua, Wisconsin. "Don't stand up for more than half an hour at a time, and take breaks in which you elevate your legs."

Support Yourself

"Activities that improve your muscle tone and general health can help improve varicose veins," says Sarah Johansen, M.D., medical director of emergency services at New London Hospital in New London, New Hampshire. "Exercise, such as moderate walking or running, can be especially helpful by toning your legs and helping them to support the veins."

Don't Strain Those Veins

Don't increase the pressure on those already-stressed veins. "Avoid chronic straining with a bowel movement, which increases intra-abdominal pressure and aggravates varicose veins," Dr. Johansen advises. If constipation is a problem for you, increase the fluids and fiber in your diet. Cruciferous vegetables such as brussels sprouts, broccoli, and cabbage are high in fiber. So are salad mixings, bran muffins, and apples.

Give It a Rest—And a Lift

Sometimes all other treatments may be in vain. "If the vein becomes palpable (you can feel the raised, cordy vein under the skin), painful, and inflamed, you may be developing thrombophlebitis," Dr. Johansen says. "That's best treated with bed rest, local heat, elevation, and aspirin."

VOMITING

Toss your cookies?
Catch these remedies

Throwing up is no fun, but it's a pretty efficient way to get rid of your stomach contents, says Hugh P. Hermann, M.D., a family doctor in Woodstock, Vermont, and the health of-

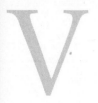

ficer for Pomfret, Vermont. "The body will induce vomiting to get rid of an unwanted substance such as a poison. Your stomach muscles contract, and the valve at the bottom of the stomach closes up, so that the contractions force the contents upward."

Sometimes the part of your brain that controls vomiting hits the Eject button on your stomach, even when throwing up doesn't do it any good. "A fever or a bad reaction to a drug can signal the vomiting center in the brain," Dr. Hermann says. "Other causes include viruses and infections, appendicitis, gallstones, a blockage in the intestines, and motion sickness." Even a bad fright, such as a near-miss on the highway, can make you lose your lunch, he says.

An eighteenth-century cure was to hold a hot toasted nutmeg to the belly—a cure that doctors don't recommend today. Here are some old and new treatments to try instead.

Replace What's Lost

"The main thing to concentrate on when you're vomiting is to stay hydrated," says David Sigelman, M.D., a pediatrician with Holyoke Pediatric Associates in Holyoke, Massachusetts. "Look in your drugstore or grocery store for a pre-mixed formula that replaces what your body has lost through vomiting. One formula is Kao Lectrolyte, put out by the makers of Kaopectate. Kao Lectrolyte comes in small packages like Kool-Aid, and you just mix it with water. Because it comes in a powder, you don't have to pay for the water and the high cost of shipping it. It's really the best thing out there."

Make Your Own

The World Health Organization recommends a formula that you can mix at home to replace the fluids lost through vomiting or diarrhea. "The whole secret is the ratio of ingredients," says Dr. Sigelman. "Too little glucose won't replace what's lost, and too much can cause diarrhea." Start with 1 liter water (use an empty soda bottle to measure the amount) and stir in 1 teaspoon salt and 8 teaspoons sugar.

Keep downing the mixture, and you'll help to keep your fluid level on target.

Stay Abreast of Nature's Cure

If you're a breastfeeding mother, you're already carrying the best treatment for your vomiting baby, according to Dr. Sigelman. "Breast milk is an ideal source of fluids," he says. "And the great thing is, the baby can't drink it too fast. Too much fluid taken at one time can cause a tendency to vomit again."

Remember the Boiled Milk Cure? Forget It

"AN OLD cure for vomiting is boiled skim milk," says David Sigelman, M.D., a pediatrician with Holyoke Pediatric Associates in Holyoke, Massachusetts. "I'd steer clear of that remedy. You boil away nearly all the water, and what you end up with is a whole lot of sodium—salt. You can actually cause sodium intoxication with this 'cure.'"

Open Your Trap

"When children are vomiting, I have them breathe through their mouths between bouts," says Susie Tann, R.N., an elementary school nurse in Bradford, Vermont. "Mouth breathing helps calm them down, and it gives them something to think about other than their vomiting."

Just Leave

"In the South, people make a tea from peach tree leaves to relieve nausea and vomiting," says Corinne Martin, a certified clinical herbalist in Bridgton, Maine. "Up here in New England, we use ginger. You can take fresh ginger, buy ginger capsules at your health food store, take ginger tea, or just drink ginger ale, the kind made with real ginger. It works on the brain to convince the body that you are not nauseous."

Ease Back In

"Once you feel ready for solid foods after you've been vomiting, go easy," says Laurie Duncan, M.D., an internist who moved from Cooperstown, New York, to Washington, D.C. "Try something mild like toast, rice, mashed potatoes, a banana, squash, or chicken broth."

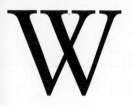

WARTS
The bumpy road to smooth skin

Don't jump to any conclusions about frogs and toads. The real cause of warts in people is the human papillomavirus. Coming in more than 60 varieties, the papillomavirus is spread on the surface of the skin—either from person to person or from contact with an object that an infected person has touched. You can have the virus without any warts. Scientists are unsure why the virus touches off some skin, while other people seem unaffected by it. For some reason, kids get warts more often than adults do.

Different viruses cause different kinds of warts. The common wart, which often appears on the hands and elbows, has a rough surface. The flat wart is smooth. It can show up in clusters wherever people shave, such as a woman's legs or a man's face. Then there is the plantar wart, which hangs out on the feet and can get painful as it rubs against a shoe.

The common wart (A) often appears on hands, the flat wart (B) on the face or legs. The plantar wart (C) is trouble afoot.

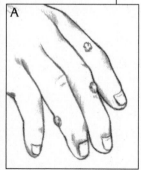

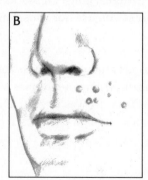

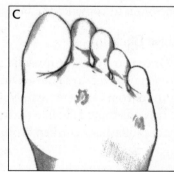

Why Many Princes Are Wart-Free

THE old folklore that toads cause warts comes from the fact that toads themselves have warty skin," says Scott Jackson, a herpetologist and conservation specialist at the University of Massachusetts Extension service in Amherst. "It was thought that if you handled them, you'd get warts, too."

Jackson says that although handling toads won't give you warts, you still might want to take care before petting one of these creatures.

"Those warty bumps on the back of a toad are part of its defense system," Jackson says. "If you handle a toad roughly, the warts can exude a toxic substance that has the consistency of white glue. If you rub your nose or eyes after handling a toad, it can cause a burning sensation in your mucous membranes."

What should you do if a toad slimes you? "Just wash your hands," Jackson says. "That should prevent the burning."

Time is the best cure, doctors say. Most warts go away on their own within two years. "Eventually, your body's immune system will get rid of warts," says Charles Hammer, M.D., a dermatologist with the North Country Outreach Program of the Lahey Hitchcock Clinic in St. Johnsbury, Vermont. If a year or two seems too long to live with warts, try these remedies.

Smear on Some Aspirin and Don't Call in the Morning

"Dermatologists are often asked about wart therapy because nothing works well for everybody," Dr. Hammer says. "Patience is key. Nothing works overnight." Dr. Hammer recommends over-the-counter wart remedies such as Wart-Off and Compound W, which contain varying concentrations of salicylic acid—the main ingredient in aspirin. The higher the concentration, the better, he says—unless the wart is near the eyes or mouth or anywhere on the face of a child. "And you should be very careful, because these products can cause blisters or ulcerations," Dr. Hammer adds.

Apply the salicylic acid remedy every night until the wart goes away. Then keep applying it for a week afterward for good measure, Dr. Hammer advises.

Give a Wart a Bath

"Soak the wart in warm water for 10 minutes," says Kathryn A. Zug, M.D., a dermatologist at the Dartmouth-Hitchcock Medical Center in Lebanon, New Hampshire. "The soaking will moisten the wart and make it easier for the over-the-counter preparation to reach the virus. Repeat soaking the wart and applying the salicylic acid remedy every day for six to eight weeks. Remember, getting rid of a wart is a marathon."

Watch the Nerve

Warts are extremely sensitive to the body's immune system—and the immune system is closely tied to a person's feelings, notes Gerard Bozuwa, M.D., a retired family physician in Wakefield, New Hampshire. "Teenagers under stress often get warts on their hands," Dr. Bozuwa says. "The warts disappear when the stress goes away. So if you have a child with warts, look for signs of stress in her life, and deal with the cause of the stress."

WINDBURN

When cold makes your skin feel fiery

You'd think that winter would be the one time you and your skin would be safe going outdoors. Clothing blocks the weak winter sun, and your bathing suit lines are fading. But suddenly your face turns red and slightly swollen.

Don't blame the sun. You have windburn.

Doctors say that, despite appearances, windburn is not a real burn but an irritation of the skin. "Windburn is the reddened, irritated eruption of the skin of the face," says Mark Quitadamo, M.D., a dermatologist at the Lahey Hitchcock Clinic in Bedford, New Hampshire. "You can get windburn in the summer, but people are more prone to it when they're exposed to dry winter winds. You get windburn when your skin is deprived of moisture." Here's how you can keep the moisture in your mug.

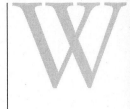

Try Ruffing It

"I wear a parka hood with a fur ruff," says Dudley Weider, M.D., an otolaryngologist at the Dartmouth-Hitchcock Medical Center in Lebanon, New Hampshire. Weider is a founding member of the Geriatric Adventure Society, a group of older outdoorsmen who venture north of the Arctic Circle every year. "Below that I put on ski goggles, and below the goggles I put on a ski mask. I look a lot like Darth Vader, and it may look more appropriate for the Arctic than for the city, but all that gear is excellent for stopping the wind."

"You need a good fur ruff around your face," agrees George Wenzel, Ph.D., associate professor of geography at McGill University in Montreal. "The fur traps in your own warm air and keeps the cold air out. Also, if you have a good ruff, you can prevent frostbite on your cheeks and nose."

Avoid High Winds

"It's not the wind itself that's the problem," Dr. Wenzel says. "The wind amplifies the cold." An expert on Arctic native peoples, Dr. Wenzel notes that even the Eskimo, also called Inuit, stay indoors when the wind is free. "The Inuit don't go out at all in the winter if the wind is more than 15 kilometers, or 10 miles, per hour, because the resulting windchill makes it much harder to keep warm."

Put a Coat on Your Face

"Pretreat your skin with a bland lotion that contains sunscreen with a sun protection factor of 15," says Robert Averill, M.D., a dermatologist in western Massachusetts and northern New Hampshire. When you come back indoors from the cold, "apply plain emollient lotion." Dr. Averill recommends Eucerin Facial Moisturizing Lotion or Neutragena

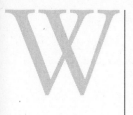

Moisture facial moisturizer, both of which are available at most drugstores.

As an alternative to expensive lotions, "give yourself a good coating of petroleum jelly," says Jorge Crespo, M.D., a former New England dermatologist who works with the Clark & Daughtrey Medical Group in Lakeland, Florida. "It works just as well as the fancy stuff."

Get a Gaiter When the Wind Bites

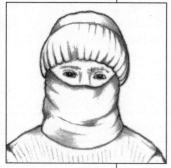

A doughnut-shaped neck gaiter and a hat will keep most of your skin protected from those burning winter winds.

One of the best wind blocks is a neck gaiter—a doughnut-shaped scarf made of polyester pile material—according to Michael Pelchat, an emergency medicine instructor who has taught emergency first-aid to the weather researchers atop New Hampshire's windblown Mount Washington. "Also wear a hat, and pull it down so that just your eyes are exposed," Pelchat says.

WINTER DEPRESSION
Ways to lighten up the darkest time of the year

If people were bears, the wintertime blues would be no problem. When your energy level dropped during the cold, dark months, you could just snuggle up in a warm den and sleep until springtime. We humans have unbearlike obligations—jobs and friends, for instance—and the urge to hibernate comes across as a sign of depression. Lots of people feel a bit draggy during the winter months, especially if they live in northern climes. One out of five Americans gets the blues big-time in the winter. If you're one, you feel unaccountably sad starting in the fall. You might also find food and sleep irresistible, while losing interest in sex.

Psychiatrists call the problem seasonal affective disorder, which has the perfectly appropriate acronym SAD. Women are three times as likely as men to suffer from winter depression. SAD tends to set in when people are in their twenties, but kids can get it, too. Winter blues tend to run in families.

People with this disorder respond to light less efficiently than other people. "There are genetically determined differences in sensitivity to seasonal reduction in light," explains Charles Ravaris, M.D., Ph.D., emeritus professor of psychiatry at Dartmouth Medical School in Hanover, New Hampshire. "Some folks start to feel awful in late August and continue feeling bad until March. Others will be fine until the first of December and only suffer until the first of February. The more your light sensitivity is reduced, the earlier SAD will occur, and the more severe the symptoms are likely to be."

The good news for everyone comes in the spring, when the lengthening days cheer people up. No one is entirely sure what light has to do with it, except that sunshine seems to affect the hormones melatonin and serotonin, which help regulate the sleep cycle. "People with SAD have their daily sleep-wake rhythms messed up," Dr. Ravaris says. "They feel as if they're jet-lagged all the time." If you feel this way in

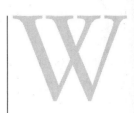

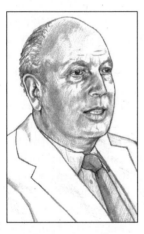

A House for My Calling

You know the old expression "Doctor, heal thyself"? My neighbors are healers for me. Being part of my town is important to my mental health.

Apparently, some of my predecessors have felt the same way. In front of my 1780 farmhouse in Wakefield, New Hampshire, is a big stone with a plaque that says "The Doctor's House." The plaque names the three doctors who have lived in the house since 1849—including me. "This historic marker was dedicated in heartfelt appreciation for Dr. Gerard Bozuwa's 36 years of service to the community," the plaque says.

I bought the house in 1958. Now, as far as I'm concerned, it's priceless. And so, of course, are my neighbors.

GERARD BOZUWA, M.D., *retired after 36 years as the sole family doctor for the town of Wakefield, New Hampshire.*

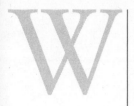

the winter, here's how you can gain altitude in your seasonal moods.

Get out of Your Cave

"Going outdoors is very important if you have SAD," Dr. Ravaris says. "No matter how overcast the day is, outdoor light energy is stronger than most indoor lighting. Midday is best because it's the time of maximal light."

Install Extra Light in Your Tunnel

"You need to get your entire indoor environment set up so that no matter where you turn, you get a full blast of light energy," Dr. Ravaris says. He recommends installing fluorescent lighting with a rating of 2,500 lux (a unit of light energy) wherever possible. "One of my patient's neighbors told her that in the winter, her house looks like a meteor streaking across a dark sky," Dr. Ravaris says.

Put Your Blues in a Box

Dr. Ravaris recommends buying a light box from a medical supply store. Taking up the space of a medium-size television set, a light box has a bank of fluorescent lights that imitate the sun. "Buy phototherapy lights with a full spectrum of color, from ultraviolet to ultrared," Dr. Ravaris says. "That means your lights should have the critical wavelength of 400 to 660 nanometers." Most light boxes are more powerful than ordinary fluorescent lighting, offering a blast of 10,000 lux. Expose yourself to the light by sitting a couple of feet away from it twice a day, morning and evening, for 30 to 45 minutes at a time. Many patients use the time to catch up on their reading. Within a week of starting this treatment, most people with SAD start to feel better.

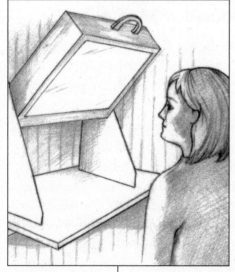

A light box brings the cheering effects of the sun indoors.

Wake Up, You Sleepyhead

"You must try to force yourself to get out of bed in the morning and get to a fluorescent light," Dr. Ravaris says. Studies on light treatments show that they're most effective in the morning, he says. "Be sure to set your alarm."

Don't Wait for Summer

"I recommend what is called situation manipulation," says Gerard Bozuwa, M.D., who is retired after 36 years as a family doctor in Wakefield, New Hampshire. "Get a break from your winter routine. Take a vacation if you can. Depending on the person's pocketbook, I have been known to write on the prescription pad: 'One week in Bermuda.'"

Stay Away from the Tube

"Don't sit and watch TV if you suffer from winter depression," Dr. Bozuwa says. "Most people do that in a dark room," which doesn't help their depression any. "Read a book in a well-lighted room—your mother was right about that," he says. Long-term use of computers also can be a problem for people with winter depression. "The light from the computer screen isn't very bright," Dr. Bozuwa says. "Take frequent work breaks and go outside."

Get Your Misery Some Company

Dr. Bozuwa also recommends "joining something." A sense of belonging to a group is often effective in treating depression, he says. "Here in Wakefield, we have a group called Active Older Adults who walk together. It gives them exercise and that sense of belonging."

WINTER ITCH
Get repose when the cold wind blows

In northern climes, cold, dry air can zap your outermost layer of skin, disrupting the natural oils that hold in moisture. So what do you do? You go inside, where the air can be even drier—desertlike 15 percent relative humidity in an unhumidified, heated room. "Water!" you cry, and you treat yourself to a hot, soapy shower. And so you manage to scrub away the skin's last remaining defenses against the dry blasts of winter: dead skin cells.

"The body has a highly evolved, preprogrammed cell death pattern," says Jorge Crespo, M.D., a dermatologist who left New England to work with the Clark & Daughtrey

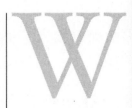

Take My Advice

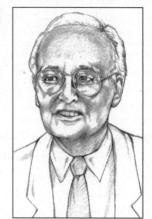

BEFORE I retired, I spent as much time on preventive medicine as I did treating illnesses. Sometimes the time you give patients is more important than the pills.

People in Chelsea must hear my voice whenever they think of their health, because I always told them the same things.

- Exercise at least three times a week.
- Drink lots of water, at least eight 12-ounce glasses a day.
- Don't smoke.
- Don't be a pig at the dinner table, and avoid fried and fatty foods.

Those patients who paid attention to my advice are benefiting from longer, more active lives than those who didn't. I'm convinced of that. After all, I followed my own advice, and I'm well into my seventies.

BREWSTER MARTIN, M.D., *a retired family doctor in Chelsea, Vermont (population 1,166), and cofounder of the Chelsea Family Health Center. He was named Vermont Doctor of the Year in 1991.*

Medical Group in Lakeland, Florida. "The dead cells on top of your skin help seal moisture in the living cells." Get rid of the dead cells in the bath, and your watery interlude can cause water in the live cells to evaporate 50 times more rapidly than normal. Result: the dry, itchy skin that physicians call simple xerosis.

"Winter itch becomes increasingly prevalent with aging. It's a big problem with the elderly," Dr. Crespo says. "In addition, genetics plays a role in dry skin. People with a Celtic heritage—Irish, Scots, English, and the like—have far more of a problem than those with, say, Mediterranean roots."

If you're one of those whose itchiness rises as the temperature falls, get some relief from these country cures.

Hold the Baths

"Most seniors remember when the Saturday night bath was an institution," says Robert Averill, M.D., a dermatologist in western Massachusetts and northern New Hampshire. "Some folks seem to have thought that even once a week was too much. The old joke was that some folks took a bath each spring whether they needed it or not. Now it's not uncommon for people to bathe daily, or even twice a day. Even though we use milder soaps and abstain from scrub brushes, winter itch is still with us. That's because our frequent baths strip skin of lipids—natural oils—causing loss of water from the skin."

Dr. Averill's advice? "Bathe in warm—not hot—water, and limit your bath or shower to five minutes," he says. "Pat yourself dry with a towel immediately after you finish bathing. Waiting too long to dry off will allow the water that has filled your cells to evaporate. As soon as you've patted yourself dry, apply moisturizer to lock in the water your skin soaked up during the bath or shower."

Mush Away the Itch

"If you have itchy winter skin, try taking an oatmeal bath," says Donald Dickson, R.Ph., owner of Dickson's Pharmacy in Colebrook, New Hampshire. He recommends using Aveeno, a special colloidal oatmeal made to coat the skin. You can buy it over the counter at drugstores.

Have a Moisturizer Handy

"Keep a bottle of lotion near the sink so you can use it after washing your hands," Dr. Averill advises.

Avoid Drying Liquids

Be especially careful to avoid drying agents such as astringents and alcohol in clarifying lotions, aftershaves, and splash-on fragrances, Dr. Averill notes.

Use the Lower-Priced Spread

"As a dermatologist, I say the heavier the moisturizer the better," Dr. Crespo says. "Crisco is great, and it's very cheap. I tell my patients to shower at night and put on the Crisco— the regular kind, not butter-flavored. If you're embarrassed about putting shortening on your body, put it in a fancy jar so no one will know what you're using." Dr. Crespo adds that in the daytime, you might want to use a lighter, less sticky remedy such as Lubriderm or Eucerin.

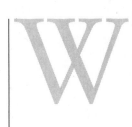

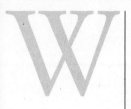

Prepare the Air

"While you're thinking about moisturizing your skin," Dr. Averill says, "don't forget to add moisture to your environment." Use a room humidifier, he says. "More water is lost from your skin through evaporation in dry air than in moist air."

Wear Soft Clothes

"Wear cotton against the skin," recommends Lawrence H. Bernstein, M.D., a former family doctor who is the medical director at Jewish Geriatric Services in Longmeadow, Massachusetts. "Avoid wool. It will just make the itching worse."

Take Allergy Medicine

"If itching is intolerable at bedtime, you can take Benadryl," Dr. Bernstein says. "Available over the counter, Benadryl reduces itching while making you sleepy. You usually don't feel like scratching when you're asleep."

Moisten Your Innards

"To prevent winter itch, you need to keep the skin wet from the inside out," says Nancy Bronstein, D.C., a chiropractor and homeopath in Great Barrington, Massachusetts. "Flaxseed oil, taken as a capsule or in a smaller pearl, is the least expensive essential fatty acid. It works well." You can buy flaxseed oil at health food stores.

Look Into Estrogen

"Winter itch is an especially big problem with elderly women," Dr. Crespo says. "A woman's skin can be abnormally dry in the postmenopausal years. If you're trying to decide whether or not to use hormone replacement therapy, put your skin in the pro column. Your skin needs estrogen."

WORMS
What to do when your skin isn't the only thing crawling

Worms are a serious problem in poorer countries, where they can make children terribly ill. In this country, worms are much rarer, but kids do occasionally show up at the doctor's

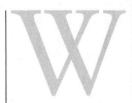

office with pinworms—tiny creatures that look like pieces of white sewing thread half an inch to an inch long and that first make themselves known through stomachaches and anal itching.

"Worms enter the body in egg form, through the mouth," says Brewster Martin, M.D., a retired family doctor in Chelsea, Vermont. "An infected child scratches his itchy anus, getting eggs on his hands. He passes the eggs by touching another child or a playing surface, and that second child then puts his hands—and the worm eggs—into his mouth. It's a common cycle. A simpler version of it, seen mostly in Third World countries, is the simple fecal-oral route: A child touches worm-infested feces or dirt and then puts his hands to his mouth." The eggs also can get passed from one person to another through bedsheets, clothing, and toys.

How do you know when your child has worms? "If a child has recurrent stomachaches, I'll call home and see if he is having anal itching at night," says Susie Tann, R.N., an elementary school nurse in Bradford, Vermont. "The worms become active at night, which is when the itching is at its worst."

Here's what you can do when you discover signs of the creatures.

Heat Fabric

"While the worms themselves should be treated with a prescription medication from your doctor, you can avoid their spread by cleaning your bedsheets thoroughly," Dr. Martin says. "Washing alone won't do it, though. In my mother's day, sheets were washed, dried on a line, and then ironed. The heat from the iron would kill the eggs. The best thing to come along for combating worms—since permanent-press sheets eliminated the need for ironing—was the clothes dryer, which also kills the eggs. Make sure you set the cycle on Hot."

Clean Those Hands

"To reduce the chance of a worm infestation, make sure your family gets into the early habit of washing their hands regularly," says Laurence Bouchard, D.O., an osteopathic family physician in private practice in Narragansett, Rhode Island.

Index

to formaldehyde, 96–97
hay fever, 236–41
to latex, 148, _181_, 217, 377
to medications, 217
Aloe vera, for burns, 83
Altitude sickness, 7–9, _8_
dangerous conditions with, _9_
Ammonia, for bee stings, 44–45
Anemia, 10–11
from menstruation, 177–78
nosebleeds from, 348
Angina, 254
Animal bites, preventing, _12_
Animal scratches, 11–13
preventing, _12_
Time to See the Doctor, _13_
Anise seeds, for treating
bad breath, 35
belching, 46
flatulence, 188
Ankle sprain, 13–15
Time to See the Doctor, _15_
from unbalanced gait, _14_
Antacids, for treating
heartburn, 255–56
nausea, 334
side stitches, 394
stomachache, 418
Anterior cruciate ligament, injured, 309
Antibiotic ointment
for preventing scarring, 386
for treating
blisters, 56
cuts and scrapes, 136
dermatitis, 147
nosebleeds, 348
skin infections, 54–55
snakebite, 403
toenail fungus, 445
Antibiotics
effects of
indigestion, 292
nausea, 333–34
yeast infections, 215
for Lyme disease, 317
Antidepressants, effects of
fainting, 174
gum problems, 224
impotence, 286

Antihistamines
gum problems from, 224
for preventing sneezing, 404
for treating
bee stings, 44
bloodshot eyes, 60
dizziness, 159
hay fever, 239–40
hives, 274
insect bites, 298
itchiness from haying, 243
shingles, 389
urination problems and, 289
Anti-inflammatory drugs. _See_ Aspirin;
Ibuprofen
Antioxidants, for preventing eye
problems, 341–42
Antiperspirants, avoiding, 62
Antivenin, for snakebite, 403
Anusol, for hemorrhoids, 262
Anxiety
attacks, 283–84, 339–40, _340_
stomachaches from, 418–19
Apnea, sleep
afternoon slump from, 5–6
bed-wetting and, 40, _40_
drowsiness from, 159
snoring and, 406
Appendicitis, _128_, 417
Apple juice, cavities from, 94
Aquaphor, for cuts and scrapes, 136
Arch supports, for treating
calluses and corns, 91
flat feet, 186
knee pain, 311
Arm & Hammer Tooth Powder, for
preventing gum disease, 379
Arthritis, 15–20
treatment of, 16–20
types of, 15–16
Artificial tears, for dry eyes, 162
Aspirin
avoiding, for treating children,
103
effects of
acid reflux, 254
ear noises, 167
stomach upset, 334
ulcers, 452

Underscored page references indicate boxed text. **Boldface** references indicate illustrations.
Prescription drug names are denoted with the symbol Rx.

Underscored page references indicate boxed text. **Boldface** references indicate illustrations.
Prescription drug names are denoted with the symbol Rx.

Underscored page references indicate boxed text. **Boldface** references indicate illustrations.
Prescription drug names are denoted with the symbol Rx.

Celery seeds, for treating
  belching, 46
  flatulence, 188
Cerebral edema, from altitude sickness,
      8, 9
Cervical pillows
  for neck pain, 337
  for snorers, 408
Chafing, 94–97
Chamomile, for treating
  indigestion, 292, **292**
  ulcers, 454
Chapped hands, 97–98
  old-time treatment of, 98
  preventing, 97
Chapped lips, 99–100
  old-time treatment of, 100
  Time to See the Doctor, 99
Charley horse, 101–2
Cheek bites, 445–46
  preventing, 446
Cheese, for preventing cavities, 94
Chest pain
  causes of, 253–54
  from exertion, 349
  with heart attack, 255, 259, 363, 394
Chewing gum
  in hair, 228
  jaw problems and, 303
  sugar-free, for preventing cavities, 94
Chewing tobacco, mouth sores from, 330
Chickenpox, 102–5, **103**
  shingles from, 387
  vaccine, 104
Chicken soup, for treating
  colds, 114
  diarrhea, 155
Children
  conditions affecting
    bed-wetting, 39–42
    colic, 110–12
    cough-variant asthma, 20
    cradle cap, 126–28
    crossed eyes, 130–33
    croup, 133–35
    diaper rash, 151–53
    diarrhea, 155, 156
    fever, 180
    fractures, 15, 73

headaches, 244–45
hyperactivity, 279–83, 281
knee pain, 311–12
nausea, 333
nursemaid's elbow, 75
pinkeye, 358
stomachaches, 419
stress, 422
stuttering, 424–27
swollen glands, 433
  nightmares of, 344–45
  night terrors of, 345–46
  teeth flossing in, 379–80
  thumb sucking in, 440–42
Chinese restaurant syndrome, 193
Chlorine buildup, on hair, 228
Chocolate
  acne and, 53–54
  breast aches and, 66
  cravings for, 191, 192
  indigestion from, 291
  as stimulant, 176
  teeth grinding and, 437
Cholesterol
  HDL vs. LDL, 267–69
  high, 266–69
    Time to See the Doctor, 267
Chondromalacia patella, 309–10
Chronic fatigue syndrome, 176
Circulation, poor, 363–65
  Time to See the Doctor, 363
Citric acid, for kidney stones, 308
Clicking, jaw, 302–4
Clotrimazole, for treating
  athlete's foot, 25
  nail infections, 181–82
  ringworm, 399
  toenail fungus, 445
Clots, blood, phlebitis from, 356–57
Clover tea, red, for colds, 115
Cloves, for gum pain, 223
Cobalt, for preventing chapped hands, 98
Cocoa, as stimulant, 176
Codeine, in cough syrup, 125
Coffee
  indigestion from, 291
  for treating
    afternoon slump, 7
    asthma, 24

Underscored page references indicate boxed text. **Boldface** references indicate illustrations.
Prescription drug names are denoted with the symbol Rx.

<u>Underscored</u> page references indicate boxed text. **Boldface** references indicate illustrations.
Prescription drug names are denoted with the symbol Rx.

Cucumbers, for bags under the eyes, 36
Cuticle oil, for brittle nails, 72
Cuts, 135–37
    barbed wire, 37–39, <u>37</u>, **39**
    homemade salve for, <u>37</u>
    old-time treatment of, <u>136</u>
    Time to See the Doctor, <u>135</u>
Cystitis. *See* Urinary tract infections
    (UTIs)

D

Dairy foods, diarrhea and, 157
Dandelion, for breast aches, 66, **66**
Dandruff, 138–40
    shampoo, 139–40
        for cradle cap, 126–27
    Time to See the Doctor, <u>139</u>
Dark circles under the eyes, 140–41
    Time to See the Doctor, <u>140</u>
Deafness. *See* Hearing loss
Decongestants, for treating
    colds, 114
    earache, 166
    flu, 190
    postnasal drip, 367
    sinus problems, 397
Dehydration, 142–44, <u>143</u>
    diarrhea, as cause of, <u>153</u>, 155
    effects of
        fatigue, 178
        headaches, 245
        side stitches, 394
        teeth grinding, 437
    hangover, as cause of, 235, 236
    in winter, <u>142</u>
Dental implants, 145–46
Dental problems
    cavities, 92–94, **92**
    gum pain, 222–24
    receding gums, 378–80
    teeth grinding, 436–37
    tooth stains, 448–50
Denture problems, 144–46
Deodorant, <u>61</u>
    for foot odor, 198
Depression
    food cravings with, 191–92
    summer, <u>88</u>
    winter, 87–89, 468–71

Dermatitis, 146–49
    from haying, 242
Detergents
    dermatitis from, 149
    rashes from, 377
Deviated septum, <u>367</u>, **367**
Diabetes, 149–51
    boils and, <u>63</u>
    food cravings with, 192
    foot problems with, 195–96
    old-time treatment of, <u>150</u>
    thirst as sign of, <u>148</u>
Diaper rash, 151–53
    Time to See the Doctor, <u>152</u>
Diaphragm, side stitches from, 393, **393**
Diarrhea, 153–57
    with dyspepsia, 163
    Time to See the Doctor, <u>153</u>
Diet
    for diabetics, 151
    for diarrhea, 156–57
    low-fat
        for lowering cholesterol, 268
        for preventing impotence, 287
        for preventing sore muscles, 412
        after vomiting, 463
Dieting
    fad, <u>351</u>
    gallstones from, 213
Digestive problems. *See* Gastrointestinal
    problems
Dill seeds, for bad breath, 35
Diphenhydramine, for bee stings, 44
Discipline, for calming children, <u>281</u>
Disk, slipped, 26, 27
Diuretics, gout from, 219
Dizziness, 157–59
    with Ménière's disease, <u>158</u>, 168
Domeboro, for poison ivy, 362
Doorknob covers, childproof, for
    sleepwalkers, 401, **401**
Douching, genital irritation from, 216–17
Dramamine, for treating
    motion sickness, 326–27
    nausea, 334
Dressing, for preventing
    cold hands and feet, 106–8
    frostbite, 208
Drowsiness, 159–60

<u>Underscored</u> page references indicate boxed text. **Boldface** references indicate illustrations.
Prescription drug names are denoted with the symbol Rx.

<u>Underscored</u> page references indicate boxed text. **Boldface** references indicate illustrations.
Prescription drug names are denoted with the symbol Rx.

Eyedrops, for treating
  bloodshot eyes, 59–60
  dry eyes, 162
  foreign object in eye, 203
  pinkeye, 358
Eyeglasses
  cleaning, <u>171</u>
  for eyestrain, 172
  frostbite with, 208
  for improving night vision, 343
Eyelashes, head lice on, 247–49
Eye(s)
  bags under, 35–37
  black, 51–52
    preventing, <u>52</u>
    Time to See the Doctor, <u>51</u>
  bloodshot, 57, 59–60
    Time to See the Doctor, <u>59</u>
  crossed, 130–33, <u>131</u>
    Time to See the Doctor, <u>130</u>
  dark circles under, 140–41
    Time to See the Doctor, <u>140</u>
  dry, 161–62
    preventing, <u>161</u>
    Time to See the Doctor, <u>161</u>
  foreign object in, 201–3, <u>202</u>
  infection, pinkeye, 59, 357–59
  itchy, from hay fever, 240
  patch, for crossed eyes, 132
  puffy, 370–71
    Time to See the Doctor, <u>371</u>
  sties on, 427–28, **427**
  vision problems
    eyestrain, 170–72, 245
    night blindness, 341–43
    snow blindness, 408–9

F

Fabric softener sheets, allergy to, 149
Fainting, 173–75
  position for preventing, 174, **174**
  Time to See the Doctor, <u>174</u>
Farsightedness, crossed eyes and, 133
Fat, dietary, gallstones and, 213–14
Fatigue, 175–78
  afternoon slump, 5–7
  drowsiness, 159–60
  overexertion, 349–50
Feet. *See* Foot problems

Fennel seeds, for treating
  bad breath, 35
  belching, 46
  flatulence, 188
Fertility, signs of, <u>117</u>
Fever, 178–80
  Time to See the Doctor, <u>179</u>
Fever blisters, 328, 329, **329**
Feverfew, for migraines, 323, **323**
Fiber
  hemorrhoids and, 263
  sources of, 120, 290, 461
  for treating
    constipation, 120, 290
    high cholesterol, 269
Fibromyalgia, <u>410</u>
Fingernails
  brittle, 71–72
  infections of, 181–82
    preventing, <u>181</u>
  removing blood from under, 231, **231**
Fingers, fractured, 230–31
Fishhook caught in skin, 182–85, <u>183</u>,
  184, 185
Fish oil
  for arthritis, 17–18
  for lowering cholesterol, 268–69
  for preventing asthma attacks, 24
Flat feet, 185–87
  exercises for, <u>186</u>
Flatulence, 187–89
  colic from, 110–11
  side stitches from, 394
  Time to See the Doctor, <u>188</u>
Flaxseed oil
  for preventing gallstones, 214
  for winter itch, 474
Flossing, teeth
  in children, 379–80
  for preventing
    cavities, 93–94
    gum pain, 222
  technique for, <u>32</u>, **32**, 34
Flu, 189–91
  Time to See the Doctor, <u>190</u>
Fluorescent lighting
  for reading, 172
  for seasonal affective disorder, 87–88,
    470

<u>Underscored</u> page references indicate boxed text. **Boldface** references indicate illustrations.
Prescription drug names are denoted with the symbol Rx.

Underscored page references indicate boxed text. **Boldface** references indicate illustrations.
Prescription drug names are denoted with the symbol Rx.

Glacier goggles, for preventing snow
   blindness, 409, **409**
Glands, swollen, 433–35
   from animal scratches, 13
   preventing, 433
   Time to See the Doctor, 434
Glasses. *See* Eyeglasses
Gloves, for preventing cold hands, 108,
   108
Glycerin, for earwax removal, 169
Gout, 217–19
   old-time treatment of, 218
Grape juice, for constipation, 122
Graying hair, 220–21
Grinding, of teeth, 436–37
   Time to See the Doctor, 436
Growing pains, 312
Guaifenesin
   for bronchitis, 76
   for increasing fertility, 119
Guarana tea, for fatigue, 178
Gum, chewing
   in hair, 228
   jaw problems and, 303
   sugar-free, for preventing cavities, 94
Gums
   bad breath from, 31, 32–33
   painful, 222–24
   receding, 378–80
      Time to See the Doctor, 378
Gyne-Lotrimin, for treating yeast
   infections, 458

H
HACE, from altitude sickness, 9
Hair problems
   chlorine buildup, 228
   graying hair, 220–21
   gum stuck in hair, 228
   hair loss, 225–27
      male pattern baldness, 226, **226**
      Time to See the Doctor, 226
   ingrown hairs, 293–94
   mineral buildup in, 227
   with permanents, 228
   tangles, 229–30
Hammered thumb, 230–31
   Time to See the Doctor, 230
Hammertoe, 232–33, **232**

Hands
   chapped, 97–98, 98
      old-time treatment of, 98
      preventing, 97
   cold, 105–10
      Time to See the Doctor, 107
   dermatitis on, 148
Hangnails, 233–34
   Time to See the Doctor, 233
Hangover, 234–36, 236
   preventing, 235
HAPE, from altitude sickness, 9
Hay fever, 236–41
Haying or lawn-mowing discomfort,
   241–43, 242
HDL cholesterol, 266, 267, 269
Headaches, 243–46
   migraines, 322–23
      preventing, 323
   old-time treatment of, 244
   Time to See the Doctor, 245
Head lice, 246–49, **246**, 248
   old-time treatment of, 247
Hearing aids, 252, **252**
Hearing loss, 249–53
   Time to See the Doctor, 250
   treatment of, 251–53
Heart attack
   mimicking indigestion, 163, 255
   signs of, 255, 333, 363, 394
Heartburn, 253–56. *See also* Indigestion
Heart disease, signs of, 112, 259
Heart palpitations, 256–57
Heat, for treating
   ankle sprain, 15
   backache, 31
   boils, 64
   bursitis, 84–85
   earache, 165–66
   joint pain, 306
   menstrual cramps, 321
   muscle cramps, 129
   neck pain, 336–37
   shinsplints, 390
   shoulder pain, 392
   side stitches, 394–95
   sinus problems, 397
   sore muscles, 410
   swimmer's ear, 433

Underscored page references indicate boxed text. **Boldface** references indicate illustrations.
Prescription drug names are denoted with the symbol Rx.

Underscored page references indicate boxed text. **Boldface** references indicate illustrations. Prescription drug names are denoted with the symbol Rx.

Underscored page references indicate boxed text. **Boldface** references indicate illustrations.
Prescription drug names are denoted with the symbol Rx.

Underscored page references indicate boxed text. **Boldface** references indicate illustrations.
Prescription drug names are denoted with the symbol Rx.

Underscored page references indicate boxed text. **Boldface** references indicate illustrations. Prescription drug names are denoted with the symbol Rx.

Naps
  for afternoon slump, 7
  insomnia and, 300
Narcolepsy, drowsiness from, 159–60
Nasal sprays, for treating
  hay fever, 241
  sinus problems, 396–97
Nausea, 333–35
  morning sickness, 324–26, _325_
  motion sickness, 326–28
    Time to See the Doctor, _327_
  Time to See the Doctor, _333_
Neck gaiter, for preventing windburn,
    468, **468**
Neck pain, 335–39
  preventing, _336_
  stretching for, _338_, **338**
  Time to See the Doctor, _335_
  treatment of, 336–39
Needle
  for draining blisters, 56–57, **57**
  for removing
    ingrown hairs, 294, **294**
    splinters, 415–16
Nervousness, 339–41
Night blindness, 341–43
Nightmares, 343–46
  old-time remedy for, _345_
  Time to See the Doctor, _344_
Night sweats, in menopause, 278
Night terrors, 345–46
Nipple infections, from breastfeeding,
    69
Nix, for head lice, 247, 249
Nodules, vocal, hoarseness from, 276
Noises, ear, 166–68, _167_
Nonsteroidal anti-inflammatory drugs
    (NSAIDs). _See also_ Aspirin;
    Ibuprofen
  for preventing gallstones, 214
  ulcers from, 452
Nosebleeds, 346–48, **347**
  old-time treatment of, _348_
  preventing, _347_
Nose blowing, technique for, _396_
Nose picking, preventing, _347_
NSAIDs. _See also_ Aspirin; Ibuprofen
  for preventing gallstones, 214
  ulcers from, 452

Nursemaid's elbow, in children, 75
Nursing. _See_ Breastfeeding

O

Oatmeal, colloidal, for treating
  chickenpox, 104–5
  dermatitis, 149
  genital irritation, 216
  poison ivy, 362
  rashes, 376–77
  winter itch, 473
Obesity. _See_ Overweight
Ocuvite, for preventing eye problems,
    342
Odor
  body, 60–63
  foot, 197–98
Oil
  for removing gum from hair, 228
  for treating
    chapped hands, 98, _98_
    cradle cap, 127–28
    earache, 165–66, **165**
Omega-3 fatty acids, for preventing
    gallstones, 214
Opcon-A, for bloodshot eyes, 60
Orabase, for mouth sores, 329
Orthostatic hypotension, fainting from,
    175
Orthotic devices, for bunions, 80
Osgood-Schlatter disease, 312
Osteoarthritis
  overweight and, 18
  symptoms of, 15–16
Overeating, indigestion from, 291
Overexertion, 349–50
  Time to See the Doctor, _349_
Overweight, 351–55
  effects of
    gallstones, 213
    knee problems, 312
    osteoarthritis, 18
    phlebitis, 357
    snoring, 406
  heat exhaustion and, 260
  old-time treatment of, _351_
Ovulation, pain from, 129
Ovulation predictor kit, for conception
    problems, 119

Underscored page references indicate boxed text. **Boldface** references indicate illustrations.
Prescription drug names are denoted with the symbol Rx.

492   INDEX

P

Pain(s)
  arthritis, 15–20
  back, 26–31
    preventing, 27, 30
    stretching for, <u>28–29</u>, **28–29**
    Time to See the Doctor, <u>30</u>
    treatment of, 30–31
  birthing, 47–50
  from boils, 64–65
  breast, 65–67
    from breastfeeding, 67, 69–70
    Time to See the Doctor, <u>65</u>
  from bursitis, 84–86, 270, 309, 391
  chest
    causes of, 253–54
    from exertion, <u>349</u>
    with heart attack, <u>255</u>, 259, <u>363</u>, <u>394</u>
  cramping, 101–2, 128–30, 320–22
  earache, 164–66
  engagement, before childbirth, 48, 50, 50
  growing, 312
  gum, 222–24
  headache, 243–46, 322–23
  hip, 269–72
    preventing, <u>270</u>
  joint, 304–6
    Time to See the Doctor, <u>305</u>
  knee, 309–12
    preventing, <u>311</u>
    Time to See the Doctor, <u>310</u>
  leg, 101–2
  muscles, 410–12
  neck, 335–39
    preventing, <u>336</u>
    stretching for, <u>338</u>, **338**
    Time to See the Doctor, <u>335</u>
    treatment of, 336–39
  ovulation, 129
  from shingles, 386–89
  from shinsplits, 389–91
  shoulder, 391–93
    Time to See the Doctor, <u>391</u>
  from tendinitis, 437–40, **438**
  from walking, <u>363</u>
Palpitations, heart, 256–57
Panic attacks, 283–84, 339–40, <u>340</u>

Paper clip, for removing blood under nail, 231, **231**
Parasites
  teeth grinding from, <u>436</u>
  ticks (*see* Ticks)
  worms, 474–75
Parkinson's disease medication, fainting from, 174
Paroxysmal atrial tachycardia (PAT), 256–57
Parsley, breastfeeding and, 69
PAT, 256–57
Patch, eye, for crossed eyes, 132
Peanut butter, for removing gum from hair, 228
Pectin, for diarrhea, 163
Pedialyte, for diarrhea, 155
Penis
  impotence and, 285–88
  preventing frostbite of, 210
Pepcid AC, for treating
  heartburn, 255–56
  nausea, 334
Pepper, red, for preventing cold feet, <u>109</u>
Peppermint, for treating
  indigestion, <u>291</u>
  stomachache, 418
Pepto-Bismol, for diarrhea, 155–56
Permanent waves, protecting, 228
Permanone, as tick repellent, <u>443</u>
Petroleum jelly
  preventing scarring with, 386
  for treating
    blisters, 56
    brittle nails, 72
    burns, 81–83
    chapped hands, 98
    chapped lips, 100
    cuts and scrapes, 136
    dermatitis, 148
    lice on eyelashes, 248
    windburn, 468
Pets
  as asthma trigger, 22
  for relieving stress, 422–23
  ringworm from, 399
Phlebitis, 356–57
  preventing, <u>357</u>
Phobias, 340–41

Underscored page references indicate boxed text. **Boldface** references indicate illustrations. Prescription drug names are denoted with the symbol Rx.

Phytoestrogens, for preventing hot flashes, 279
Pillows
  cervical
    for neck pain, 337
    for snorers, 408
  contoured, for preventing teeth grinding, 436–37, **437**
Pimples. *See* Blemishes
Pineapple, for canker sores, 330
Pinkeye, 357–59
  bloodshot eyes from, 59
  Time to See the Doctor, <u>358</u>
Pinworms, 475
Plantain, for treating
  cuts, 137
  insect bites, 298, **298**
Plaque
  gingivitis from, 222
  tooth stains from, 450
PMS, 368–70, <u>368</u>
PMS Escape, for PMS symptoms, 370
Poison ivy and oak, 359–63, **359**, <u>361</u>
Pollen masks, for allergy sufferers, 239
Poor circulation, 363–65
  Time to See the Doctor, <u>363</u>
Popcorn hulls, mouth sores from, 330
Postherpetic neuralgia, 387–88
Postnasal drip, 365–67
  Time to See the Doctor, <u>367</u>
Postural hypotension, during pregnancy, 326
Posture, for preventing hip pain, <u>270</u>, 272
Powder, baby, for preventing body odor, 62
Pregnancy
  chickenpox and, <u>104</u>
  morning sickness during, 324–26, <u>325</u>
Premenstrual syndrome (PMS), 368–70, <u>368</u>
Preparation H, for blisters, 56
Presbyopia, 172
Prescription drugs. *See also* Medications; *specific prescription drugs*
  generic, <u>273</u>
Preventive medicine, guidelines for, <u>472</u>
Prickly heat, 260–61
  preventing, <u>260</u>
Pudding, for constipation, <u>122</u>

Puffy eyes, 370–71
  Time to See the Doctor, <u>371</u>
Puncture wounds, 371–73, <u>372</u>
Purple coneflower, **115**. *See also* Echinacea

Q
Q-tips, earwax and, <u>169</u>, 251
Quinine, for treating
  charley horse, 101
  muscle cramps, 101, 129
  restless legs, 384

R
Raisins, gin-soaked, for arthritis, 19
Rash(es), 374–78
  diaper, 151–53
    Time to See the Doctor, <u>152</u>
  from haying, 241, 243
  heat, 260–61
    preventing, <u>260</u>
  hives, 272–75, **274**
    Time to See the Doctor, <u>275</u>
  Lyme disease, 316–18, **317**
  poison ivy and oak, 359–63, **359**, <u>361</u>
  Time to See the Doctor, <u>375</u>
Raynaud's disease, <u>107</u>, 363–64
Receding gums, 378–80
  Time to See the Doctor, <u>378</u>
Rectal thermometer, for stimulating infant bowel movement, 121–22, **122**
Red clover tea, for colds, 115
Red eyes, 57, 59–60
  Time to See the Doctor, <u>59</u>
Red pepper, for preventing cold feet, <u>109</u>
Reflux. *See also* Heartburn; Indigestion
  croup with, 134
  effects of
    hoarseness, 276, <u>276</u>
    sore throat, 412
Refresh, for pinkeye, 358
Rehydralyte, for diarrhea, 155
Relaxation
  for preventing ear noises, 168
  for stress, 423–24
Repetitive motion injury, 380–83
  Time to See the Doctor, <u>381</u>
Restless legs, 383–84
  Time to See the Doctor, <u>383</u>

<u>Underscored</u> page references indicate boxed text. **Boldface** references indicate illustrations.
Prescription drug names are denoted with the symbol Rx.

Underscored page references indicate boxed text. **Boldface** references indicate illustrations.
Prescription drug names are denoted with the symbol Rx.

Underscored page references indicate boxed text. **Boldface** references indicate illustrations.
Prescription drug names are denoted with the symbol Rx.

Underscored page references indicate boxed text. **Boldface** references indicate illustrations.
Prescription drug names are denoted with the symbol Rx.

Underscored page references indicate boxed text. **Boldface** references indicate illustrations.
Prescription drug names are denoted with the symbol Rx.

Underscored page references indicate boxed text. **Boldface** references indicate illustrations.
Prescription drug names are denoted with the symbol Rx.

<u>Underscored</u> page references indicate boxed text. **Boldface** references indicate illustrations.
Prescription drug names are denoted with the symbol Rx.